Management Concepts for the New Nurse

Management Concepts for the New Nurse

KATHERINE W. VESTAL, R.N., Ph.D.
Associate Executive Director
Hermann Hospital, Texas Medical Center
Houston, Texas

WITH 19 CONTRIBUTORS

J. B. Lippincott Company
Philadelphia
London   Mexico City   New York   St. Louis   São Paulo   Sydney

Sponsoring Editor: Paul Hill
Manuscript Editor: Lorraine D. Smith
Indexer: Ann Cassar
Design Director: Tracy Baldwin
Designer: Susan Hess
Production Manager: Kathleen P. Dunn
Production Coordinator: Kenneth G. Neimeister
Compositor: University Graphics, Inc.
Printer/Binder: R. R. Donnelley & Sons Company

1 3 5 6 4 2

Library of Congress Cataloging-in-Publication Data

Management concepts for the new nurse.

   Includes bibliographies and index.
   1. Nurses—Life skills guides.   2. Nursing services—
Administration.   I. Vestal, Katherine W.   [DNLM:
1. Leadership—nurses' instruction.   2. Nursing,
Supervisory.   3. Professional Competence—nurses'
instruction.   WY 105 M2663]
RT82.M22   1987   610.73'068   86-27618
ISBN 0-397-54629-7

The authors and publisher have exerted every effort to
ensure that drug selection and dosage set forth in this text
are in accord with current recommendations and practice
at the time of publication. However, in view of ongoing
research, changes in government regulations, and the
constant flow of information relating to drug therapy and
drug reactions, the reader is urged to check the package
insert for each drug for any change in indications and
dosage and for added warnings and precautions. This is
particularly important when the recommended agent is a
new or infrequently employed drug.

To my parents and friends,
whose unconditional support
helped make this book
possible.

Contributors

RICHARD W. ASHTON, R.N., J.D., M.P.H.
Vice President, Patient Services
Riverside Methodist Hospital
Columbus, Ohio
Adjunct Assistant Professor
College of Nursing
Ohio State University
Columbus, Ohio

HARRIETT S. CHANEY, R.N., Ph.D.
Associate Professor
University of Texas School of
  Nursing
Galveston, Texas

MARILYN B. CHASSIE, R.N., Ph.D., C.N.A.A.
Assistant Dean, Nursing Practice
Associate Professor
University of South Carolina College
  of Nursing
Columbia, South Carolina

EULA DAS, R.N., Ph.D.
Vice President, Baylor University
  Medical Center
Dallas, Texas
Adjunct Assistant Professor
University of Texas
Arlington, Texas

MARIANNE DIETRICK-GALLAGHER, R.N., M.S.N.
Gynecology Chemotherapy Clinical
  Specialist
Hospital of the University of
  Pennsylvania
Philadelphia, Pennsylvania

NANNETTE L. GODDARD, R.N., M.S.
Senior Partner, Goddard
  Management Resources
Houston, Texas
Assistant Professor
University of Texas School of
  Nursing
Galveston, Texas

LINDA C. HODGES, R.N., Ed.D.
Acting Director, Graduate Nursing
  Program
University of South Carolina College
  of Nursing
Columbia, South Carolina

JOYCE E. JOHNSON, D.N.S.
Associate Administrator
Division of Nursing
Washington Hospital Center
Washington, D.C.
Professor in Nursing
Marymount University of Virginia

School of Nursing
Arlington, Virginia

KARLENE M. KERFOOT, R.N., Ph.D.
Senior Vice President, Nursing
St. Luke's Hospital
Adjunct Professor
Texas Women's University
Houston, Texas

NANCY R. KRUGER, R.N., D.N.S.
Director, Nursing Services
University Hospital
Milton S. Hershey Medical Center
Pennsylvania State University
Hershey, Pennsylvania
Clinical Professor
Thomas Jefferson University
Philadelphia, Pennsylvania

J. ELIZABETH OTHMAN, R.N., M.S.
Assistant Director, Nursing
Mott, Women's Holden Hospitals
University of Michigan Medical
  Center
Adjunct Instructor
University of Michigan School of
  Nursing
Ann Arbor, Michigan

GAYE W. POTEET, R.N., Ed.D.
Director, Graduate Nursing
  Program
University of Texas School of Nursing
Galveston, Texas

SUSAN C. ROE, R.N., M.S., D.P.A.
Executive Director of Nursing
  Programs
University of Phoenix
Phoenix, Arizona

**DONNA RICHARDS
  SHERIDAN, R.N., M.B.A., Ph.D.**
Director, Nursing Continuing
  Education and
  Management Consultation

Stanford University Hospital
Stanford, California

DEBORAH J. TEASLEY, R.N., M.S.N.
Associate Executive Director
West Jersey Health System
Camden, New Jersey

LINDA CARRICK TOROSIAN, R.N., M.S.N.
Clinical Director, Surgical Nursing
Hospital of the University of
  Pennsylvania
Clinical Instructor
University of Pennsylvania School
  of Nursing
Philadelphia, Pennsylvania

BETH TAMPLET ULRICH, R.N., M.S.
Director of Renal Services and of
  Nursing Research and
  Development
Hermann Hospital
Assistant Professor
University of Texas School of Nursing
Houston, Texas

KATHERINE W. VESTAL, R.N., Ph.D.
Associate Executive Director
Hermann Hospital
Professor of Nursing
University of Texas School of
  Nursing
Galveston, Texas

MARGARET M. VOSBURGH, R.N., M.S.
Clinical Nursing Director
Cedars-Sinai Medical Center
Los Angeles, California

WILLIAM M. WARFEL, R.N., M.S.N., C.N.A.A.
Associate General Director
Albert Einstein Medical Center
Northern Division
Philadelphia, Pennsylvania

Preface

In the complex arena of health care today, the new nurse enters a job world filled with expectations of professional competencies. Initially, these expectations center on clinical responsibilities, but by nature the expectations must also include some managerial, educational, and research responsibilities. Many nurses think that nurses in management, manage, and that nurses in clinical practice, practice. This attitude can no longer be supported.

This book addresses the managerial issues and responsibilities of the new nurse. In the role of a new graduate, whether in a hospital, long-term care, home health care, or other delivery site, a nurse must both recognize and contribute to the managerial aspects of the job. In a constant struggle to be efficient and productive, organizations today expect that all employees will contribute to the managerial function of the services provided. The organizational environment attempts to foster a sense of achievement, loyalty, efficiency, and job enthusiasm.

"Management Concepts for the New Nurse" describes the issues related to the management focus in complex organizations, the issues related to being a good employee, and the issues related to contemporary professional nursing practice. Examples are drawn from a variety of organizations—both union and nonunion. It is designed to provide a practical as well as theoretical base to the managerial focus of the new nurse. Each chapter contains (1) behavioral objectives for the major concepts included; (2) presentation of theory and applications; (3) a summary of major ideas in the chapter, and (4) references that are cited in the chapter.

The book is not intended to provide the in-depth managerial knowledge needed by a middle manager in nursing. It is clearly designed for the newcomer to nursing, as a tool to increase her competence and confidence in the managerial aspects of an entry-level nursing position. Nursing must provide a setting in which the new graduate can thrive, not merely survive, and in which she can come to appreciate her total role in today's health care arena.

Katherine W. Vestal, R.N., Ph.D.

Contents

Management
Concepts
for the
New Nurse

SECTION I

FOCUS ON MANAGEMENT

Chapter 1

The management role of the new nurse

KATHERINE W. VESTAL

This book is based on the premise that all nurses, regardless of their primary role, must assume responsibility for managerial roles. These managerial roles may differ, but will always include effective communication, human relations, and the management of time, the change process, and resources. For decades, nursing has rigidly categorized nurses as clinicians, or educators, or managers, or researchers. The expectation was that if a role were defined as one of these four, activities related to the other three were not appropriate.

The time has come in health care to blur the lines between roles. The purist role cannot meet the demands of the complex care-delivery systems, and changes must take place to ensure survival of the nursing base. The person who often initiates this change is the new nurse who is entering professional practice for the first time.

The new nurse is under intense pressure to perform at a level acceptable to the hiring organization. An effort is made to prescribe clearly the level of competence needed to work in the organization, and to have these competencies met as quickly as possible. If a nurse is not functioning at 100% of productivity, it is costing the organization money to compensate for the lost percentage of work.

So, experiencing this pressure, the new nurse concentrates on learning and performing clinical activities—the primary role she was hired to perform. If the role were purely clinical, this concentration would result in a clearly directed effort. However, other factors immediately begin to emerge. Not only must the nurse apply a Band-Aid, she must also charge for it, chart the procedure, and/or direct others to do the task. For each simple nursing activity, there are innumerable compounding issues to be addressed.

The next scenario is usually a frustrated new nurse, who proclaims that she was hired to be a *nurse,* that is, a clinician, not an accountant, secretary, or housekeeper. Reality has set in and it is obvious that the role of a clinical nurse encompasses much more than clinical care, and it is often the accomplishment of the peripheral tasks that ensures good patient care.

In addition, the new nurse does not work in a vacuum, isolated from everyone but her patients. She finds a vast array of allied health personnel—physicians, managers, families, and others—who demand her time and energy in coordinated events. In addition, she finds that, despite her own lack of job experience, she is expected to manage the work flow and activities of other personnel who have less formal preparation, but usually more practical experience. This human resource management is critical to the total care of patients.

It is evident that the new nurse must have a sound management basis from which to operate. This aspect of the clinician's role cannot be delegated or relegated as a lower priority. The issue becomes one of managing both aspects of the job—clinical care and managerial tasks—with equal consistency. As with most tasks, it is easier to start with the simple and move to the complex. The new nurse can identify the simple managerial behaviors needed and practice those until mastery is achieved. Then she can move toward the more complex tasks that may ultimately result in a change in her primary role from staff nurse to supervisor.

Obviously, becoming proficient at managerial activities is not easy. However, it becomes easier when the managerial roles frequently assumed by staff nurses are defined, the theory related, and examples of activities given. This book will approach the managerial activities in this manner. Later, when more complex managerial resources are required, they will be available.

Human Effectiveness

An individual's behavior stems from his interpretations of what he *thinks* he perceives. Other perceptions influence and help crystallize these individual values and behaviors. In time these behaviors operate as a person's individual theories, and govern his actions as though they were law. Theories in general are guidelines for behavior, and there are many that govern human effectiveness. Management books devote great attention to the theorists who founded the managerial practices followed today.

Busy managers are understandably impatient with theory, preferring to devote practical application in a crisis mode. Kurt Lewin has said that "there is nothing so practical as a good theory," especially when the manager wants to improve things and needs a useful method of doing so.

The application of theory requires that there be an awareness of a problem, and an understanding of the need to change, a commitment to change where practice differs from theory, and an establishment of new habits as the theory is applied. Thus application of the managerial theory that is a part of this textbook will require an intellectual conditioning experience as well as an active process of behavioral changes.

The theories of leadership, motivation, and values clarification are all important as the new nurse assumes managerial responsibilities. If a nurse believes that, as a clinician, she is also assuming managerial responsibilities for her job, then the acquisition of a theory base is essential. These theories, then, can be translated into practical methods of enhancing human effectiveness. Health care is undeniably a complex business and the care-delivery system supported by nurses is in itself a mesh of complexity.

Just as some persons choose complex or simple lifestyles away from the job, so do individuals differ in their preferred vocational roles on the job. At one extreme, some desire complex and continuously challenging positions; at the other extreme, some prefer simple routine jobs. However complex or simple the job, nurses have one desire in common, the freedom to choose the kind of work they prefer and relate to it in a way that is compatible with their own personal values. Hence, the concept of "every employee a manager" can have meaning for persons at all levels of talent, though their preferred job roles may differ substantially in terms of scope and variety.

In fact, "every employee a manager" is a universally applicable concept, but one that depends on appropriate job conditions for its fullest implementation. Every nurse has the potential for managing some jobs, but not all jobs. However, every nurse has the potential for managing certain components of any job, or combinations of several jobs. The realization of this potential depends on matching the nurse's talents and aspirations with the appropriate job, which includes not only the work itself but also the style of supervision, procedural constraints, peer relationships, and other climate factors in the workplace.

The New Kid

Every nurse is a new kid on the block at least once in her career, and probably many times. The feeling of being a neophyte recurs with each new job or new role. It is never easy to handle although, as experience builds, the feeling dissipates more rapidly. Being a new nurse breeds multiple issues to be considered. First, you are a new kid because, clinically, you are new to the profession. Second, you are a new kid because, as a professional nurse, you will automatically be expected to assume some leadership and managerial roles, thus making you a "manager" before you are even comfortable being a nurse.

So it is helpful to consider carefully the dilemma of the new kid structure and ways to deal with it. Generally, your fellow employees will react in one of three ways when you begin working with them. Some will be glad you are there, others will resent you for varying reasons, and others will test you before making any decision about you. Hopefully, the majority will adopt a wait-and-see attitude by not condemning or praising you until they see how you perform. The latter attitude is healthy and all that you can reasonably expect.

You will be measured initially against your predecessor in the position. If that person's performance was miserable, you will seem far better by comparison. If you follow a highly capable performer, your adjustment will be more difficult. In any event, you will have to be you, and decide just how you can best integrate yourself into the work setting.

It is a time to move slowly with changes, to communicate effectively downward as well as upward, and to listen intently to what others tell you. Make it a point to have a personal conversation with each of the persons working in your area sometime within the first 60 days on the job. Do not do it the first week or so, but once you have begun to know your colleagues, find a way to know them better. You must be genuinely interested in people, care about them as individuals, and help them achieve their goals. As time goes on, your "human" abilities will prove to be more important than your technical abilities.

In time, you will expand your influence from the formal group to the informal group as you become an accepted member of the team. Soon you will lose your status as the new kid, and others will step into that role. At that point, you are well on your way to assuming more managerial responsibilities because your increasing seniority will dictate such activities. Still a new nurse? Yes, but growing, both clinically and managerially.

THE HONEYMOON IS OVER

Fortunately, most new jobs have a honeymoon period. That is the time you have to adjust to the new setting and begin to reach full productivity. This adjustment period is undefined in length, and in some organizations may be several days, while in others it may be several months. It is during this time that the phrase "I don't know, I'm new here" holds a valid place in your communication.

Predictably, the honeymoon will come to an end and the real marriage between you and the organization will begin. You will see clearly good aspects, bad aspects, and puzzling aspects of the work setting. It is comforting to realize that there is no employee utopia, that every work setting has its pluses and minuses, so you can begin fitting in, as effectively as possible.

Once the honeymoon is over, the difficult decisions that might have been deferred, surface for action. As a new nurse you are concentrating on becoming clinically competent, learning the expectations of physicians, bosses, and colleagues, and finding your way in the complex organization. But as a professional nurse, you are in the spotlight to provide some managerial supervision to other employees, either newer R.N.'s, licensed practical nurses, or nurse attendants. In addition, you are required to coordinate the activities of many persons and processes from other departments. You will begin to understand fully why health care is considered one of the most difficult settings to manage, because it is a people business. People dealing with people in an atmosphere of great stress and confusion can only lead to one thing—a difficult role to fill.

As a new nurse, you will find your managerial responsibilities quite frequently relate to *people*. You will discover personalities you would like to change, persons who do not give positively to the organization, who do not get along with the group, as well as those who consistently *do* give their very best. While specific approaches to these situations are discussed later in this text, initially, the real need is to develop priorities for your own role.

Quite obviously, the process of developing priorities begins with determining what *is* most important. As a new graduate you probably feel that it is *all* important. This places you in the position of deciding what should be done at what time. Subtle shifts repeatedly occur when defining the workload and its importance, and you will find yourself constantly juggling your priorities as well as those of your subordinates. The pressure of juggling activities is a major source of frustration for new nurses, because inevitably some things must go undone, leading to feelings of guilt and inadequacy.

During the initial phase of a new job, sit down with the supervisor and have a private discussion about priorities. Relate your needs, learn the needs of the unit, and understand the needs of the organization. Then, in concert with the supervisor, set realistic goals for the next few weeks. Frequent reappraisal is important, and the resetting of priorities will follow as you increase in competence and confidence.

BUILDING CONFIDENCE

Building confidence is a gradual process that is usually the result of successes. As you experience success, you build mastery, and mastery leads to confidence. The learning curve of a new nurse is steep, with almost each encounter with patients, families, and employees becoming a new learning experience. It is important to take the time each day to review your successes. What did you do well, how did that feel, and how can you do even better tomorrow?

At the same time, as a professional nurse, you will need to develop the confidence of your fellow employees, both in their own ability and in your performance. They must have confidence that you are competent in your job and that you are fair. Following the same process, as you review your successes, consider the successes of your employees. Especially when dealing with new employees, assign them tasks they can master and so build in them the habit of being successful, starting small with small successes.

Occasionally nurses will perform a task incorrectly or incompletely. Handling such situations is a delicate issue that has great impact on the confidence of employees. "Praise them in public, criticize them in private" is a good credo to follow and is a basic managerial concept. Even when you talk to a nurse in private about an error, your function is to train that person to recognize the nature of the problem so that the error will not be repeated. This is not a personal judgment intended to make the nurse feel inadequate, but rather to isolate the incident and to correct it.

The fact is, nurses are not perfect. Expecting perfection may, in fact, defeat your own purposes, because persons will become so self-conscious about making a mistake that they will slow down their performance to a crawl to make absolutely sure they do not make a mistake. As a result, the volume of work cannot be completed. As a new nurse, being correct as much of the time as possible is important but, by the same token, mistakes will happen. Handle the error with as much attention as needed, and then move on. Nobody is perfect, but the odds for success should be made as high as possible.

Another area that affects the building of confidence is the issue of power. In today's workplace, there are many, many qualified and experienced individuals. They tend to question instructions and decisions and associate power with leaders who are persuasive rather than dictatorial. When you are in a leadership role your own attitude will be important in building confidence. The persons working with you will sense your mood, and determine your trigger points. Consequently, one of the most important and powerful attributes you can develop is consistent behavior so other personnel are not continually surprised by your fluctuating attitudes and actions.

You will find that your concern and efforts toward building your fellow employees' confidence will do a great deal in fortifying your own self-confidence. You can also build self-confidence by making correct decisions. Each time you make a good, sound decision, confidence in your ability to make judgments is reinforced.

Decision making in nursing is a crucial component of self-confidence because the majority of decisions you make will be a matter of public record. Your decisions will be discussed with colleagues, reviewed at report, and recorded in the patient record. New nurses agonize over every decision to be made because they are not sure they have all the information necessary to make that decision; second, they are afraid of making a mistake and possibly causing further injury to a patient.

It is unlikely that you will ever have 100% of the information that might apply to a given situation. If you have made a reasonable and prudent search for data, then use the 95% of information that you have to make a judgment, and move on. As you acquire more experience, you will find that you are making correct decisions 99% of the time, because in most situations the answer is obvious or you are being asked to reinforce someone else's judgment. Many problems will be brought to you because a colleague wants your agreement and approval before proceeding. This simple act by others will continually reinforce your confidence in your own abilities.

Building confidence in yourself and for yourself by others is an important process for a new nurse. You will not be able to depend on someone else to do it for you. Think in terms of the things you do well, the activities you did right, and the amount of new information that you are learning daily. A continuous review and evaluation will reinforce the competencies you are gaining and will become the framework of self-confidence that will support you for years to come.

PREPARING AND IMPROVING YOURSELF

As a new nurse, one of your major interests is to do well and be successful. It is difficult to determine exactly how to accomplish these tasks because of the complexity of your role as a professional nurse. But when you look around it is easy to identify many nurses who are successful and from whom you can learn.

One aspect of success is to feel comfortable with your own self-image. Having a fairly high opinion of yourself is a positive step in beginning a professional career. If you think success, if you look successful, if you are confident of being successful, you greatly increase your chances of reaching that goal. It is primarily a matter of attitude that is reinforced by a series of building blocks of achievement.

This success model must be tempered by reality. Realizing that you do *not* know everything, avoiding the impression of arrogance, and handling mistakes well will be important parts of your image. Identifying your learning and practice needs is equally as important. Be willing to admit these needs and do all you can to reinforce them. For example, very frequently the things you do not do well are also the things you do not like to do. That can hardly be a coincidence. But recognize your shortcomings and objectively determine a course of action to become proficient. View yourself as honestly as you can and help yourself to move ahead. Planning your future and your career is critical to designing a reasonable career path. While mastery of your current job is the number one priority, the second priority should be working on the path to your future development.

Other aspects of your improvement program may relate to communicating more effectively, managing your time more effectively, and participating successfully in organizational groups and efforts. These activities will, in time, lead to chairing committees, public speaking, and a highly visible profile. Any preparation you make along the way that can ultimately boost your future visibility will pay off later on.

Managing Innovation

All management involves the management of innovation. Without innovation, the workplace is stagnant and cannot possibly survive in the turbulent times that health care is experiencing today. Creativity is a form of spontaneity that finds expression in an atmosphere of freedom. Thus, an effective organization encourages its members to assert themselves as individuals in such a way as to meet the organizational goals. In order to ensure that anarchy does not reign, a certain degree of managerial guidance is always required so that individuals function within the framework of the organization.

In the past, innovation was often regarded as the exclusive realm of the managerial group. Today's nurse expects and accepts involvement as her just due, and responds counterproductively to constraints that limit creativity. Staff nurses, in fact, probably still remain the greatest reservoir of untapped resources in the health-care field today.

Innovation can thrive if the work climate supports and promotes it. Certain requirements, such as good job design, group participation, employee involvement, and supervisors whose roles are to advise, consult, and coordinate, must be met before a nurse can actually accept a role as manager of her own area of responsibility. It is this final level of involvement that ensures a commitment to successful change, when change is introduced.

Working in groups is also a key factor in innovation. Natural work groups are the primary work systems through which creativity can find expression. These systems consist of a group of peers who work together with their common leader. Moreover, because of its established relationship to other parts of the organization, a natural work group channels creativity toward the attainment of organizational goals.

This points up the need for the supervisor to include team building as a component of her job. And in turn, it identifies the need for the new nurse to learn to be a team player, team member and, eventually, team manager. While that may sound easy, as a new professional, new hire, and new team member, defining and enacting your role may take a good deal of thought, work, and sheer guts to carve out a place for yourself.

It is clear that innovation is essential to organizational growth and development. Providing a framework on which practices and systems for innovation can be built is one of the managerial roles of the professional nurse.

Quality of Work Life

During the 1960's, managerial journals emphasized the concept of job enrichment as the key to happy workers. In the 1970's, this concept was enlarged to that of "life enrichment" or "quality of working life." This broadened emphasis was the result of the realization that work itself, important as it is, is not the only medium through which meaning is given to life in the workplace. Systems peripheral to the work itself also needed modification. Both the work itself and the peripheral systems are influential in shaping attitudes and improving performance.

Moreover, life-enrichment programs cannot be seen as paternalistic or manipulative ploys if they are to have a positive impact on the work force. If supervisors feel that job-enrichment efforts for staff result in erosion of their already diminished and ambiguous responsibilities, they are not likely to support the efforts. It is clear then, that any attempt to improve the quality of work life for nurses must be supported by the nurses and their supervisors, and must not be done at the expense of the organization's success. In short, the long-term success of an organization is dependent on the pursuit of organizational goals that are synergistically related to the needs of its members.

Examination of the quality of work life usually begins with a review of Maslow's hierarchy of needs (see Chapter 4). When living is precarious, man devotes most of his attention to survival. As security increases, he is free to set his own standards and goals and to examine the rewards of achievement. This simplistic view of Maslow's model must be coupled with the managerial theory that evolved from scientific management, through the human relations era, to emerge into the organizational democracy that institutions strive for today.

Organizational democracy is a model based on the free society that exists outside the hospital doors. This model is a matrix of conditions in the workplace in which all members of the work force have an opportunity to participate in the democratic processes—creating profit, establishing systems for equitable sharing, changing the climate of the organization, and enabling nurses to take charge of their own careers.

This establishes a set of conditions in which responsible, creative, and productive individuals and groups reap higher rewards than the less effective members of the organization. Moreover, these conditions result in a competitive advantage in the business sector, and cost effectiveness in the public sector.

The quality of work life for nurses may be improved by ensuring meaningful work, reducing the management-labor dichotomy (we-they) and improving the peripheral work system that seems to encumber nurses in their jobs. Then the issues of organizational climate can be addressed.

Every organization is said to have a climate that colors the perceptions and feelings of persons within the work environment. A company's climate is influenced by innumerable factors such as its size, the nature of its business, its age, its location, the composition of its work force, its management policies, rules and regulations, and the values and leadership styles of its supervisors. Many of the factors influencing an organization's climate are dynamic and interactive, resulting in ever-changing "weather" within the organization. However, some factors remain relatively constant, and this tends to stabilize the characteristic climate for the organization. These pivotal factors are such things as growth rate, delegation tendencies, innovative processes, communication patterns, and stability of the organization. These variables can be analyzed individually for any organization and can provide guidance to new employees when determining what to expect.

The new nurse must concern herself with the quality of work life. Health-care organizations are neophytes in the process of converting from the outdated organizational styles to the more contemporary managerial models. The complexity of this change is compounded by the numerous factions that must be coordinated into a new model. This change will not be easy, but it will be essential to the survival of the organization. The new nurse today will be the change agent for this process.

Changing Roles of Management

Managerial roles are the key to coordinating effort and technology. The responsibility is not new, of course, but is becoming increasingly complicated by the accelerating rate of change in health care. Because change requires adaptation at all levels of the organization, the new nurse is confronted with the circular problem of encouraging innovation, and then introducing change in a manner that will not threaten the innovator. Being human, the new nurse, too, is vulnerable to the threats of change and must be able to monitor and evaluate her own effectiveness and take measures to prevent her own obsolescence. Through capable supervisory style, management systems, and other factors affecting organizational climate, the source of influence must shift from official authority to people power so that the initiative and freedom at all levels of the organization will find responsible expression.

The environment in which every employee is a manager provides a realistic opportunity for each employee to be responsible for his job. Though many jobs in their present form cannot be fully enriched, most can be improved, or fused with others, or more uniquely matched with individual aptitudes and attitudes. Whether the supervisor's mission is to modify the job or to match it to the right persons, it is best achieved by utilizing the talents of those she supervises.

The nurse in a managerial role must be able to understand the conditions promoting and inhibiting the expression of talent among the team members. This requires a close look at the new responsibilities and activities with which she should be involved and an equally close look at which of the traditional roles must be modified to accommodate the ever-evolving changes.

It has been said that the most valuable characteristic for those who want to succeed is flexibility. This is certainly true for nurses today. As the health-care industry has changed so dramatically in the past few years, so have the roles of nurses. These changes have led to a good deal of role ambiguity as nurses search for models that will meet the demands. The managerial roles being assumed by clinical nurses are the result of requirements to push decision making lower in the organization and to encourage the staff nurse to become the determinant of ways in which the delivery system can best function.

The contemporary supervisor is finding that the pure managerial role is also changing. No longer an authoritarian order-giving manager, today's supervisor concentrates on providing a climate in which individuals have a sense of working for themselves. Thus the role of the supervisor should be to

- Provide visibility for organizational goals
- Provide resources and define constraints
- Mediate conflict
- Stay out of the way, in order to let individuals manage their work

This redefinition of the supervisor's role to provide opportunity for persons to manage their own work gives clear direction to the staff nurse to assume responsibility, whether that be clinical or managerial.

Thus, the new staff nurse must be prepared to see examples of all types of management. Some managers have made the transition to newer styles and others have not. But keep in mind that the requirements for change and organizational growth will always be with us and, in the future, those nurses who are flexible and competent will emerge as leaders. Also keep in mind the ultimate goals you have and work toward them.

Summary

Managerial concepts needed by the new nurse focus on how to deal with people, how to manage resources, and how to manage one's own job. No resource of this type can be all inclusive, but it can offer insights that offset the unknown. This is important in making that first job more meaningful and understandable.

Your own attitudes, how you view yourself, and exactly where your successes or failures lie will be determined by *you*. It is important to recognize where you are and what you feel capable of accomplishing so that you do not become controlled by events. Rather, *you* will control how you think and what you think and thereby control your reaction to these events.

It is not enough to expect that, if you work hard, you will rise to the top. The process is so complex that predictability is difficult, but it is certain that if you follow some basic concepts of managing yourself, you have a better chance of success.

You must make a commitment to grow, both as a total person and as a nurse. Your attitude is the key element, as was beautifully stated by Abraham Lincoln: "Most people are about as happy as they make their minds up to be."

It is possible to be incredibly happy and satisfied in nursing. Over time you will not necessarily become smarter, but you will become more experienced. This experience leads to more effective behaviors and outcomes. Your success as a nurse starts with you and your attitude toward that responsibility. If this book is of some value to you in that process, then the editor will be deeply gratified.

Bibliography

Belker L: The First-Time Manager. New York, American Management Association, 1978
Myers M: Every Employee a Manager. New York, McGraw-Hill, 1981

Chapter 2

Assessing the organization

KARLENE M. KERFOOT
JOYCE E. JOHNSON

One of your tasks as a newly employed nurse is to understand the behavior of individuals with whom you work. The way in which your coworkers respond to requirements of the job may be a reflection of the organization itself and its expectations of employees. Each organization has a purpose as well as a unique manner in which that purpose is put into action. That plan of action is the organizational "culture" or "character" and it will be clearly and rapidly transmitted to you and to those with whom you work.

Although formal rules and regulations create the organizational culture, so do informal expectations. In some instances informal expectations can be more powerful than formal rules, and they can have an impact on your performance—either positively or negatively. Because the character of an organization affects you as a professional nurse, understanding the formal and informal structure and functions of organizations can assist you in choosing the health-care facility where your role as a professional nurse and the organization's expectation of you coincide and complement each other.

In order to choose the health-care facility where you can best "fit," you must be able to understand and assess the organization. This chapter will enable you to

1. Identify theoretical concepts that can facilitate your assessment of the organization.
2. Describe the history of organizational theory and relate it to the health-care setting.
3. Discuss some of the variables used in assessing an organization.
4. Define organizational behavior in terms applicable to all health-care facilities.
5. Identify ingredients key to the success of an organization.
6. Identify key strategies in assessing the organization.

Classic Organizational Theory

Classic organizational theorists suggested that the size, structure, division of labor, number of supervisory levels, and span of control were key variables in determining the success or efficiency of an organization.[1] Figure 2-1 is an example of this organizational structure used by many health-care facilities today. It is based upon the belief that breaking down the operation into *specialized* components is necessary for the assignment and completion of responsibilities. Creating these specialized segments demands coordination that is best handled by *delegation of authority* to supervisory personnel such as the nursing administrator or a head nurse. *Structure* is essentially the height of the organization as compared to its width, while *span of control* defines the number of employees controlled by the supervisor. A flatter organization (depicted in Figure 2-2) may increase the span of control while levels of authority decrease. Many health-care facilities have moved in the direction of a flatter organizational design.

Classic organizational theory also defines staff and line relationships. Those with *line* roles, such as the head nurse, have direct responsibility for employees and services. Line authority has traditionally been defined

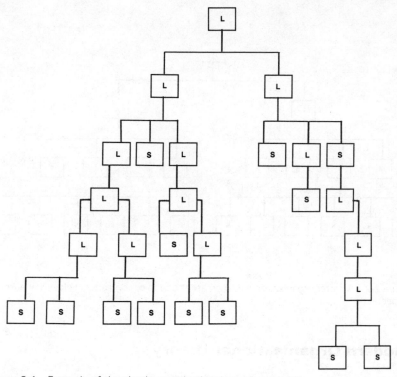

Figure 2-1   Example of the classic organizational structure used by many health-care facilities today.

as the right to hire and fire. In contrast the *clinical specialist* has traditionally held a *staff* position, indirectly responsible for the same services through employee education, consulting, and role modeling. Figures 2-1 and 2-2 depict both line and staff positions.

One of the biggest criticisms of the classic organization theory is that the lack of participative decision-making opportunities for employees is a function of the structure itself.[2,3,4] Often the individual who *makes* the decisions and the individual who *implements* the decisions occupy different positions on the organizational chart. This criticism has formed the basis for studying the psychology of work behavior that focuses on the importance of involving individuals in the decision-making process.[5] Participation by employees has been researched extensively as a means of increasing employee motivation and goal commitment.[6,7,8,9]

Most organizations, including health-care facilities, have progressed beyond the "classic" model to one that reflects the modern approach to organizational structure and design.

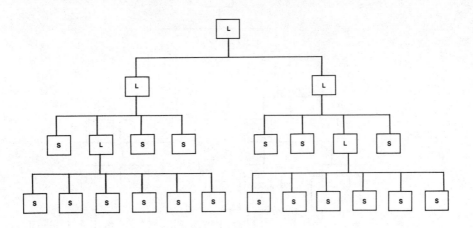

Figure 2-2 A flatter organization may increase the span of control while levels of authority decrease.

Modern Organizational Theory

Modern organizational theorists depart from organizational structure and suggest that an essential element in understanding or predicting organizational behavior is the ability to predict the behavior of the *persons* who make up that organization.[3,10]

Modern organization theorists contend that motivation, satisfaction, leadership, and the manner in which conflicts are resolved are key to organizational harmony and success. This approach maximizes the value of the individual, whereas in classic organizational theory, structure and function are of key importance. It also recognizes that each employee has a certain set of unique processes, feelings, and thoughts that may not "fit" with those of the company. If they do not, then tension exists between the employer and employees. It becomes the role of the supervisor to initiate activities that assist both the individual and the company to succeed together.

Assisting employers and employees to "work together" has been the focus of a variety of theorists who are convinced that the "structure and process of an organization is a single phenomenon."[5] For instance, in 1960 Douglas McGregor developed two fictional supervisory belief systems, labeled *Theory X* and *Theory Y,* to describe relationships between supervisors and their employees.[11] Supervisors who believed in

Theory X controlled and directed the behavior of employees, whereas those who believed in *Theory Y* provided an atmosphere that encouraged participation in decision making by controlling not the employee but the surrounding work environment.

While McGregor attempted to integrate the goals of the organization with those of the employees, Argyris contrasted the way in which organizational structure restricts employee development.[10] For instance, one nurse may be better suited to work in the technical atmosphere of the operating room, while another achieves and succeeds as a professional in psychiatric nursing care. A mismatch in either case would inevitably lead to tension between the nurse and the health-care facility, which is demanding that certain actions take place to achieve harmony. These actions could involve areas such as absenteeism, turnover, and the role of labor unions. The employer may suggest that the employee relocate to another section of the organization where the employee might have a better chance of succeeding. Perhaps the most important belief in defining modern organizational theory is that the individual must "fit" with the organization and the organization with the individual.

ORGANIZATIONAL CHARACTERISTICS

Identifying health-care facilities where you can find the best organizational "fit" for yourself is dependent upon your ability to define factors that you value in a work situation. Factors that have been identified as "key" in many organizations include: 1) organizational size; 2) formalization, and 3) centralization of authority.[12] Organizational size refers simply to the number of employees and related services. Formalization is the degree to which communications and procedures in an organization are written. It includes the extent to which rules, instructions and communications are documented.[13] Centralization of authority means the amount of power given to subunits or departments. It is the delegation of responsibility from top management, such as the nurse administrator, to the middle manager or, in most cases, first line supervisor or head nurse.[14]

You should be able to assess organizational characteristics during your interview process or early in your employment. Suggested methods of assessment are discussed later in this chapter.

ORGANIZATIONAL CLIMATE

During your interview process or early in your employment you will formulate an impression of an institution. You may perceive a large health-care facility as "busy or cold," whereas a small community hospital may appear to have a "quiet, calm, and homelike atmosphere."

The *personality* of an organization constitutes the climate. It is the perception of the climate that ultimately describes the organization as efficient, bustling, cold, easygoing, or human, to list some descriptive terms. Although difficult to conceptualize and quantify, this variable has the most impact in affecting rates, productivity, and job satisfaction.[12]

ORGANIZATIONAL EFFECTIVENESS

The ability of an organization to achieve its mission or goals or the degree of its "success" is called its organizational effectiveness.[12] The ability of an organization to be effective is dependent upon communication patterns, centralization of authority, supervisory styles, employee morale, and productivity. But perhaps the most important central concept is the ability of the organization to define its mission and related goals. If these are clear and understood, the direction in which an organization is moving will be visible as will the activities engaged to reach the ultimate mission.

Health-care institutions historically have proclaimed in mission statements a commitment to delivering *quality patient care.* Goals that include the introduction of new programs and services broadly define ways in which a hospital expects to achieve the stated mission.

ORGANIZATIONAL CONFLICT

Tension within the organization creates conflict. The idea of "conflict" may mean feelings of hostility on the part of one person or group toward another or others.[12] It may also mean intentional efforts on the part of one person or group to prevent others from achieving goals and thus ultimately decrease the chance for success by the organization.

More important than the fact that conflicts do and will continue to arise is the manner in which conflicts are resolved within an organization. March and Simon identified several approaches to conflict resolution.[3] The most commonly used of these include problem solving and persuasion.[5]

Problem solving encourages individuals to identify one common objective. They then gather information and devise and implement a plan to achieve that objective. Participation is encouraged in an atmosphere that focuses on the problem, not on the conflict arising between individuals or groups. An example of problem solving is the addition of a new patient population to a nursing unit. The nursing personnel might believe they lack the clinical experience needed to provide care to the new patient population while management believes they are prepared. In order to resolve the conflict, the nursing staff together with the management personnel develop and implement an educational program designed to provide the appropriate care to the new patient population.

Persuasion is the process in which conflicting individuals or groups can be brought together. Two groups can believe that they share the same beliefs; however, *at some level,* they work toward goals that are specific to their level of agreement.[5] For instance, employees and management may disagree on the percent of wage increase needed to achieve equity in the marketplace. Both groups do, however, believe in the need for a raise. The amount is then determined, based on each group testing its respective rationales associated with salary increases, such as salaries attached to a clinical ladder for advancement versus an "across-the-board" wage increase. Problem solving and persuasion techniques focus on encouraging individuals to participate in decisions designed to resolve the problem. Further, they are less disruptive to the organization since problems are dealt with as close to the point of origin as possible.

How to Define and Use the System

In the American health-care facility, nursing is usually the largest division or department. The placement of the nursing department in the hospital structure should be of utmost importance as you begin to assess the organization in which you are employed or are pursuing employment. Be certain to review the hospital and nursing organizational charts. This can be accomplished during your interview with the personnel department or your prospective supervisor. Structures that are "flat" usually permit decentralized participative decisions to occur and less bureaucratic "red tape" to pursue in implementing decisions.

Keep in mind that the health-care facility's chief nursing administrator *should* be on peer level organizationally or formally with the hospital's chief medical director and the director of all major service departments and should report to the chief hospital administrator. This permits direct representation of nursing's interest to those responsible for delineating the institution's mission and goals.

THE NURSE EXECUTIVE

As part of this analysis, it is important to understand the nurse executive's role within the context of this particular institution. Nurse executives assume a variety of roles throughout the United States, depending on the environment in which they find themselves, their background and level of expertise, their beliefs about what is good administration, and so forth. Nurse executives have many different roles, depending on the size of the hospital, the philosophy, and other variables. A person new to an organization needs to analyze this role thoroughly to better understand what is expected, and what is acceptable and unacceptable professional behavior. Part of being a successful professional is developing the ability to understand and meet the expectations of a particular setting.

A nurse executive's philosophy of administration can be rated on a continuum from a centralized to a decentralized management style. Centralized management systems will appear on paper as very "tall" organizational structures, with many layers between the staff nurse and the nurse executive. Most of the decision making is centralized in the nurse executive and there are no forums and councils for staff nurses and head nurses to participate in the working of the nursing department. If there are councils/forums in a centralized structure, these will not be decision-making bodies and will instead be information delivery systems for the nurse executive. Decentralized structures, by contrast, will be "flat" and there will be very few levels between the staff nurse and the nurse executive. The role of the staff nurse will be expanded in this structure and there will be greater expectations for participation by staff nurses in the governance of the organization. In a decentralized structure, persons in administration are seen as those who can bring the resources to the staff nurse to facilitate the work of the professional staff nurse as opposed to directing the work of the staff nurse in a centralized structure. Decentralized structures work from a "bottom up" style of organization versus the "top down" style seen in a more centralized organization. The power over clinical decisions in the decentralized organization resides in the highly developed role of the professional nurse rather than in the nurse executive. Decisions about nursing care are delegated to the professional nurse and supported by the nurse executive.[15,16] In a centralized style of management, the power resides in the nurse executive. Patient care decisions are made at this level and implemented by the staff nurse whose role is seen as that of a doer and not a thinker.

There are many gradations of these two models. In reality, it is virtually impossible to find the pure form of either the centralized or decentralized model. Most nursing organizations are a combination of both styles but can usually be characterized as having more components of one style than the other.

The nurse executive determines the culture of the nursing organization, based on many factors. She must design the nursing organization within the limits of the particular setting. So although the nurse executive might favor one style of management, this might be compromised because of variables such as sophistication of the nursing staff, management style of the chief executive officer, beliefs of the board, and other defining situations.

In reality, therefore, one often sees a confusing picture of management style on the part of the nurse executive. In some issues, she will react as if one style is supported and in another situation will react another way. The professional nurse learns to analyze effectively the role of the nurse executive and determine how that role will affect her practice at the particular institution and predict reactions based on this analysis.

MIDDLE MANAGEMENT

The next position to analyze is that on the first level down from the nurse executive. These positions are called assistant directors in some settings, vice presidents in other settings, clinical coordinators, divisional directors, and so forth. These positions usually have a collection of clinical units that are for the most part related in either a medical model classification or in a functional classification.

How the person in this position implements the role is dependent on a variety of factors similar to the factors under which the nurse executive operates. In some settings, the organization is decentralized to the point that persons in this position have great freedom to perform in a variety of management styles. In other organizations, behaviors are more standardized and this role carries with it less responsibility and accountability. In both models, one will see great variation in the way in which persons in this position perform. Some individuals are well prepared by education and experience for this position and fulfill the role quite well. Others have very different perceptions of the way in which this role should be performed. Depending on the influence of the person in this position, he will or will not have great impact on the every day functioning of the unit. The responsibility of the staff nurse in the institution is to analyze how this role is performed on her clinical division and react accordingly within that framework.

THE HEAD NURSE

At this point in time, the position traditionally known as the head nurse role probably has more titles than any other in nursing organization. The individual is variously called unit manager, nurse manager, clinical coordinator, and many other equally nondescript titles. This role can be categorized on a continuum from being a simple charge nurse role to that of being a department manager with 24-hour accountability and a mandate to manage a budget, to hire and fire, and in general run an autonomous unit. In this latter model, the need for persons in assistant director positions is minimized and the expertise of the head nurse is maximized. This role can also be placed on a continuum from being involved in direct patient care at one extreme to performing no direct patient care at all, and variations between.

Unfortunately in nursing, we have no consistent standards for credentialing required for the role of head nurse. Some institutions require master's degrees in clinical or administrative nursing and others require only excellent performance in the role of the staff nurse as a prerequisite. The head nurse's philosophy of administration can be quite varied. Some believe in decentralizing the governance of the unit to the staff nurse, while others keep tight centralized control of management functions. Some head nurses have a keen interest in patient care and others emphasize the management part of their role. A key to successful administration of a unit is the communication of expectations by the head nurse to others on the unit. Analyzing these expectations and understanding the "lay of the land" determine the success or failure of the staff nurse on that unit. Expectations are usually not communicated directly. The staff nurse must infer from the actions of the head nurse the beliefs that person holds.

Be alert to the number of employees under the control of one supervisor. Although management theory varies regarding the "correct" span of control,[5] a head nurse who is responsible for 50 nursing personnel may not be able to provide individual guidance unless assistant supervisory staff is available. Ask how many and what categories of personnel report to the head nurse. Are assistants provided in her absence?

STAFF POSITIONS

Assess the role of those holding "staff" positions, such as clinical specialists, nursing researchers, and educators. Determine how you will be expected to interact with them in the delivery of patient care or in committee and/or project activities. In some settings, persons in staff positions are intimately associated with the nursing staff and are expected to provide direction to the nursing staff. In other settings, they have less contact with the staff.

THE STAFF NURSE

The staff nurse also plays a variety of roles in various institutions. In some very sophisticated systems, the staff nurse is seen as the professional with the greatest amount of decision-making power concerning clinical practice. A share governance system supports this belief and staff nurses are involved in the control of clinical practice through a system of peer review and credentialing.[17,18] Councils or forums provide the vehicle in which information and decisions flow from the bottom up. On the opposite extreme, a more technical model views the staff nurse as more of a "worker bee" who carries out the directives of the head nurse and assistant director.

Defining the nursing care delivery system in which you will work will be key in assessing your organizational role. This can be done with both the head nurse and staff nurses. There are many variations of primary nursing as well as modular or team or functional care delivery. Within nursing, many types of persons work to provide patient care in addition to professional nurses. Aides, technicians, licensed practical (vocational) nurses, and unit secretaries are just some examples of unit-based staff. Pharmacists, laboratory technicians, volunteers, and many other persons come into direct contact with the nursing staff. Directing the work of patient care through these persons demonstrates that professional nurses must know how to train, motivate, and monitor ancillary staff and develop collaborative relations to ensure that nursing care standards are being met. The wide variety of patient needs has demanded that the nurse learn effectively to meet these needs by coordinating the work of others.

Cultural differences often account for problems between the professional and the ancillary staff. The ancillary staff must accept the cultural norms of the hospital as their own and support the professional nurse. Professional nurses spend a significant amount of time in school learning the concepts of professionalism such as altruism, justice, and so forth. Ancillary staff come to us without this education and consequently often do not understand what is expected of them. In some settings ancillary staff have been known to "test" new nurses, rather than support them. Nurses who are tested least are the ones who remain in control and are able to be good managers of this group.

ROLE EXPECTATIONS

Part of the adjustment to the management aspect of the nurse's role is adjusting to the expectations of what that role demands. For example, if the nurse is put in "charge" of a unit, she must think above the individual care of patients and learn how that role should be defined to provide patient care. The person who is role oriented knows the expectations of that role, the patient care outcomes that result from the full enhancement of that role, and how that role fits into the scheme of the entire institution. When they are first in practice many nurses confuse role expectation with their own personal needs, and the personal needs of others. For example, a nurse can place her personal need to be liked above the requirement of the professional nurse role of requiring performance from others that produces quality care for patients. The nurse's needs are met but patient care suffers. When people prioritize the personal aspects of the job the role is fraught with inefficiencies and ineffectiveness. The basic function of any role is to get the task completed. Individuals who cannot determine what the tasks and expected outcomes are (inherent in a role) are doomed to failure. Individuals who can get the job done (complete the tasks inherent in the role) and have their personal needs met through the accomplishment of these tasks are valuable staff members. The nurse needs to examine the expectations of this role and work to make sure her output matches those expectations.

Establishing professional relationships is the key to effective management for the nurse. Professional relationships differ from personal relationships in that the care of the patient is the ultimate reason for the relationship and this is never forgotten. When personal relationships become more important than the care of the patient, then the professional relationship is lost and the quality of patient care is reduced. If the nurse can remember that she is entering a relationship to improve patient care and not to meet her own social needs, there will not be a problem with defining how that relationship must develop. It is when social relationships and professional relationships are mixed up that the quality of patient care suffers. It is very easy to negotiate with another department when one keeps in mind that the outcome is quality patient care. It is very difficult to negotiate with a department when social and personal needs take priority above the needs of patient care.

INFORMATION SOURCES

The need for information within a nursing department is great. People in management positions must be informed of potential and actual problems. The ability to prioritize information and to keep others informed is a very sophisticated skill that is learned through experience and through mentoring. Individuals in various positions have differing needs for information. It is imperative that the new nurse analyze information and communicate effectively within the particular structure. Many institutions have unwritten rules concerning with whom a particular staff member does and does not communicate. For example, a nurse in one institution can send a memo to the chief of radiology without copies to her head nurse and assistant director. In other institutions, this would not be allowed and only the nurse executive could communicate with the chief of radiology. The best way to understand the communication structure in a particular setting is to find someone who is willing to take the time necessary to discuss communication and to provide guidance and feedback. A person who will help one learn the communication structure in a particular setting is invaluable. Understanding communication structures and learning to use them well can make the new nurse very effective in her role.

CONFLICT COMMUNICATION

Occasionally the staff nurse must determine how to handle the situation when she has a disagreement with her immediate supervisor. Again, this varies among institutions and it is very important for the nurse to understand the protocol within that particular nursing department. As a rule of thumb, it can be assumed that the nurse must thoroughly exhaust all possibilities for compromise with the immediate supervisor. If a resolution cannot be found, the nurse may request that she and the immediate supervisor meet together with the person who is above the supervisor in the chain of command. It is seldom, if ever, appropriate for a staff nurse to circumvent her immediate supervisor and go to the next level without discussing the situation thoroughly with her supervisor. It is appropriate to inform your supervisor that you would like to take the matter to the superior and that you would like the supervisor's support in this matter. The nurse can ask the immediate supervisor to accompany her or she may request to go alone. The aggressive person often places the supervisor in an untenable position by operating in a demanding mode and escalating the problem. One must be well versed in conflict management and be willing to enter the conflict with a positive frame of mind and believe a solution will be reached that will be for the benefit of all. Entering a conflict with an attitude that "I must win and you must lose" will doom the situation to failure. Both persons in a conflict must emerge the winner.

DELEGATION

One of the most difficult skills to learn is that of delegation. Throughout school, nurses are taught that they are ultimately responsible, they cannot shirk their duty, they must take care of everything themselves, and they cannot depend on anybody else for help. When they move into the world of work and are involved in the management aspect of their role, this does not hold true. Being able to work through others, to delegate appropriately and effectively, and to establish monitoring systems to make sure that what was delegated is accomplished at the level of quality expected and on time is very important. If clear directions are given, a time stated for completion of the task, and appropriate coaching and monitoring has taken place, delegation will be effective. Inherent in this process is the ability to assess the strength and weakness of each person with whom one works. An individual can delegate effectively only when she is thoroughly familiar with the capabilities of every person. If any of these principles is ignored, effective delegation will not occur and the quality of patient care will be lessened. In management, work is accomplished only through other persons. Learning to delegate effectively will accomplish this quite efficiently.

SUPPORT OUTSIDE THE NURSING DEPARTMENT

In addition to the positions with direct responsibility to nursing, the nurse must be very adept at analyzing the roles of members outside the department of nursing. In some situations, other departments are seen as totally supportive to the professional nurse and these departments see themselves as serving the main function of the hospital, which is to provide nursing care. In other settings where strong belief about nursing is not present, departments are seen as more autonomous units; they can be self-serving and exist for reasons other than providing the resources enabling nurses to take care of patients.

The successful nurse is able to analyze accurately the roles in a particular institution, and to work with them effectively. In order to deliver the best kind of nursing care possible, one must understand all the roles inherent in the institution and optimize each one of them to the point where the best service is made available for nursing. If one is able to work effectively with other departments, the goal of excellence in nursing care will be easily reached. The most effective work groups are those that feel a sense of cohesion and define the norms of the group as high output and quality care. The nurse fosters cohesion and team spirit by paying attention to interpersonal relations and by emphasizing similarities between persons and reflecting on the common goal—excellence in patient care. Nurses can take on the role of cheerleader and can support staff and reward individuals for excellence. By contrast, some nurses choose roles of constantly criticizing, gossiping, emphasizing differences rather than similarities, providing negative feedback, and initiating conflict. Each nurse is an important factor in creating the climate of the work group and its productivity, depending on the behavior chosen.

INSTITUTIONAL MISSION

Once you have reviewed the hospital and nursing department structure and associated roles, review the hospital mission statement, its short- and long-range goals. Compare the goals with those of the nursing department, especially at the unit level. Determine from the head nurse the unit goals. You should be able to identify readily a united commitment toward the achievement of the overall mission, from top management to the nursing unit. If this is lacking, the institution may have communication difficulties and/or organizational uncertainty causing employees to be out of step with management expectations. Review policy and procedure manuals, taking note of revision dates and those who, by signature, assume responsibility for their contents. Peruse newsletters and general hospital publications. The personnel department is an appropriate place to gain access to such materials. You should obtain a clear sense of where the institution is heading and how it intends to reach selected goals. Clarity of goals will enhance your productivity.

In some situations, the new nurse will find that her philosophy does not match that of the institution and therefore a poor "job fit" exists. When this goes unchecked, a situation may develop in which the nurse, who can be quite good clinically, is ostracized because she does not meet the realities of the institution. The nurse has either to alter her perceptions of what nursing should be, work to change the mores of the institution to be more compatible with her own, or leave the institution and find a place that complies more completely with her belief system about nursing. It is unfortunate, indeed, when a nurse does not realize that delivering excellence in patient care depends on the coordination of many persons and involves the synthesis of a variety of personalities in a way that assures good patient care. There is no perfect place to deliver patient care. All institutions have their good points and their bad points. It is imperative that the nurse be able to analyze these accurately and work to actualize the positive potential of the institution.

As a professional you should be interested in opportunities made available by the organization to participate in institutional decisions. Review the committee structures, activities, and reporting relationships focusing on how input from employees reaches the nursing and/or hospital administrator.

You might assess just how the organization values its employees. Is the institution unionized? If so, does an open or closed shop exist? Has the institution conducted surveys to assess employee satisfaction? Are educational programs made available to both management and nonmanagement personnel? Is a clinical ladder in place? Better yet, does the organization value nursing education and research? If so, how is this value demonstrated? You should be interested in the process routinely used to resolve conflicts. Does the supervisor unilaterally settle disagreements or is an attempt made to develop a cohesive team atmosphere or an esprit de corps? How often have the supervisory or higher management positions turned over?

Organizations that are open and interested in their employees usually have mechanisms in place where outstanding individuals are recognized. Seniority, high performance, and low absenteeism are valued. Are employee recognition programs in place, such as Employee of the Month or Year? Are merit increases tied to performance or are they "automatic?"

Answers to these questions can assist in determining if you and the institution will organizationally "fit" together. You can determine the opportunities that exist for your present and future growth and you can also determine if the institution is a "pleasant" place in which to work.

ADDITIONAL RESOURCES

There are many resources available to nurses within the institution. For example, clinical specialists in nursing can offer expertise about specific clinical problems. Institutions with nurses on an advanced level on the clinical ladder can offer invaluable expertise and knowledge about the system and patient care. Probably the most important relationship for the new nurse to develop is with a mentor. In order to do that, the new nurse must be open and available for feedback, must want to learn about herself, and must be constantly looking for suggestions for improvement. A mentoring relationship does not have to be formal. It can be quite informal. It is a relationship in which the new nurse learns the style that is appropriate to the institution and the ways in which nursing care can be performed in that setting. Mentors do not have to be supervisors. Mentors are the individuals who can teach you how nursing can be done best within the particular organization and how you can develop your personal skills. Persons who have good mentors have good coaches. Nursing is entirely too complex to learn it all by yourself.

Determining the various roles and developing resources for personal support are two key activities that will determine the success of the new nurse in the role of staff nurse.

Summary

Nursing is a complicated profession that involves much more than the direct "hands-on" care of patients. Many very competent clinicians have failed as nurses because of their inability to master the management aspects of the clinical role; as a result the highest quality of nursing care has not been provided. By the nature of their work, nurses are placed in an environment in which they must work with others to accomplish their goals. Consequently, knowing how to work most effectively with others is crucial to the success of the staff nurse.

Nursing is an exciting career that can bring many rewards. The key is developing the ability to work effectively in many varied situations and with a variety of persons.

References

1. Weber M: The Theory of Social and Economic Organization. Henderson AM, Parsons T (trans, ed). New York, Oxford University Press, 1947
2. Lowin A: Participative decision making: A model, literature critique and prescriptions for research. In Organizational Behavior and Human Performance 3(1): 68–106. New York, John Wiley & Sons, 1968
3. March JG, Simon HA: Organizations. New York, John Wiley & Sons, 1958
4. Taylor FW: Principles of Scientific Management. New York, Harper & Brothers, 1947
5. Landy F, Trumbo D: Psychology of Work Behavior. Homewood, IL, The Dorsey Press, 1976
6. Vroom VH: Work and Motivation. New York, John Wiley & Sons, 1964
7. Lawler EE: Motivation in Work Organizations. Monterey, CA, Brooks/ Cole Publishing, 1973
8. Coch L, French JRP: Overcoming resistance to change. Human Relations 1:512–532, 1948
9. Whyte WF: Money and Motivation: An Analysis of Incentives in Industry. New York, Harper & Brothers, 1955
10. Argyris C: The Applicability of Organization Sociology. New York, Cambridge University Press, 1972
11. McGregor D: The Human Side of Enterprise. New York, McGraw-Hill, 1960
12. Champion DJ: The Sociology of Organizations. New York, McGraw-Hill, 1975
13. Litterer JA: The Analysis of Organizations, 2nd ed. New York, John Wiley & Sons, 1973
14. Blau PM: A formal theory of differentiation in organizations. Am Sociol Rev, April 1970
15. Althaus JN et al: Nursing Decentralization: The El Camino Experience. Rockville, MD, Aspen Systems, 1981
16. Porter-O'Grady T: Shared Governance for Nursing: A Creative Approach to Professional Accountability. Rockville, MD, Aspen Systems, 1984
17. Peterson ME, Allen DG: Shared governance: A strategy for transforming organizations, Part 1. J Nurs Adm 16(1):9–12, January 1986
18. Peterson ME, Allen DG: Shared governance: A strategy for transforming organizations, Part 2. J Nurs Adm 16(2):11–16, February 1986

Bibliography

deLodzia G, Greenhalgh L: Creative conflict management in a nursing environment. Super Nurse 4:33–41, July 1973
Dickelmann NL, Broadwell MM: How to get the job done . . . by someone else. Nurs 77:110–116, September 1977

Doona ME: A nursing unit as a political system. J Nurs Adm 7:28–32, January 1977

Douglas LM, Bevis EO: Predictive principles for delegating authority. In Nursing Management and Leadership in Action, 3rd ed. St. Louis, CV Mosby, 1979

Drucker PF: The Practice of Management. New York, Harper & Brothers, 1954

Heimann CG: Four theories of leadership. J Nurs Adm 6:18ff, May 1976

Kast FE, Rosenweig JE: Organization and Management, New York, McGraw-Hill, 1979

Lewis JH: Conflict management. J Nurs Adm 6(10):18ff, October 1976

Marriner A: Decentralization versus centralization. In Hanson R (ed): Management Systems for Nursing Service Staffing, pp 45–53. Rockville, MD, Aspen Systems 1980

McClure M: Managing the professional nurse, Part 1. J Nurs Adm 16:83–86, February 1985

McConnell EA: Delegation—myth or reality? Super Nurse 10(10):20ff, October 1979

Rotkovitch R: The head nurse as a first-line manager. Health Care Super 1(4): 14–17, 1985

Shoemaker H, El-Ahraf A: Decentralization of nursing service management and its impact on job satisfaction. Nurs Adm Q, Winter, 1983

Stagnitto MREB: Nursing supervision: Leadership or police work? Super Nurse 10(1):17–18, January 1979

Sullivan E, Decker P: Effective Management in Nursing. Menlo Park, CA, Addison-Wesley, 1985

Chapter 3

Communication in complex organizations

WILLIAM M. WARFEL

Individuals are able to obtain undergraduate and graduate degrees in the field of "communications." With such a broad and diverse subject that *could* require years of study, it may seem futile to attempt to discuss the topic in one short chapter. But in our highly complex society and profession, and in an ever increasing environment of technologic expansion, the need for more effective ways to communicate is clear. It is apparent that nurses in particular must develop the necessary communication skills to be able to perform their jobs effectively. The problems associated with the flow of information are very evident in large, complex organizations.

When an unforeseeable outcome occurs the problem most frequently cited as the cause or source is "poor communications." One frequently hears the old retort, "It's a communication problem," as a reason why something went wrong. It is not unusual that certain medication or treatment incidents or policy implementation issues are labelled as communication problems. Given the highly diverse backgrounds and work settings in which the modern nurse practices, it is incumbent that today's nurse have the necessary repertoire of skills to reduce the communications deficit. As a nurse, there is no aspect of your position that cannot be analyzed, in part, as a communications process. In their role as professionals, nurses are constantly communicating with their environment—their patients, colleagues, superiors, and subordinates. Effective communications can improve both the quality of patient care and your working relationships and that will ultimately lead to higher job satisfaction.

This chapter will enable you to

1. Identify the basic elements of the communication process.
2. Identify barriers to effective communications.
3. Identify strategies for effective listening.
4. Become familiar with a variety of nursing activities as they constitute a communications process.

The Communications Process

If nurses are to enhance the communications in their work setting, they must understand the communications theory and process. While many theorists have described models to explain how individuals communicate, it is generally accepted that there are a few elements basic to any communication process. Communication is the exchange of meanings between and among individuals through a shared system of symbols that have the same meaning for both the sender and the receiver of the message. These symbols include both verbal and nonverbal forms of communication.

In the process, the message may be affected by feedback from the receiver to the sender. The channel that carries the message carries the spoken or written word, and includes other aspects of communications such as nonverbal gestures and pictures. The message is surrounded by many other variables, the "climate" in which the transmission occurs. The climate includes the environment or circumstances under which the communications take place. A particular message may be interpreted differently by the same receiver, depending on the circumstances surrounding the transmission. Moods, weather conditions and temperature, and timing, as well as many other considerations, are part of the climate. If a person initiates a message while under stress, there may be distortion in the message transmission. The same is true if the receiver is experiencing a stressful situation—the likelihood of hearing the message clearly is affected. Effective communications are far more than clearly sent messages.

Consideration of the climate surrounding the message transmission is equally important. Transmission of messages must take place in an environment or "climate" that permits clear transmission of the message. Disturbances in the environment, frequently called "noise," need to be considered seriously in order for effective communications to take place. Just as atmospheric disturbances can create static or distortion in radio or television reception, disturbances in the climate surrounding the message transmission can seriously distort the communication attempt. Many of the elements of the climate may be controlled. For example, visiting hours may not be the time for the nurse to give discharge instructions if the patient is enjoying a visit from relatives or friends. If the patient is preoccupied with the happiness of a given moment, this distraction may affect the information the patient hears. Because of its numerous distractions and interruptions, the nurses' station may not be the place to talk with the patient's primary nurse about the patient's response to nursing interventions. The only way to communicate effectively may be to leave the station and find a quieter spot for the discussion. The study of communications includes all of these considerations, as well as an analysis of the barriers to effective communications.

The Flow of Communications: Upward, Downward, and Lateral

In large, complex organizations, such as the ones in which nurses work, skills are required in writing, speaking, and listening *effectively*. Because communications involves the transmission of information from a sender to a receiver, and because the formal structure of an organization has a powerful effect on communication between workers, it is helpful to study the direction in which the communications flow in complex organizations. In this context all communications can be thought of as falling into one of three categories: upward, downward, or lateral communication. The direction of the communications then refers to one's superiors in the organization, their subordinates, and their peers. This framework is particularly appropriate for analyzing the transmission of messages within complex organizations. The directional flow of communications is important because different strategies are required for different segments. It is evident that the way in which you communicate with your superior will involve different considerations than the way in which you communicate with a nurse colleague. The same distinction is true when you are communicating with ancillary staff members. Your position in the organization will, to a degree, determine the way in which you communicate. Planning care with the ancillary staff will require a completely different repertoire of strategies than communicating to your nurse manager your need to take some time off on a scheduled work weekend.

Gillies (1982) states that downward communications in a line organization consist mostly of commands in authoritarian terms. An example would be how you would delegate aspects of care to the ancillary staff. However, it is clear that delegating in authoritarian terms may be perceived in a negative manner. Including staff in planning the assignment communicates a more participative approach that can promote a more satisfactory outcome.

Communications laterally tend to be more consultative or coordinative and are delivered in terms of equality. Communications with nurse colleagues will be on an equality basis where there is cohesiveness and a sense of trust and respect within the work group. Effective lateral communications, then, will be partly affected by the atmosphere of collegiality that exists in your work unit.

When you communicate upward in the organization, to your nurse manager or to a member of administration, the communication is much more carefully filtered and is often delivered in apologetic or defensive terms. It is a fact that by virtue of your position in the organization, you will be more cautious about communicating upward. However, in a properly structured work environment, one that fosters openness and creativity, a person is more comfortable with upward communications. The outcome can be less defensive posturing and more comfort in keeping your superiors informed and seeking consultation. Obviously, the choice of a work place with a "climate" that values individual contribution is as important as how to communicate messages clearly.

An interesting question occurs. How do you communicate with doctors—upward, downward, or laterally? There has been a good deal written about collegial relationship between doctors and nurses. This implies lateral communication relationships that can benefit patient care. It will take some time to establish your credibility so that communications are truly lateral. Some nurses "talk down" to doctors—downward communications—and many will view the physician as "above them" in the organization that, we have said, "filters" the information exchanged. Lateral communications that are accomplished on a basis of mutual respect and trust will have the most benefit for you and your patients. It is hard work to establish that type of trust but it is achievable.

The Nurse's Credibility as Sender of the Message

A person's ability to communicate a message is related to a person's credibility as a source for that message. A large part of one's success is based on whether the receiver believes or trusts in a person as a credible source. If the source is considered knowledgeable, truthful, and reliable, then the person has enhanced her opportunity to influence the receiver.

Lack of credibility will interfere with the receiver's ability to read or hear the message. When a credibility gap exists between the nurse and the receiver, this contributes to the "noise" or distortion in the message.

It is the nurse's responsibility to communicate the patient's needs to the physician, the goals for nursing care to peers and ancillary staff, and appropriate information to the nurse manager. The professional nurse who operates from a base of knowledge and confidence will increase the likelihood of accurate transmission of messages. One's credibility then rests on what has to be said and how it is stated. Conveying uncertainty ("I'm not sure why but . . . ") or making statements that cannot be supported by a good rationale will diminish one's credibility in the eyes of the receiver. Keane (1981) states that one can be more persuasive if

1. One is perceived to know what she is talking about
2. One believes in what she is saying
3. One presents herself in a convincing manner

The nurse's credibility can facilitate or act as a barrier to positive communications. Because the responsibility for making the message understood is primarily the responsibility of the sender, the nurse needs to evaluate her credibility as sender of the message.

Listening

A sometimes underplayed and unappreciated aspect of the communications process is that of listening. It is generally accepted that the receiver actually hears or retains only a small part of the message that was sent. The average person spends 70% of her time listening, but only one third of the message is retained. Given the inefficiency of our listening skills, coupled with the busy "climate" in which most nursing communications take place, the nurse cannot passively absorb the spoken word. She must try to grasp the facts and feelings of what is being said.

To be able to concentrate on what is being communicated is not easy. There are many barriers to effective listening. This is particularly true for today's nurse who is constantly reestablishing her priorities in order to accomplish daily activities. Many distractions and apparent excessive demands on her time can interfere with the concentration necessary to be a good listener.

The good news in terms of one's ability to be an active listener is that it is possible to improve one's listening skills through a variety of activities. Munn (1980) has identified the guidelines listed here that can be employed to improve one's listening skills.*

To improve listening skills

1. You should prepare yourself physically by standing or facing the speaker. Making sure you can hear physically is essential for good listening. You thereby tell the sender that you are ready to listen and are able to hear the verbal messages and also see the nonverbal messages the speaker is sending. This face-to-face attention also shows that you are interested in what is being said. People tend to avoid and look away from people and things in which they are not interested. Attention and interest are synonymous. You pay attention to the things you are interested in, and you are interested in the things you pay attention to.

2. You should learn to watch for the speaker's nonverbal as well as verbal messages. Everyone sends two messages. One message is sent verbally and the other is sent nonverbally through inflection in the voice or through facial expression, bodily action, or gestures. Sixty-eight percent of all messages are sent nonverbally. The nonverbal message conveys the speaker's attitude, sincerity, and genuineness. To miss the nonverbal message is to miss half of what is being said.

3. You should not decide from the speaker's appearance or delivery that what he or she has to say is worthwhile. When you start to focus on the speaker's delivery or appearance, you become distracted from the purpose of communication, receiving the speaker's ideas! You should be more interested in what people have to say than how they say it or what they look like.

4. You should listen for ideas and underlying feelings. Again, the purpose of good communication is to be able to reflect upon and exchange ideas. For example, if I were to meet you on the street and give you a dollar and you gave me a dollar, and you then went your way and I went mine, neither of us would be better off because of the exchange. But if I gave you an idea and you gave me an idea, then both of us would be better off as result of the exchange.

5. You should try to determine your own biases, if any, and allow for them. Communication gets blamed for many things. Whenever something doesn't go right, you might say you have a communication breakdown. But many times you don't have a communication breakdown at all. In fact, you might have very good communica-

*Munn HE Jr: The Nurse's Communication Handbook. Germantown, MD, Aspen Systems, 1980. Reprinted with permission.

tion; you both know what has been said, and there is a common understanding. But you don't like what you have heard. If the nurse, physician, or surgeon could learn to recognize such differences, better relationships would be formed. You will not always agree with everyone. The trauma in such situations develops when you discover you are no longer talking about the issues, but about each other.

6. You should attempt to keep your mind on what the speaker is saying. Don't allow yourself to become distracted. Too many times people fake attention and like the little dog in the back of the car window just keep nodding their heads up and down without hearing a word of what is being said.

7. You should not interrupt immediately if you hear a statement that you feel is wrong. Indeed, if you listen closely, you may be persuaded that the statement is right. Sometimes you may fail to listen just because of this fear of something different, of the possibility that you may have to forsake some sacred position you have held for years.

8. You should try to see the situation from the other person's point of view. This doesn't mean that you always have to agree. However, there is no way that you can change other people's perceptions until you can see how they have formulated those perceptions.

9. You should not try to have the last word. Listen to what is being said and then think about it. This reflection may take some time, but you need time to think before you communicate. Sometimes, in order to solve problems, you have to walk away from the problem for a while and think about it from different points of view, and about the advantages and disadvantages of possible solutions.

10. You should make a conscientious effort to evaluate the logic and credibility of what you hear. Our mind functions at some 500 words a minute, but we normally speak at 125 words a minute. In other words, we can think four times faster than we can speak. Rather than letting our minds become bored, we can take advantage of this time differential between thinking and speaking. We can attempt to anticipate the speaker's next point, attempt to identify and evaluate supporting material, and mentally summarize what the speaker has said: What has thus far been said that I can use?

The nurse who is able to use these suggestions to improve her listening skills will begin to realize how important active listening is as part of the communication process. The average nurse spends more time listening than she spends speaking or writing. When you begin to realize how much information can be gleaned through active listening, it will become apparent that it deserves considerable attention as an aspect of communication because good listening skills are the antithesis of barriers to effective communications.

Nursing Activities as Communication Processes

The remainder of this chapter will focus on communication activities in which nurses commonly engage. The focus will be on these activities as communication processes, which implies the need for careful analysis of the many dynamics in order to ensure a favorable outcome. Such activities are predominantly a matter of communicating. Reflecting on these activities as a communication process can provide new insight for better results.

CHANGE-OF-SHIFT COMMUNICATIONS

An excellent example of an area in which communications may or may not work is the change-of-shift report. Depending on the length of your shift, this routine typically occurs 3 times each day. Nurses who provide care in the home report to others regarding patient status, but on a less frequent basis. In this age of primary nursing, the need effectively to communicate patient needs seems essential in a system designed to encourage individualized care planning and continuity.

What sometimes happens is that nurses ritualistically report on the patient using the Kardex, their work sheets, or tape recorders. The emphasis is on what needs to be done for the patient. While that may be essential information to communicate, it is frequently retrievable from the source of the tool being used to "give report." Effective communications for improving continuity of care would include exchange of information not readily available in other ways. Why read the Kardex to one another? It is far more productive to spend this relatively brief time communicating about the patient's condition and response to nursing interventions. Consistent with previous statements, it is well worth considering the idea of "walking rounds" as a way to maximize the exchange of information, by actually observing the patient. Rather than having the charge nurse make out assignments before actually observing the patient, this approach will enhance the communications process by focusing on meaningful information from specific observation. By looking critically at what kinds of information will be most beneficial, you can actually improve the change-of-shift report and enhance communications. The change-of-shift report can become an integral part of the nursing process by using the opportunity for observing and assessing the patient's condition and by planning and evaluating nursing interventions.

INTERVIEWING AS A COMMUNICATIONS PROCESS

One of the communication sessions most important to you personally is the job interview. You have probably had or will have many different job interviews. You wanted some of those jobs because they were in your area of interest or expertise, the work hours were desirable, the institution was appealing and provided the opportunities for professional nursing practice, and so forth. Whatever your reason for wanting the job, the interview is an opportunity to communicate your interest and knowledge.

There are many considerations to be made in preparing for the interview. Attire, makeup, and other considerations are important and will nonverbally communicate your suitability for the position as perceived by the interviewer. But the importance of being able to clearly convey your thoughts is imperative during the interview process as stated so succinctly by Rose S. LaRoux:

> You can have expert knowledge; but if you cannot communicate your ideas clearly, forcefully, and fluently, you will have little influence. You can have expert skill; but if you cannot demonstrate your skills to others and move them to action, you will have little power.*

Interviewing is something that nurses do over and over again. You interview patients, families, physicians, coworkers—you spend a large part of your day interacting with others for the purpose of gathering information. Interviewing is purposeful communication. It focuses on a specific subject. It is one of the most controlled or structured types of communication experiences. Because it is so planned, it would seem that the information obtained would be as accurate as possible. The reality is that even formal interviews are subject to the same considerations and opportunities for miscommunication as are other human interactions.

One thing that nurses do frequently is to go on job interviews. The employment interview is an opportunity for you to apply principles of communication for the purpose of achieving a favorable outcome. A review of some of these considerations is worthwhile and applicable to interviewing generally.

*Communication and influence in nursing. In Huntsman AJ, Ringer JL (eds): Communicating Effectively, p 11. Wakefield, MA, Nursing Resources, 1981

The employment interview would appear to be mostly a verbal communications effort. Decisions regarding your employment will be made on the basis of the information exchanged. The important point is that the interview is two-sided—both parties attempt to gather as much information as possible in order to make an informed decision.

Presume you are in a job interview. Are you the interviewer or the interviewee? Well, that all depends! If you presume that you are there to be interviewed, then you have assumed a passive position and will not obtain the information you need to make a decision. You may be able to assess the environment to a degree by the nature of the questions you are asked, but you will not receive the necessary clarification in order to accept or reject an offer.

But if you assume a more active approach, you, too, will have a set of questions you need answered. In this way, the communications flow both ways. At any point, you may be the interviewer or the interviewee. It's a good idea to remember that you are not the person who arranged the interview and you should not attempt to "take over" the communications process. At the same time, you have an obligation to yourself to obtain the information you need to make your decision.

Basically there are two ways to ask questions during an interview. Two theorists who have most influenced the way in which questions are phrased are B.F. Skinner and Carl Rogers. Skinner, the well known behaviorist, believed that behavior that is rewarded tends to be repeated. What rewards can you give? You can listen as a form of positive feedback, you can look interested, and you can nod approvingly. The Skinnerian line of questioning is directive and provides the opportunity for you to answer a question honestly and factually.

Rogerian questioning assumes a contrasting viewpoint—one in which the questions are open-ended or nondirective. These types of questions allow for your creative and intellectual expression and are more thought provoking.

Your employment interview is likely to include both types of questions. When the opportunity arises to address some of your concerns, you would be wise to tailor your line of questioning according to the information you desire. For example, questions about employment conditions and benefits could be more directive, while your questions about nursing philosophy and other more esoteric issues may best be approached in a nondirective way.

There are many opportunities to maximize this communication opportunity. Consider the nonverbal communications that go on if you are late, if you are not neatly dressed, or if you are chewing gum. The same nonverbal communication goes on with your patients—they expect you to appear and behave in a certain way and when you do not meet these expectations, the communications may be hampered.

In interviewing, there are many other positive considerations that will enhance the information imparted. Again, the principles are applicable whether it is an employment interview or another interaction, including nurse-patient interactions.

1. Avoid being too formal or too cold. Conveying a warm, friendly demeanor will encourage positive communications.

2. Avoid distractions. Communication is an active process that requires you to focus on the line of questioning and devote your attention to the interview. One should minimize the environmental distractions by providing adequate space, quiet, and comfort.

3. Avoid "yes" and "no" responses. These may be appropriate to a very directive line of questioning but usually these responses discourage further communication.

4. Do not monopolize the conversation. While "yes" and "no" answers are poor, so is the interviewee who digresses and fails to respond to the specific question. Answers should be succinct; lengthy answers will be viewed unfavorably.

5. Avoid your personal biases. Be aware that our personal values, beliefs, and biases may interfere with successful communications. Awareness is the first step in assuring that biases do not interfere with information exchange.

The well planned interview, with principles properly applied, affords the nurse the opportunity to maximize the communications process. When interviewing for a job, you have the opportunity to decide whether you want the position. A poor choice on your part could result in unhappy employment circumstances. At the same time, the perspective employer is making a decision about you, mostly as a result of verbal and nonverbal communications. Understanding the dynamics of this process can enhance the opportunity for a favorable outcome.

COMPUTER COMMUNICATIONS

The use and potential for computer applications in nursing communications systems is well substantiated. The application of computers to the health-care industry has been predicted but, in part, lagged behind the technology for many agencies. Now, in the wake of prospective payment, the need for better data management systems has hastened the installation of terminals and printers, and the nurse has become one of the "users." The need to be able to communicate by means of the computer is a reality that every nurse will face in the near future.

Unfortunately, many nursing school curricula have not been any more ambitious about the possibilities of computer automation than the

health-care facilities that have postponed installations. Schools of nursing that are forward thinking have included computer literacy considerations and are preparing for present realities. The computer will
enable the nurse to handle an increasing volume of information in forms
that can be readily applied to practical patient care or management
problems.

An example of how you will communicate with the computer for
improved patient care includes sophisticated patient scheduling systems. Without automation, it is not unusual to have conflicting therapies
and tests scheduled for the same patient, that is, the patient is in physical therapy when he is called to go to radiology. Automated scheduling
will discourage such conflicts and even print a work order that informs
you of the appropriate patient prep.

The communications opportunities that computers afford are very
exciting and scary at the same time. The opportunity for nurses to
reduce uncertainty in decision making and to ensure more timely and
effective care delivery can present a positive opportunity. But, traditionally, nurses have not been schooled in such technologies. Resistance to
automation is, in large part, a result of the nurse's acculturation. In this
case there is no truer saying than "the only thing to fear is fear itself."
The fear is quickly overcome when nurses begin to use computer hard-
ware and software to maximize information and patient care. They find
that much of the mystique surrounding computers is more imagination
than fact. Automated patient information systems in which the patient's
medical records are filed in computer memory and nurses add information to each file on a real-time basis are currently available. The goal for
computer systems is the elimination of planning and documentation *as
we know them today* and movement toward a "paperless" system. What
dramatic implications these changes will have for the ways in which
nurses communicate with patients and other members of the health-care
team! The challenge is clear but nurses will need to acquire new skills in
order to communicate successfully in the near future.

CONFIDENTIAL COMMUNICATIONS

While nurses have infrequently been challenged for disclosing personal
information they learned about a patient during the provision of care,
the possibility does exist that it may happen. Nurses are not usually protected by the law as are doctors and lawyers, where the court gives them
information under the condition that it may not be disclosed (Gillies,
1982). The danger for nurses, though, is the possibility of divulging to
others information that the other person should not have. Patients come
into a health-care institution and place their confidence and trust in the

institution's employees. Nurses walk a delicate line between what is appropriate to communicate and what is not.

Suppose Miss Smith from another floor informs you in the cafeteria that she heard her neighbor, Mrs. Green, is a patient on your floor and then asks you "What's she in for?" Presuming you know the answer, would you stop to think twice before responding? This is a sensitive communications issue. Is it a violation of Mrs. Green's confidence for you to answer Miss Smith? The answer is clearly yes. But what do you say to Miss Smith? "You'll have to ask Mrs. Green"? Maybe! It is clear that Miss Smith would not have to try very hard to get the answer she wants.

Miss Smith's desire to know why Mrs. Green is in the hospital is not the real issue here. The fact is that nurses are continually exposed to confidential, sensitive information. As a nurse, you will continually be in situations in which you are trying to decide what and what not to communicate. There is a fine line between these two extremes. The mistake nurses make is presuming that information they have about a patient is part of a common body of knowledge other members of the team share the right and need to know. The point is that it is the patient's right first and the patient can expect that only necessary information will be shared.

Why not give Miss Smith the answer to her question? You give the very same information to other nurses who are working on the unit. The decision is based on who has the need for the information in order to provide Mrs. Green with the care she needs during her hospital stay. These are not always easy decisions. But the realization that certain information you have is confidential will help you be aware there is the potential for a violation of a patient's right if you communicate certain information. Your employing agency should also have a policy on confidentiality. Familiarize yourself with these guidelines. Like many others, they will not tell you specifically what you may and may not communicate, but they will provide you with the framework to make reasonable decisions when faced with such matters.

COMMUNICATING THROUGH TOUCH

The use of human touch in nurse-patient interactions has received a fair amount of attention in the nursing literature. It is generally accepted that the use of touch may have a beneficial response for patients in developing nurse-patient relationships and in their recovery. But have nurses really viewed touch as a major form of nonverbal communications? Most publications focus on whether or not touching makes a difference in establishing relationships or in promoting recovery. If we begin to view touch within the framework of communication forms, then it follows that the principles of effective communications will apply.

A knowledge of when touch can be "therapeutic" and when it may actually be more of a barrier can help the nurse to decide how to practice effective communications through touch. To begin with, we may presume that touch can sometimes be an effective form of communications, but not always. Research by Witcher and Fisher (1979) serves to illustrate how touch may or may not be a good form of communications. Their experiment focused on some implications of interpersonal touch by studying the value of touch in nurse-patient interactions. Specifically, they assessed the effects of nurses touching patients during preoperative teaching, considering many variables. Their results suggest that touch led to positive effects for female patients but had a reverse effect for male patients.

Touch for females resulted in lower anxiety and more positive behavior preoperatively, and these results were associated with more favorable postoperative physiological responses. In the experiment by Witcher and Fisher, touching was a beneficial form of communication for female patients but not for male patients. The experimenters' results support a sex difference hypothesis. This hypothesis predicts that when dependency cues are pervasive, such as in touching, male and female patients will respond differently. Their rationale is that males and females are acculturated in American society so that males are more uncomfortable with dependency situations than females. Therefore, the experience of nurse-patient touch is perceived by male patients as a threatening gesture that communicates inferiority and asserting dominance. This leads to negative reactions.

The nurse needs to be sensitive to the message she as the sender transmits by touching the patient as receiver. All the same principles of effective communications apply. For example, the barrier to effective touch communications may be male/female acculturation. However, the touch response to touching may be improved through consideration for timing, the environment, and so forth. Like other forms of communication, whether touch is experienced positively or negatively by the receiver depends on the meaning and evaluation that the patient receivers ascribe to touching. Touching as a form of communications can transmit many things—positive messages such as concern or empathy, or negative messages such as dominance or a desire for intimacy that can make some patients uncomfortable. Touch messages may be expected to have a negative response to the degree that they overstep the boundaries the patient has defined as appropriate. They will be positively received to the extent that they are appropriate to the situation, do not impose a greater level of intimacy than the patient desires, and do not communicate a negative message.

DOCUMENTATION AS A FORM OF COMMUNICATION

Documentation is one of the most frequently used forms of communicating that nurses perform. Documentation is meant to validate the care you deliver, to provide a means of communicating care between health-care providers, and to create a permanent record of that care. Despite the increased emphasis on the importance of good documentation, nurses frequently assign a low priority to documentation. Because of the many activities they are expected to perform for patients in the course of a normal work day, they feel that the time spent documenting patient care takes away from the precious time they have to deliver that care. Nurses need to rethink this reasoning because you have probably heard it said that "if it isn't documented, it wasn't done." What is meant by this statement is that the only way to verify the care given to patients is through a record of process and outcomes. Nurses become really tired of being told to "document it" in response to an issue they identify. For a variety of reasons, documentation takes a low priority for many nurses. But the fact remains that documentation as a written communication form is a necessary part of the professional nurse's role.

The patient's record is the most obvious example of documentation. It is full of entries that attempt to establish the assessment and plan for the patient. But few really seize the opportunity to use the record for the intended purpose of communicating between various members of the health team—the opportunity to share observations, concerns, plans, and findings.

The patient's record will serve the goals of effectively communicating patient care when those who record entries seize the opportunity. Some of the rules for nurses in communicating through documentation include clear and concise messages that are legibly written and properly endorsed. Nurses need to follow hospital policy, such as by observing the use of abbreviations that are on the approved agency list. Health-care providers are notorious for formulating new abbreviations but unless we observe the rules, we may destroy our ability to communicate effectively, which requires that we speak the same language. Creating your own language through unapproved abbreviations is not acceptable.

Accuracy and truth in documenting is a must. Legally speaking, you should put the whole truth and nothing but the truth on the medical record. Purposely omitting information from the chart or making inaccurate entries can result in legal penalties or loss of license. The courts consider lack of truthful documentation as strong evidence that proper care was not given (Bernzweig, 1985). The importance of the medical records as evidence in a court of law cannot be overemphasized. The accuracy and completeness of nurses' entries have been receiving increasing attention as malpractice issues rise and as nursing is becoming increasingly recognized as a profession accountable for its own practice. Following established, accepted procedures for altering an entry in the medical record can provide you protection. Observing rules such as never erasing anything, and following generally accepted practices for the proper way to document can help to protect you. All entries, including changes, should include the date, your name, and your title.

The same concerns for communicating properly apply to other forms of nursing documentation. The nurse's plan of care has become a permanent part of the patient's record and a recording of the nurse's assessment of the patient's needs/problems and nursing interventions. One of the issues that surfaces in nursing documentation centers on the fact that communication may not be effective because nursing has not sufficiently developed its own language. While still a long way from standardization, the nursing diagnosis may serve as a common vocabulary for the nursing profession because it identifies precisely what nurses do. The development of a common vocabulary is essential to improved communications.

Another problem that frequently occurs in documentation is the lack of consistency in format within a particular agency. For example, the problem-oriented approach to documentation is favored by some and discouraged by others. It would be nice to think that the opportunity for creativity and self-expression occurs when nurses are allowed individual ways of approaching the matter. The unfortunate truth is that nurses do not always communicate effectively because they do not speak the same language. It is incumbent that all providers decide on which format they will use in order to ensure proper communications concerning patients.

Another pertinent example is the topic of integrated progress notes. All providers are expected to document on the same progress note. It is apparent that this should be a positive step toward improved communications. But, tragically, some like it and some do not. Many physicians are offended when others make entries on "their" progress notes. They argue that there may be a conflict between the nurse's entry and their entry. How sad this argument is! It is very clear that such conflicts between entries already exist. If nurses were to use the integrated notes approach, the possibility of eliminating such conflicts would be increased through better communications. Nurses can help the system to move in the right direction by continually improving the documentation, regardless of which approach is used. Clear, concise documentation of patient assessments and response to nursing interventions will eventually lead to improved communications in the medical record.

NURSE-PHYSICIAN COMMUNICATIONS

According to Prescott and Bowen (1985), "When physicians and nurses work together optimally, relationships are positive, disagreements are collaboratively resolved to the benefit of the patient and patient care flows smoothly and efficiently." Considerable attention has been given to nurse-physician relationships in the literature and there seems to be agreement that there is room for improvement.

It is clear the articles and research on nurse-physician relationships could also have been entitled nurse-physician communications. Clearly, there has been a breakdown in communications between the two groups that may be attributed to a variety of social, economic, and political changes. Changing scopes of practice and redefining relationships have frequently led to what is perceived to be a competitive rather than collaborative posture. This agenda will not serve to benefit patient care.

What exists appears to be a communications breakdown that is manifested by attitudinal responses. This is different from semantic communication disorders that are more easily corrected. Communication failures due to poor attitudes are more difficult to remedy but they can be improved through training and effort.

Although there should be no desire to return to former styles of accommodating behaviors—those in which physician dominance and nurse deference are maintained—there should be an opportunity to communicate effectively. The establishment of collaborative practice models, primary nursing models, and nurse-physician forums are attempts, in part, to establish mechanisms that promote improved communications. Given the complex and acutely ill patients for whom nurses provide care today, there is no room for the errors that can result from poor communications. Doctors comment that "the nurse never makes rounds with me anymore." Nurses respond that "I'm too busy." The patient suffers. The need for effective teamwork that fully uses the potential contribution of *all* care-givers is apparent. Teamwork is really all about communicating effectively to the patient's advantage.

NURSE-PATIENT COMMUNICATION

Within the nurse's realm of management possibilities, no other area affords the nurse so much opportunity for application of theory as when she is interacting with patients. Most of the time nurses are engaged in some form of nurse-patient interaction. This represents the most significant part of what nursing is, and is actually a form of continuous communications between you and your patients. Every word and every gesture give the nurse and the patient more and more information about each other. The frequency with which you interact, the tone of your voice, and how you appear all transmit messages that are perceived differently by different patients depending on a variety of influencing variables—the patient's age, sex, race, religion, and many other environmental considerations.

Excellent nurse-patient communications requires sensitivity to the patient's needs and a well developed and carefully thought-out plan to meet the assessed needs. What are you communicating if your plan includes visiting the patient briefly at least once an hour because your assessment concludes that the patient is very lonely? Your plan includes frequent interactions to show interest. But what message are you communicating to the patient? That depends on a variety of considerations. You may very well be communicating what you intended *or* the patient may become concerned with the frequency of your visit, which he perceives to be necessary because of his serious condition. An unappropriate alarm reaction could result rather than your well-intended plan to decrease the patient's sense of isolation and loneliness.

One message nurses frequently give patients is that they do not have time. This may be transmitted nonverbally by standing near the doorway when talking to the patient or by confiding to the patient how busy they may be.

Consider further another example, the difficulty in establishing effective communications with patients in complete isolation. Patients may feel inadequate and estranged. Verbal communications to the patient may sound different as a result of being filtered through the mask you are wearing. You bathe the patient while wearing rubber gloves that serve as a physical barrier to tactile communication. The ritualistic way you need to handle linen and fomites further reinforces the patient's sense of alienation. Most of what you must do to protect yourself and the patient communicates to the patient that he is "dirty" or at extreme risk of becoming infected because of his immunosuppression. The example of the "completely isolated" patient requires that the nurse-patient communications be well planned in order to be effective.

If it is accepted that effective nurse-patient communications can positively affect outcomes, then it suggests that the corollary should also be considered. Ineffective communications may have either desired or deleterious effects. Because blood pressure and heart rate are significantly affected while speaking (Thomas, 1984), nurses need to consider the cardiovascular response they invoke when communicating with patients. A nurse who approaches a patient when stressed or in a brusque manner may elicit higher blood pressure measurements that would not generally be a desirable psychological response.

The most important realization is that communications between nurses and their patient is the essence of nursing practice. Through your understanding of the communication process and the barriers to effective communications, you will have the skill to look beneath the surface of nurse-patient communications for meanings and implications. Among the techniques available to you are interviewing, reading, consulting with others in developing your plan of care, including nurse specialists, doctors, and the patient's family, and by educating patients and their families through the use of materials that are available for teaching. The nurse is the one who is best prepared to assess and respond to patient needs. Effective communications are synonymous with effective nurse-patient interactions.

Summary

Communication is the core of all of the elements of nursing practice. Nurses practice in complex organizations where networks of communication are established. Organizational structures may facilitate effective communications or provide barriers that inhibit communications. The nurse's understanding of the dynamics involved can increase the nurse's effectiveness in communicating.

When communicating, the nurse will be sending or receiving information. The sender-receiver channel is influenced by many variables that determine the "climate" in which the interaction is occurring. The feedback loop further influences the form of the communications. Generally, the sender should be aware that the way the message is interpreted by the receiver is largely determined by the receiver's systems of thought. If the message is to be clearly understood, it must be stated precisely, under the appropriate circumstances, and it must be recognized by the receiver as valid to the situation. The receiver has the responsibility for working actively to understand and interpret the content of the message. While communicating is a complex process with many variables that influence the transmission of the message, there are opportunities, too, for the nurse to increase her ability to communicate effectively through the development of communication skills.

Bibliography

Bernzweig EP: Go on record with nothing but the truth. RN 4:63–64, 1985

Gillies DA: Nursing Management: A Systems Approach. Philadelphia, WB Saunders, 1982

Keane CB: Management Essentials in Nursing. Reston, VA, Reston Publishing, 1981

Prescott PA, Bowen SA: Nurse–Physician relationships. Ann Intern Med 7:103–110, 127–133, 1985

Thomas SA, Friedmann E, Lottes LS, Gresty S et al: Changes in nurses' blood pressure and heart rate while communicating. Res Nurs Health 6:7-2, 119–126, 1984

Witcher SJ, Fisher JD: Multidimensional reaction to therapeutic touch in a hospital setting. J Pers Soc Psycho 1:37–1, 87–96, 1979

Chapter 4

Leadership and motivation

BETH TAMPLET ULRICH

Often thought to be a function only of those in supervisory positions, leadership and motivation are, in fact, necessary abilities for *every* nurse. If your position includes the responsibilities of primary nurse, team leader, charge nurse, staff nurse on a unit with licensed practical nurses or aides, or of patient care, you need to understand how to lead and how to motivate other persons.

This chapter will enable you to

1. Identify the necessary ingredients of leadership.
2. Understand the role of a leader.
3. Understand the basic characteristics of motivational theories.
4. Understand when and how to delegate.

Leadership

The essence of leadership is the relationship between an individual and either another individual or a group of individuals. For every leader, there must be those who are willing to follow. This relationship develops over time and results in one person (the leader) having influence over others (the followers). Having followers is one thing, however, and being an effective leader is quite another. General Custer was a leader, but his last followers would certainly question his effectiveness.

It is also necessary to differentiate leadership from management and supervision, although the terms are often used interchangeably. Zalenik (1981) offers several distinctions. Managers, he says, are problem solvers who tend to be *reactive* rather than *active*. Managerial goals arise out of necessity rather than desire, with the manager viewing work as an enabling process. The manager is a negotiator, continually coordinating and balancing to maintain the existing order of affairs. Leaders, on the other hand, are risk takers with an active approach to problem solving and goal setting. They look for new ways to solve problems and create excitement in others. Leaders work in organizations, but never totally belong to them. Think of the leaders in nursing. Florence Nightingale certainly chose a new and unique path for a woman of her time. Since then, nursing leaders have developed both the art and the science of nursing through taking risks and opening new territories for professional nursing.

While it is certainly possible to be both a good manager and a good leader, good managers are not always good leaders and good leaders are not always good managers. Likewise, not every good manager or leader matches all of the description given by Zalenik. As you progress through your nursing career, try to determine the difference between managers and leaders. Then look at yourself. What characteristics do you have that would enable you to manage or to lead effectively? What abilities do you need to develop? The challenge as you progress through your career is to find a match between what you enjoy doing and what your abilities will enable you to do. There is and will continue to be a need in nursing and health care for both managers and leaders. You need only to choose a path.

WHAT MAKES A LEADER?

The challenge to define what makes a leader has plagued researchers since the early 1900's. The question has not yet been answered conclusively, but many concepts have been proposed.

Trait Concept

The trait or "great man" concept was popular in the 1930's and 1940's. It assumed that there was a finite number of identifiable traits that differentiated between successful and unsuccessful leaders. Originally, believers in the trait concept thought the traits were inherited. This gave rise to a term still used today, the "born leader." Later, however, the thought shifted to the theory that traits could be obtained through learning and experience. The traits identified most often were intelligence, attitudes, and personality measures. The problem was that the study results were not consistent and no pattern could be identified that accurately predicted a leader.

Behavioral Concepts

Given the inconclusive data obtained when researching the trait concept, investigators began to focus on analyzing just what a leader does and how the leadership function is carried out. Behavior was most often seen as a continuum, ranging from autocratic to democratic or production centered to employee centered. The move to behaviorism was accompanied by an increasing concentration on management rather than leadership, and it might better be called a management concept. As noted previously, however, the terms are often used interchangeably.

Production-centered versus employee-centered management distinguishes between an orientation to tasks and an orientation to the employee or, sometimes in nursing, to the patient. This is also known as the structure-consideration concept. Each aspect or structure-consideration is regarded independently. Attention to both can be high at the same time or low at the same time, or attention to one can be high and to the other, low. This concept paved the way for the contingency leadership concepts that followed.

Contingency Concepts

An alternative to believing that the effectiveness of a leader is based solely on traits or behaviors, the contingency approach holds that leader effectiveness is contingent on some combination of leader traits, leader behavior, and the situation itself. A number of contingency models have been proposed. The most popular is the situational leadership approach, which holds that the effectiveness of a leader is based on the task to be performed, the person or persons performing the task, the degree to which the leader is perceived to have influence, and the style of leadership that the leader employs. This means that no one way of doing things is right for every situation.

Nowhere is that clearer than in health care. A participative approach may work well, for example, when the staff is developing specific patient education programs; but it does not work well in the middle of an emergency procedure such as a code when one person must be in charge. The problem that most often causes conflict between a leader (or manager) and her followers (or employees) is when the roles and decision-making authority are unclear. It does little good to request participation if the employees feel that the decision has already been made. One should only invite participation when the participants can really contribute to the decision. It must be clear whether the participants are being asked to contribute their input and advice *only* or whether they are being asked to help make (and therefore to assume responsibility for) the decision. If you have the most information and knowledge about a subject and if you are ultimately responsible for the decision, it is reasonable for you to make the decision and to let others know that you are doing so. For example, in some patient care situations, you as the registered nurse should make the decision because your education and experience make you the expert when compared with nonprofessional health care workers. In other situations, such as when you are the primary nurse for a patient, it may be very beneficial to hold a patient-care conference in order to collect information and to establish the plan of care as a team. Whatever style you use or participate in at any given time, it is more effective if everyone involved knows her role ahead of time.

LEADERSHIP STYLES

Leadership style is the way in which a leader goes about accomplishing her goals and those of the organization. There are numerous ways of classifying leadership styles, most of which rely on some continuum of behavior patterns. While it is unusual today to see a leader who practices only one style, it is important to recognize the styles and the situations in which each may be most effective.

The most common classification of leadership styles is the continuum that ranges from autocratic to laissez-faire. Autocratic or authoritarian leadership is a style in which the manager makes the decisions and the employees carry them out. Little input is requested or received from the employees. Autocratic leadership is effective in a crisis, but it encourages dependency. Democratic leadership, in its purest form, means that everyone contributes information and input into the decision-making process and that everyone has a say in the decision that is made. It is a very people-oriented process. Democratic leadership often increases employee morale, but can decrease efficiency. Autocratic leadership has been viewed as undesirable while democratic leadership has been favored and hailed as a sign of enlightenment. The difference between the two is the degree to which the decision-making function was shared. Participative management is an outgrowth of democratic leadership. Participative management is a matter of degree rather than the all-or-nothing approach often seen in the past. While many have sung its praises, the results of participative management have not been consistently positive. In much of the research, participative management has been shown to be associated with higher satisfaction but also with lower performance. Laissez-faire leadership is at the opposite extreme from authoritative or autocratic leadership. In this form of leadership, the leader takes a "hands off" approach and lets the employees make decisions, implement plans, and so forth. While some people protest that laissez-faire leadership is no leadership at all, others note that this style can work well when the employees all work well independently and are committed to the job and the organization.

Likert (1962, 1967) proposed four styles of leadership that he described as management systems. These styles were exploitive-authoritative, benevolent-authoritative, consultative, and participative. The first two categories are both authoritative, but differentiate in the manager's approach to the employee. In the exploitive-authoritative, the manager makes the decisions and communicates them in a dictatorlike fashion. In the benevolent-authoritative style, the manager occasionally seeks some minor input from employees, but does it in a condescending manner. The manager still makes the decisions. Neither of these approaches is likely to result in a commitment by the employees to the organization or to the manager. In the consultative style, as the name implies, the manager consults the employees and decision making begins to filter into the levels of the organization below the manager. Likert is a major supporter of the participative style, in which increased communication and group decision making is the norm. It is of interest to note that Likert originally developed the now widely utilized Likert scale as a means of measuring factors related to management.

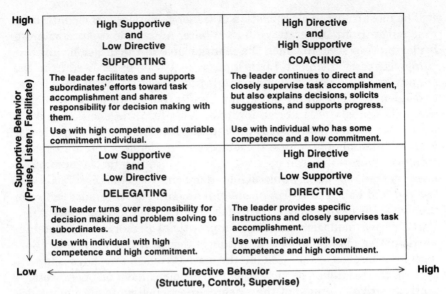

Figure 4-1   Four basic leadership styles. (From Blanchard K, Zigmari P, Zigmari D: Leadership and the One Minute Manager, pp 30, 47, 56. New York, William Morrow & Co, 1985)

Blanchard and colleagues (1985) describe the four leadership styles shown in Figure 4-1: Directing, coaching, supporting, and delegating.

These four styles are composed of various combinations of two basic behaviors, directive behavior and supportive behavior. In the early development of the situational leadership concept, these behaviors were referred to as task behavior and relationship behavior. Directive behavior involves structure, control, and supervision, while supportive behavior involves praise, listening, and facilitation. Blanchard and co-workers (1985) also note that in deciding which leadership style to employ, the leader must also assess the competence and commitment of the individual. Competence is a function of knowledge and skills ability, while commitment combines confidence and motivation.

CHOOSING YOUR LEADER AND YOUR APPROACH

It is important for you to understand yourself and how you work best. If you are someone who likes to work independently, calling on resource people only when needed, then working with a manager who is very structure-oriented would probably not satisfy either of you. However, as a new graduate, you will need more resources than nurses who have been in practice for awhile. When you interview for a position, ask questions about the person for whom you will work and the resources that are available. Aim for the best fit between your needs and an organization's needs.

You will be in a leadership position on your first day of work as a professional nurse. The patients see you as a leader and the licensed practical nurse by law works under your supervision. Think about the task to be performed, the ability of the person performing it, and the nature of the situation (life threatening or routine) before you decide what approach to take.

In addition to the formal leadership structure, you will also need to become familiar with the informal leadership of the unit and the organization. Organizational charts do not always paint a clear picture of the real world. On nursing units, there is often an informal leader among the professional staff and an informal leader among the ancillary staff. Their power may be derived from a number of sources that will be described in the following section. Regardless of the source of their power, be it knowledge, skills, length of service, or who they know, it is important for you to recognize who these leaders are. Power is not always used positively and you may not agree with their beliefs. Before you can change beliefs, you must plan, and planning involves obtaining information. An informal leadership structure is usually more evident in units or organizations without a strong formal leadership.

Power

Del Bueno and Freud (1986) note that "organizations are made up of people who are consistently vying with one another for power, status, and prestige." This statement aptly describes health-care organizations, especially as resources become increasingly scarce. Power is the ability to impose the will or desires of one person or group of persons on another individual or group of individuals, in order to influence and alter their behavior. In any discussion of power, one must first move beyond the point of seeing all "power" and those who have it or seek it in a negative way. Power and the balance of power are facts of life. Power itself is neither good nor bad. It is how an individual or group uses or abuses power that ultimately colors the perception of the power. Power is inherent in the ability to lead. How that power is used ultimately determines the effectiveness of the leader. Some power is gained from the position held by an individual and some power is derived from the leader herself. Power is in the eye of the beholder. If you feel that someone has power, then in your relationship with them, they do. Power is most often classified using descriptions developed by French and Raven (1968) that include reward power, coercive power, legitimate power, referent power, or expert power.

As its name implies, reward power is based on the ability to control the administration of incentives. The head nurse has reward power when she makes out the unit schedule or promotes someone. The staff nurse has reward power with the patient when she controls visiting hours or activity levels. The charge nurse has reward power when she makes out assignments.

On the other hand, coercive power is based on the ability to control the administration of punishment. The nurse must take care not to use coercive power with patients. "If you don't drink your fluids, we'll have to start another IV," or "If you don't stop pulling at your tube, I'm going to tie your hand down" are misuses of coercive power. In such cases, the approach of reward power may well be more effective.

Legitimate power rests on the authority given to an individual by an organization because of the position held by that individual. The R.N., assistant head nurse, head nurse, and so forth, all have power based on their positions. The head nurse, for example, has the power to reward or discipline her staff, based on their performance. She can do this with verbal feedback, formal counseling sessions, promotions or demotions.

Referent power exists either because the person in power has other positive traits and behaviors that contribute to power in other areas or because the person in power has positive connections or influence. An example of the first case would be the nurse who is good clinically and always helps her peers. This gives her more power to influence decisions than the power of a nurse who constantly complains and offers no support. An example of the second case occurs when you as a staff nurse realize that your head nurse has a great deal of influence on her boss, or your nursing director is well-known nationally. You are bestowed with a certain degree of power in the organization because you work for that head nurse, and outside the organization because of its director.

Expert power is based on being recognized as knowledgeable or skillful in a certain area. On every unit, there always seems to be one nurse who is the expert at starting IV's or one nurse who works well with a specific kind of patient. The patient may well (and should be able to) perceive all professional nurses as experts in health care. In doing so, the patient grants the nurse power. The nurse, in turn, must be careful not to abuse that power.

Because power is in the eye of the beholder, it must be used in order to be maintained and increased. A way to increase power is to form coalitions with other persons who have power. As a newcomer to the organization, you need to learn who has power and why, and what resources are valuable enough to contribute to the establishment of a power base.

You can then work to increase your own power and work more effectively with the power of others.

Delegation

Being a professional nurse does not mean doing everything yourself. In some situations tasks and duties can be delegated. The usual response to this statement from a new nurse is "but no one works for me! How can I delegate?" Just as not all power comes from the position in the organization, neither does delegation require a boss-employee relationship.

The key item to remember is that delegation of responsibility does not mean abdication of the responsibility. You are still responsible.

Delegation accomplishes several things. It gets the job done, it frees you to do the things you (but not the other person) are qualified to do, and it helps other people grow and develop. Delegation works best when the work is either routine or well-defined. As a professional nurse, you may delegate tasks to the L.P.N. or other ancillary personnel when the tasks are within the scope of their legal practice. As a primary nurse, you may delegate to associate nurses. You may also delegate certain tasks to the patient or family members if it is in their best interest. Your charge nurse, assistant head nurse, head nurse, and physicians will, likewise, delegate to you.

When you are delegating or being delegated to, you should provide or request the following:

- Clear objectives and instructions
- Checkpoints and follow-up
- An empathetic ear if problems arise
- An understanding that the person to whom the job is delegated will not do it exactly as would the person delegating the job.

The last statement is the one that often makes delegation the hardest. There is only a finite amount of time available to meet the needs of all of the patients. To be effective, a new nurse must learn to set priorities. An L.P.N., for example, can do some things a professional nurse can do but not other things. It makes sense, therefore, that if the R.N. has more tasks than time, she should delegate some of those that the L.P.N. can do. We would all like to provide each patient with professional nursing care at all times. The economics of health care do not allow that, and, in fact, each patient does not need it.

One thing to watch out for is reverse delegation. Once a job has been delegated, it should be completed by the person to whom it was delegated. Some persons are very skilled at dumping delegated jobs they do not want back onto the person who has delegated it. The patient who does not like learning to give his own insulin shot may quickly become a pro at convincing the nurses to do it. The aide who doesn't like stocking supplies can find numerous reasons why someone else should do it. As a new nurse, you must be aware that trying reverse delegation yourself will not develop a very positive image.

During your management clinical and periodically thereafter, you may wish to assess your success at delegating. Theodore Krein (1982) has developed a quick delegation self-evaluation tool shown below. Answer the questions objectively. Add up your score. A score of 72 to 90 indicates that you are not delegating correctly. This may mean that you are still trying to do everything yourself or that you expect far too much when you delegate. A score of 54 to 71 indicates the need for substantial improvement whereas a score of 36 to 53 implies the need for some improvement but indicates that you are doing a lot of things right. Any

HOW TO TEST YOUR DELEGATION HABITS

	STRONGLY AGREE				STRONGLY DISAGREE
1. I'd delegate more, but the jobs I delegate never seem to get done the way I want them to be done.	5	4	3	2	1
2. I don't feel I have the time to delegate properly.	5	4	3	2	1
3. I carefully check on subordinates' work without letting them know I'm doing it, so I can correct their mistakes if necessary before they cause too many problems.	5	4	3	2	1
4. I delegate the whole job—giving the opportunity for the subordinate to complete it without any of my involvement. Then I review the end result.	5	4	3	2	1
5. When I have given clear instructions and the job isn't done right, I get upset.	5	4	3	2	1
6. I feel the staff lacks the commitment that I have. So any job I delegate won't get done as well as I'd do it.	5	4	3	2	1
7. I'd delegate more. But I feel I can do the task better than the person I might delegate it to.	5	4	3	2	1
8. I'd delegate more. But if the individual I delegate the task to does an incompetent job, I'll be severely criticized.	5	4	3	2	1
9. If I were to delegate the task, my job wouldn't be nearly as much fun.	5	4	3	2	1
10. When I delegate a job, I often find that the outcome is such that I end up doing the job over again myself.	5	4	3	2	1
11. I have not really found that delegation saves any time.	5	4	3	2	1
12. I delegate a task clearly and concisely, explaining exactly how it should be accomplished.	5	4	3	2	1
13. I can't delegate as much as I'd like to because my subordinates lack the necessary experience.	5	4	3	2	1
14. I feel that when I delegate I lose control.	5	4	3	2	1
15. I would delegate more but I'm pretty much a perfectionist.	5	4	3	2	1
16. I work longer hours than I should.	5	4	3	2	1
17. I can give subordinates the routine tasks, but I feel I must keep non-routine tasks myself.	5	4	3	2	1
18. My own boss expects me to keep very close to all details of the work.	5	4	3	2	1
Total score					

From Krein TJ: How to improve delegation habits. Man Rev 71: 58–61, 1982 score between 18 to 36 means that you understand and correctly use your delegation skills. Now you need to share that information with your peers. It is also helpful to go back and review each item on the self-assessment, especially those you checked as a 4 or a 5. These are areas in which you need to improve.

Motivation

Think back over your years in school. Do certain courses stand out as especially good or do you remember feeling like you really learned more or better with a certain instructor? The key to your successes was probably motivation in one form or another. Sometimes you studied because you just wanted to pass the course and graduate; other times you studied because you knew a patient would be depending on you to care for him the next day, and still other times you studied because you were really interested in the topic. As a professional nurse, you will need to understand how to motivate other nurses, ancillary personnel, patients, and other health-care personnel.

HAWTHORNE STUDY

The emphasis on motivation dates back to the often quoted Hawthorne study performed in the early 1900's. The study, performed by Harvard researchers at the Hawthorne plant of Western Electric in Chicago, investigated the effects of changes of illumination on productivity. Lighting was changed for one group of employees, but remained constant for another group. As the lighting was increased for the first group, the production of both groups increased. When lighting was decreased for the first group, production continued to rise for both groups until the lights were so low that the first group could not see. The conclusion was that the attention paid to members of each group was the key factor that increased production. Additional studies at the same plant also revealed the influence of norms set by the work group. For you as the professional nurse, the message is clear. Sometimes, the only thing required to motivate people is to pay attention to them. This applies to patients, peers, and ancillary staff. As you progress in your career and move into positions of added authority, you will find that norms set by those you supervise are often much more stringent than those you would set and, at the same time, much more accepted by the group.

MASLOW'S HIERARCHY OF NEEDS

The next major concept in motivation came from Abraham Maslow, a psychologist. Maslow believed that every individual has ever-increasing needs and seeks to meet those needs. He proposed a needs hierarchy consisting of five levels presented in a pyramid diagram (Figure 4-2).

Physiological needs form the base of the pyramid and the base of the individual's existence. These needs include the survival needs of food, air, drink, clothing, and shelter. Safety needs form the next level and consist of items such as a safe working environment and personal security. Once physiological and safety needs are met, the individual moves on to fill social needs through friendships and group memberships. Ego needs are next, and are satisfied by internal feelings of achievement, recognition, and personal respect. At the apex of the pyramid is the need for self-actualization.

Maslow's hierarchy of needs underscores the concept of individuality and, therefore, of not trying to motivate everyone in the same way. It

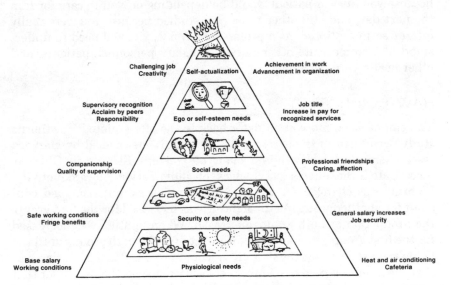

Figure 4-2   Maslow's hierarchy of needs with application to members of an organization. (Adapted from Szilagyi A: Management and Performance. Santa Monica, CA, Goodyear Publishing, 1981)

also underscores the need to work progressively with an individual rather than starting at the top. For example, in dealing with a patient, you must first reassure him that he will live before you can get on to other things such as his return to work. In your own case, you are unlikely to be motivated to be a star if you are worried about how to feed and shelter your family. To motivate, based on Maslow's concept, you need first to assess the level of the individual's need and then provide motivation at that level.

THEORY X—THEORY Y

Douglas McGregor (1960) proposed the Theory X—Theory Y concept. Theory X is based on the traditional assumptions that persons consider work as a job to be done with no pleasure involved, are inherently lazy, are productive only when they fear demotion or termination, do not want to think for themselves, resist change, and must be coerced. Theory Y, which McGregor proposed as a more successful alternative, includes the assumptions that people are inherently good and enjoy work, take personal pride in a job well done, can be self-directed, are constantly striving to grow, and will perform well if given the opportunity. Theory Y believes that if the needs of an individual, as described by Maslow, are met, then the individual will contribute effectively to the organization. Theory X can be regarded as the pessimistic approach while Theory Y is the optimistic approach.

HERZBERG'S TWO-FACTOR APPROACH

Frederick Herzberg (1968) took Maslow one step further. He looked at both job satisfaction and dissatisfaction. The result was two lists of factors, one which Herzberg termed motivation factors and the other hygiene or maintenance factors. Hygiene factors are those items which, if not met or satisfied, will lead to dissatisfaction, but whose presence will not create satisfaction. These include money, working conditions, interpersonal relations, degree and quality of supervision, and policies and administration of the organization. Motivation factors are those whose presence leads to satisfaction. Motivation factors include achievement, recognition, challenging work, increased responsibility, and growth and development (Figure 4-3).

As you can see, the maintenance factors are generally those from the lower level of Maslow's hierarchy, while the motivation factors are found in the higher levels. Herzberg does note that some persons are maintenance seekers, and will concentrate mostly on those factors, but that most individuals are motivation seekers.

Factors may change with the individual or the environment. Insurance coverage is a good example of something that was once a motivation factor, became a maintenance factor, and now seems to be a motivation factor once again. When health insurance first came into being, having it provided as an employment benefit was seen very positively by employees. After a period of time, however, persons grew to expect health insurance. They did not think better of an organization for offering it but did think much worse of the organization that did not provide it. Dental insurance then became the insurance benefit that gained "points" for the organization in the eyes of the employees. In the current economic environment, health care is once again becoming a benefit

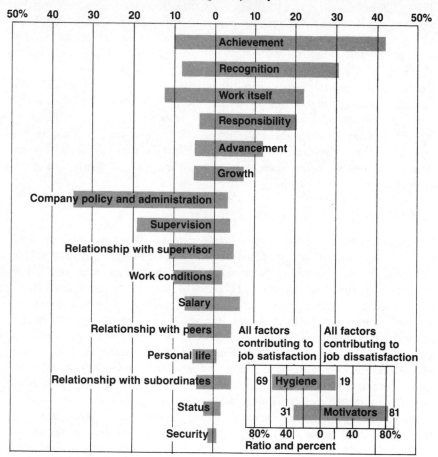

Figure 4-3   Factors affecting job attitudes, as reported in 12 of Herzberg's investigations. (Adapted from Herzberg F: One more time: How do you motivate employees? Harvard Bus Rev 46:53–62, 1968)

rather than an expectation and some persons, especially heads of households, may decide to stay with or leave an organization based on insurance plans.

EXPECTANCY CONCEPTS

Vroom (1964) proposed that the effort a person exhibits is based on her expectations of the likelihood that effort will pay off in performance and the likelihood that performances will pay off in outcomes such as money, a sense of accomplishment, promotions, and so forth. Carried one step further, this concept becomes "you get what you expect to get."

In Vroom's model, individuals are seen as being rational, intelligent, and capable of pursuing actions based on their beliefs and expectations. Motivation (and the resulting performance) is based on three dynamic processes: effort-performance expectancy, instrumentality, and valence. In the effort-performance expectancy process, the individual assesses the likelihood that a certain effort will result in a desired performance, and whether or not she has the ability to perform that effort. Instrumentality is related to the belief that a certain performance will lead to a certain outcome. Valence refers to the value an individual assigns to the outcome.

The nurse who puts forth an effort directed toward an outcome that she values will very often reach that outcome. The nurse who goes through her career putting forth a good deal of effort aimed at advancing herself usually does advance. The nurse who has realistic expectations for her patients usually sees them materialize. However, expectations can work in two directions. The nurse who expects nothing gets just that.

INDIVIDUALIZING MOTIVATION

Levine (1983) and Fitzgerald (1982) both found that there is no single motivator that works with all individuals. Rather, it is usually a unique combination of motivators that is necessary for optimum results. Just as with leadership, motivation must be situational. In this case, the style or technique employed depends on the personality of the individual, the career goals, the current job and job requirements, age, and so forth. Different strokes for different folks.

It is important for you to understand what motivates you, and to convey that information to your peers and to your boss. Do you have an identified career goal that you are working to reach? Are you motivated by positive feedback or embarrassed by it? What do you consider a reward? Until you understand your own motivational needs, it is unfair to expect your boss and peers to understand what motivates you and to contribute to that motivation.

LEADING AND MOTIVATING: FROM CONCEPT TO PRACTICE

Throughout this chapter, we have reviewed the concepts related to leadership and motivation. The practical aspects have been summarized quite well in "The One Minute Manager" by Blanchard and Johnson

(1982) and "Leadership and the One Minute Manager" by Blanchard, Zigmari, and Zigmari (1985). The highlights of these books include the following:

"People who feel good about themselves produce good results." Remember the Hawthorne effect discussed earlier? A few positive strokes and a little recognition go a long way. In an international study of factors influencing hospital employee motivation, Alpander (1985) found that the crucial motivational element in hospital employees in the United States is the degree to which a feeling of recognition is experienced!

"Help people reach their full potential. Catch them doing something right." Rather than always telling the L.P.N. or aide what she did wrong or how she could do the job better, try pointing out the things she does well. At the very least, balance the negative with something positive.

"Everyone is a potential winner. Some people are disguised as losers. Don't let their appearance fool you." Sounds like Theory Y, doesn't it? Giving people the benefit of the doubt isn't always easy, especially on typically crisis-oriented nursing units, but it is far more effective in the long run than assuming the worst. The person to whom you give the benefit of the doubt today may be in a position to do the same for you tomorrow.

"When the best leader's work is done, the people say 'we did it ourselves!'" A real leader develops the persons who work with her and then gives credit to those persons. When you as a staff nurse do a good job, it reflects on you, your head nurse, your director, the organization, and nursing in general.

Summary

The abilities of leadership and motivation, and the use of power and delegation are all a part of professional nursing. Understanding the concepts and learning to put them into practice are necessary parts of your education and the transition from student to professional. All of these concepts can be viewed from two sides. It is important for the new nurse to see herself on both sides; to recognize her needs *and* her responsibilities.

Bibliography

Alpander GG: Factors influencing hospital employee motivation: A diagnostic instrument. Hosp Health Serv Admin 30: 67–31, 1985

Blanchard K, Johnson S: The One Minute Manager. New York, William Morrow and Co, 1982

Blanchard K, Zigmari P, Zigmari D; Leadership and the One Minute Manager. New York, William Morrow and Co, 1985

Del Bueno DJ, Freud CM: Power and Politics in Nursing Administration: A Casebook. Owings Mill, MD, National Health Publishing, 1986

Fitzgerald PE: Developing the health worker's attitude inventory: A tool for assessing worker/management relations in health care institutions. Dissertation, University of Alabama in Birmingham, 1982

French J, Raven B: The basis of social power. In Cartwright D, Zander A (eds): Group Dynamics, Research and Theory. New York, Harper & Row, 1968

Levine HA: Efforts to improve productivity. Personnel 60: 4–10, 1983

Likert R: New Patterns of Management. New York, McGraw-Hill, 1961

Likert R: The Human Organization. New York, McGraw-Hill, 1967

Maslow AH: A theory of human motivation. Psychol Rev 50: 370–396, 1943

Maslow AH: Motivation and Personality. New York, Harper & Row, 1943

McGregor D: The Human Side of Enterprise. New York, McGraw-Hill, 1960

Vroom V: Work and Motivation. New York, John Wiley & Sons, 1964

Zalenik A: How to improve delegation habits. Man Rev 71: 58–61, 1981

Chapter 5

Decision making*

EULA DAS

Decision making is a process of choosing between alternatives. Within this process, the decision maker must

A. Assess the situation
    - Define the situation that has given rise to the opportunity for decision making.
B. Plan the process

    - Set criteria for the decision to satisfy personal, professional, and institutional values.
    - Determine who can make the decision.
    - Recognize possible strategies and screen them for acceptability.
    - Predict the possible outcomes of strategies and the positive and negative impact of each.
    - Weigh the risk involved.
    - Select the most satisfactory strategy.

C. Implement the decision.
D. Evaluate the outcome of the decision.

This process is applicable to any type of decision-making situation, both professional and personal. Professional decisions are made in clinical and management situations, such as when to perform CPR and when

*"Decision Making" was a joint effort of administrative, nursing education, and patient education staff at Baylor University Medical Center, Dallas, Texas. Contributors included Karen Anne Bufton, Kathleen Rice Doherty, William D. McKinnon, Jill Lenk Schilp, and Naomi White.

71

to counsel an employee. Personal decisions are those that affect your own private or personal life, such as getting married, or going into psychiatric or pulmonary nursing. Some decisions fall into both categories, as when a nurse decides to join a committee on clinical standards. She will be serving the organization and furthering her career. The process she uses to make decisions will be the same in both areas.

This chapter will enable you to

1. Identify the four components of the decision-making process.
2. Apply clinical dilemmas to the decision-making framework.
3. Discuss situations arising in a managerial role that could be solved by utilizing a structured decision process.
4. Identify risks for making decisions haphazardly.

Rationale for Process

Taking an organized approach to decision making has benefits. Following specific steps is not merely an exercise. The decision-making process presented here is a reliable method, and an effective and justifiable decision is more likely to be its result. At each step of assessment, planning, implementation, and evaluation, a decision should be justifiable and effective.

A decision-making process leads you to assess the situation thoroughly. It should help you consider most factors that will affect your decision. You can prove that a choice was made only after the relevant data was considered. However, because the system allows for orderly grouping of pertinent information, you can avoid wasting time with inconsequential details.

Creativity is an element of the decision-making process. The generation of possible strategies is a major step in planning decisions. Creative thinking can produce solutions that are not at first apparent but that are practical and effective. Outcomes predicted creatively will also reveal advantages *and* disadvantages of the various strategies, thus helping to prevent mistakes.

In the implementation phase, this model allows decision makers to be more confident in and committed to the decision. With supporting information considered in an orderly process, decisions can be made with more confidence. Confidence engenders commitment.

Group decisions in particular depend heavily on commitment. When group members have followed steps together and have seen the factors and reasons resulting in the decision, they can work harder to see that the implementation is successful.

Systematic decisions can also be analyzed. If you have followed steps you can retrace them to see how the decision was reached. When the decision is evaluated, the steps leading to success or the need for revision can be scrutinized.

Familiar Decisions

Driving a car is a familiar situation that, moment by moment, requires decisions. A brown pasteboard box tumbling into the road in front of the car requires the driver to decide what to do. The proficient driver and the new driver will differ in the way they make their decisions.

First, the proficient driver has a broader view of the situation. She has been scanning constantly, keeping a running assessment of the road conditions, positions of other cars, speed, car performance, sound of the engine and wheels, and feel of the road surface and the car's motion. These observations may be made half-consciously, but they are, nonetheless, monitored constantly, and form a continuous baseline of data. Maintaining the flow of observations, the driver is open to cues outside the usual. Then she can compare them to the baseline.

On the other hand, the new driver has a narrower view. Because her attention is filled with the very act of driving, such as clutching the steering wheel, pressing the gas pedal, and focusing on the road immediately ahead, she probably will not see the box as soon as the proficient driver sees it. The new driver may also have more preconceptions about driving. She may expect the road to be safe and clear and may not be prepared to notice changes.

Once both drivers see the box, they will assess it differently. The proficient driver will ask many questions. From what direction did it come? Did another car hit it? How did the box move? Did it roll heavily as if something were inside it, did it bounce, or did it skim over the road as if it were empty? How wide and how tall is the box? Is there anything in the car that could fly around and hurt passengers after a sudden stop or swerve?

The new driver will ask questions the proficient driver has been mentally answering all along. Is the road slick or dry? How fast is the car moving? Are there cars behind or in the left, right, or oncoming lanes?

Is there a shoulder, a ditch, or a guard rail? How good are the car's brakes and steering?

After they assess the situation, the proficient driver and the new driver may differ in their planning. Having a narrower view of the situation, the new driver may see only the option of stopping or not stopping. However, the proficient driver will take all the information she has gathered and generate the options of stopping, going around, running over the box, or slowing down to let it blow out of the way.

The proficient driver will also hypothesize the numerous consequences of each strategy she has developed. If she swerves on the slick street she could lose control. If she comes to a complete stop the car behind her may not be able to stop. The new driver may see only limited consequences of her action.

To make her decision the proficient driver must weigh the risks of each of the alternatives, gauging the effect each will have on herself, her passengers, and other drivers. The new driver may not be able to weigh risks.

Based on her assessment, her strategies and predictions of their outcomes, and weighing of risks, the proficient driver will choose her action. The new driver may react with the only alternative she sees.

Nursing Decisions

The process that nurses use to make decisions has the same elements as that of making any other decision. The steps of assessment, planning, implementation, and evaluation determine the way you view a situation and lead you to your decision.

ASSESSMENT

Assessment is the collection of data about a situation. Within the process of decision making, assessment concerns maintaining baseline data and defining the problem.

Maintain Baseline Data

Assessment is done continuously. It is often carried out unconsciously because it has many sources.

Through the senses of sight, hearing, touch, and smell, nurses assess constantly. You see skin color, drainage, and nonverbal behavior such as restlessness. By hearing heart and breath sounds and listening to the patient's concerns, you assess other areas of health status. Signs such as skin turgor, warmth, and pulse quality are assessed by touch. The smell of urine, breath, and wounds yields other information.

Still other sources of information are patient history, the physical, sociological, economic, cultural, and psychological assessment, diagnostic data, and reports from other members of the health-care team.

From all these sources you are forming a running assessment of patient status. This baseline of knowledge is the foundation for comparing information obtained in future assessments. These pieces of gathered information are cues—signs, symptoms, or impressions indicating something is within or outside the norm. When related and categorized, cues may form patterns indicative of the situation's status. The accumulation of cues and cue patterns is the knowledge you need to determine if the situation is congruent with the norm or if a discrepancy exists.

Norms are standards established by the institution's policies and procedures, by professional theory, or literature on the subject. Standards are influenced by the values and expectations of the nurse, the patient, significant others, and managers or other superiors. When cues or cue patterns are within the norm, the decision can be made either to continue with current interventions or not to act. Identifying a discrepancy between the situation and the standard may also signal the beginning of the decision-making process.

Define Problem

If the baseline assessment meets the standard and future assessments yield no deviation from the standard (no new relevant cues), then the decision to continue with present interventions or to start no new interventions may be made. However, if the presenting cues indicate a discrepancy between the present situation and the desired situation, you must decide what, if anything, needs to be done.

The first step in making a decision is additional assessment to define the situation or clearly state the problem needing resolution. A single cue is often not enough to determine if action is needed. Go back and assess the situation further. Find other cues and determine their relevance to the situation. Then group or cluster them into categories to form possible diagnoses. You may find several explanations, and cues may fit into more than one grouping. Gather sufficient information to define the problems.

The following is an example of identifying and grouping cues to formulate an explanation or nursing diagnosis for a situation.

Mary B., R.N., answers Mrs. Jones' call on the intercom. Mrs. Jones say, "My arm with the IV hurts." Mary replies that she will come and check it. As Mary walks down the hall, she mentally reviews what she already knows about Mrs. Jones and her IV.

> The IV has been in for 48 hours.
> I checked it within the last 4 hours.

It met standards for a patent IV site in that the site was not tender or edematous, and skin color around the site was undifferentiated from surrounding tissue.

Mrs. Jones was admitted for electrolyte imbalance.

Her condition is listed as good.

Her veins are small and venipuncture is difficult.

Mrs. Jones is "very afraid of needles" and becomes distraught during venipunctures.

She is receiving potassium, 40 meq in 1000 cc D5NS at 125 cc/hour.

Obviously, Mary has started the assessment process even before she enters Mrs. Jones' room. She is reviewing her baseline data, what she already knows about the situation. She will then move on to gaining new data.

Although, in assessing a situation, you identify and group cues, it is important not to be burdened with preconceptions. Make sure that the problem producing this set of cues is correctly identified. The differentiation between the cause and the symptoms is critical to making a decision. For example, Mrs. Jones may be experiencing vein irritation, phlebitis, or symptoms of infiltration in the IV site. However, she could also be uncomfortable in her strange surroundings, and may be lying in a position that has decreased circulation in that arm. Because she is anxious about having an IV, she may dismiss such a simple explanation and call the nurse. Stay open to any possible causes.

When Mary arrives she finds Mrs. Jones lying in a comfortable position that should allow good circulation. Examining the site, Mary notes the area around and above the site to be red, tender, edematous, and without return blood flow into the tubing. Mary groups the subjective and objective data into related clusters and compares them to standards for IV sites. Now Mary has identified the discrepancy between "what is" and "what should be." From the cues, her knowledge of theory, and her experience, Mary defines the problem as "infiltrated, phlebitic IV site."

Obviously, many conclusions related to nursing observations are not slow, deliberate, conscious thought processes, as those shown in the above example. These cognitive processes often occur so rapidly that they bypass conscious awareness. However, making this process a deliberate and conscious one is helpful because you can organize your approach and recognize the variables influencing the situation.

PLANNING

Once you have defined the problem, the next step in decision making is planning how to solve it. Planning includes establishing criteria for the outcome(s) of the decision, classifying it according to domain (identifying the individuals) who can make the decision, identifying possible strategies, screening them for acceptability, hypothesizing outcomes, and weighing risks of strategies.

Establish Criteria for Decision Outcome

Set the criteria for your decision. In other words, define what outcomes or effects your decision must have, regardless of what the decision is. Desired outcomes may be derived from standards such as the ones previously discussed. For example, Mary wants to relieve Mrs. Jones' pain, avoid inflicting more pain, maintain the patient's fluid balance, keep a line open for administering fluids and medications, and prevent inflammation and infection at the IV site. The standards for these desired outcomes are derived from institutional policies and procedures, nurse-patient expectations, pathophysiological theory, and personal values. Any action Mary decides to take must satisfy these criteria as closely as possible. Comparison of the desired outcomes, standards, and actual results is the basis for evaluation of decisions.

Classify According to Domain

Classify the problem by determining who has the authority to make the decision, or whose domain covers it. Your nursing license, hospital policies and procedures, and job description define your domain of decision-making authority. According to the domain of the decision, you can make the decision yourself, share the decision, or refer the decision to someone else. You must determine the domain of authority. For example, Mary must determine if the decision to discontinue and restart the IV is within her domain.

Discerning if the decision lies within your domain may be easy. If you have the legal, institutional, and moral sanctions to make the decision and the resources to carry it out, proceed to do so. In Mary's case, her nursing license and the policies and procedures of her hospital allow her to discontinue the IV and to prepare for restarting it.

At other times, however, the domain of responsibility may be quite vague. Situations will occur when nursing action is sanctioned by legal and institutional guidelines, but the means necessary to carry out the decision are lacking. These situations require decisions either to be shared or referred to someone else.

1. The nurse recognizes the discrepancy but cannot define the problem.
    Example: A patient becomes increasingly restless. The nurse recognizes the single cue of restlessness but is unable to recognize other existing cues to establish a label. As a result, she does not know the etiology and cannot intervene.

2. The nurse recognizes the discrepancy, and can label it but the required interventions and/or desired outcomes are not known.

    Example: The nurse observes bright red blood spurting from a tracheostomy. She wants to stop the bleeding and maintain a patent airway, but she does not know what to do.

3. The nurse lacks the necessary resources, that is, skills, knowledge, equipment, or time, to make or carry out the decision.

    Example: The nurse is unable to palpate a pedal pulse and does not have access to a doppler. She may collaborate with others to borrow the necessary equipment or she may delegate to a subordinate the task of obtaining it.

4. The nurse lacks the legal, moral, and/or institutional sanction to intervene.

    Example: The nurse finds a patient in acute respiratory distress. She recognizes the urgent need for intubation and mechanical support but she is not sanctioned by the institution and the state law to perform that procedure.

    Example: A nurse may believe strongly that life support systems be discontinued in a case of terminal illness but she may lack the moral sanction to intervene directly.

Identify Strategies for Problem Resolution

Next, identify possible strategies for solving the problem. This is where creativity enters the picture. Try not to make a decision until you have considered several strategies for handling the situation. Devising several strategies increases the likelihood that the decision will yield the best results. Course of action may include:

Direct Intervention: To intervene directly, you carry out physical or verbal activities. Discontinuing or restarting the IV, counseling subordinates, and teaching patients and colleagues are examples of direct intervention.

Indirect Intervention: Because you as a nurse are at the center of the communications and operations network of the health-care setting, you may intervene indirectly with interpersonal skills. If the IV was not infiltrated or rejected, allaying Mrs. Jones' fears about the IV and assuring other checks would be indirect intervention. Negotiation, conflict resolution, persuasion, and confrontation are examples of indirect intervention.

Delegation: You may delegate certain responsibilities to others who are "available, capable, and allowed to take action (del Bueno)."* Del-

*del Bueno D: Personal communication. October 1985

egation to another health-care worker is preferable when that individual can accomplish the desired outcome. For example, in assessing potential sites for restarting the IV, Mary finds that a suitable vein cannot be located. In this instance, she may elect to delegate this task to someone with venipuncture expertise, such as the IV team.

Purposeful Inaction: A conscious decision not to act is advantageous in some instances. For example, if a patient makes sexual advances, you may choose to ignore the behavior if it does not exceed certain limits. Other action may be required if the limits are exceeded.

If the decision is not yours alone to make, you also have options.

Consultation/collaboration: You may consult with a peer, a superior or a member of another discipline. This person should be "willing, available, credible"* and sanctioned by law and the institution to intervene or provide consultation. Consulting and collaborating should give you the knowledge or viewpoint to help you make the decision.

Referral: When the decision lies totally out of your domain, refer the decision to someone who is willing and mandated to intervene. This may mean referral to a charge nurse, to a supervisor, to a physician, to a minister, or to members of the other disciplines.

Screen Strategies for Acceptability

When you have identified strategies, you must screen them for acceptability. To be considered seriously, a strategy must be scientifically sound, legal, and consistent with personal and organizational value systems. Ask these questions about each strategy.

1. Do related scientific principles, research evidence or findings, and professional literature support the strategy?
2. Is it legal?
3. Does the decision fit into your value system?
4. Would your organizational structure and your managerial and supervisory environment condone the strategy?
5. Are there unit culture and environmental constraints on the strategy?

If the strategy passes this screening, it is eligible for further consideration. In the IV example, Mary can restart the IV herself or she can summon the IV team to perform the venipuncture. Both strategies pass the screening.

*del Bueno D: Personal communication. October 1985

Hypothesize Outcomes and Weigh Risks

When you have screened strategies you must hypothesize their outcomes. This will help you recognize and consider the advantages and disadvantages of each. Imagine each strategy in operation and list the problems that could arise. What are the potential risks of each alternative? Think in terms of yourself and others involved, including the patient, coworkers, and the organization.

For example, Mary imagines her two strategies, that of restarting the IV herself or calling the IV team. Mary knows that Mrs. Jones has small, deep veins. Mary's experience with difficult venipunctures is limited. She considers the outcomes of her strategies.

A. Mary restarts IV
    1. Unsuccessful venipuncture attempts resulting in excessive pain and anxiety for the patient and multiple venipuncture sites
    2. Damaging veins through unsuccessful venipuncture, making a restart more difficult for an experienced venipuncturist
    3. Increased anxiety for Mary in light of Mrs. Jones' fear of venipuncture
    4. Loss of time in attempting a difficult venipuncture
B. IV team restarts IV
    1. Successful venipuncture with fewer attempts
    2. Less anxiety and pain for patient and fewer venipuncture sites
    3. Less anxiety to Mary
    4. Time saved for Mary
    5. Higher costs for the patient/hospital

When you have considered each strategy in operation, ask the following questions about risks. To be viable, a strategy must be associated with a risk factor that is acceptable. Weigh the risks, and then rank the strategies according to their desirability, based on your answers.

1. How much effort is required for yourself or other parties involved?
2. Which alternative gives the greatest results with the least effort?
3. How much change would each alternative require?
4. Which alternative takes the best advantage of your resources?
5. How will employees be affected by the alternative and what will their reactions be?
6. How will patients be affected by the alternative and what will their reactions be?
7. What past failures or successes have you or others had with the alternative?

Of all the viable strategies, select the one most desirable, based on the lowest risk in achieving the desired outcome.

Asking these questions about both her strategies, Mary decides to request assistance from the IV team. The risk associated with that strategy is lower to the patient, Mary herself, and the organization.

Once you go through the questions, you will have examined each strategy in light of the elements that can affect your decision and its implementation. This will enable you to make your choice and defend your decisions by a rational process.

IMPLEMENTATION

To implement your decision, gather the necessary resources and carry out the action. This may be a fairly straightforward operation when you make the decision alone, implement it yourself, use resources at your disposal, and perform the action immediately.

However, the issue becomes more complicated when other persons are involved. Communication and/or negotiation become very important. When you share responsibility for a decision, delegate a task, borrow equipment or supplies, ask for assistance, or delay performance, other people are affected. They must be informed and included in the process. Negotiating with them to accept or share the responsibility for implementation makes success more likely.

EVALUATION

Evaluation is based on the degree of congruence between the desired outcome, the standard, and the actual outcome. By comparing these elements, you can evaluate the effectiveness of your decision. Dissatisfaction with the outcome leads you to reenter the process of assessment, planning, and implementation. This process should lead you to another strategy that will be more satisfactory.

Your judgment of a decision, however, can be colored by other factors. Time may be necessary to determine whether or not a decision achieves the outcome desired. You may not know until much later the outcomes of a specific decision. You must consider both the long- and short-term effects in evaluating the success of some decisions.

The judgment of decisions is also determined by values. Your values will determine how you evaluate a decision. If you value consistency and following hospital rules, you may decide to adhere to the hospital's policy of not permitting visitors under 12 years of age. However, if in some circumstances the needs of an individual supercede hospital rules, you may decide to allow a child to visit a relative.

In the delivery of health care, you will be confronted constantly with decisions that involve conflicting values. You may question the usefulness of some decisions or even disagree with them. Decisions about the allocation of limited resources such as funds, space or equipment, and services are value-laden. Patient care also entails value decisions, such as the civil rights of a patient versus your charge to protect him against himself.

Sometimes decisions are compromises in which no one is completely satisfied. If a patient is having severe pain 2 hours before he is scheduled to have more medication, you may decide to reposition him. The outcome is less effective than medication, and neither you nor the patient are satisfied. However, because the risk of medication is higher, the decision is still a good one.

Diagram: The Decision Making Process

To help you acquire the ability to make effective decisions, the "decision tree" shown in Figure 5-1 is provided. By following this step-by-step approach to decision making, you will be more likely to select the best strategy to achieve the desired outcomes.

Decisions About Priorities

Management of a patient load depends heavily on setting priorities, in other words, deciding what to do and when to do it. The new nurse tends to focus on one problem at a time rather than seeing the whole picture.

Even the nurse attending to only one patient must prioritize the needs for that patient. For example, if a patient has been subject to hourly vital signs checks, vital signs are consistently stable, and the doctor's order states that vital signs are to be checked hourly until stable, the nurse may decide to check vital signs less frequently. The cues that lead to the nurse's decision to decrease the frequency of vital signs checks are:

1. Vital signs have been consistently stable.
2. The patient has been deprived of rest because of frequent vital signs checks.

The first standard to be met is that of patient stability. Hourly assessment of vital signs reveals that this standard has been met. The nurse then focuses on the cue that reveals rest deprivation. The standard is that sufficient rest is necessary for health maintenance. The cue is deviant from this standard. The discrepancy between the cue and the

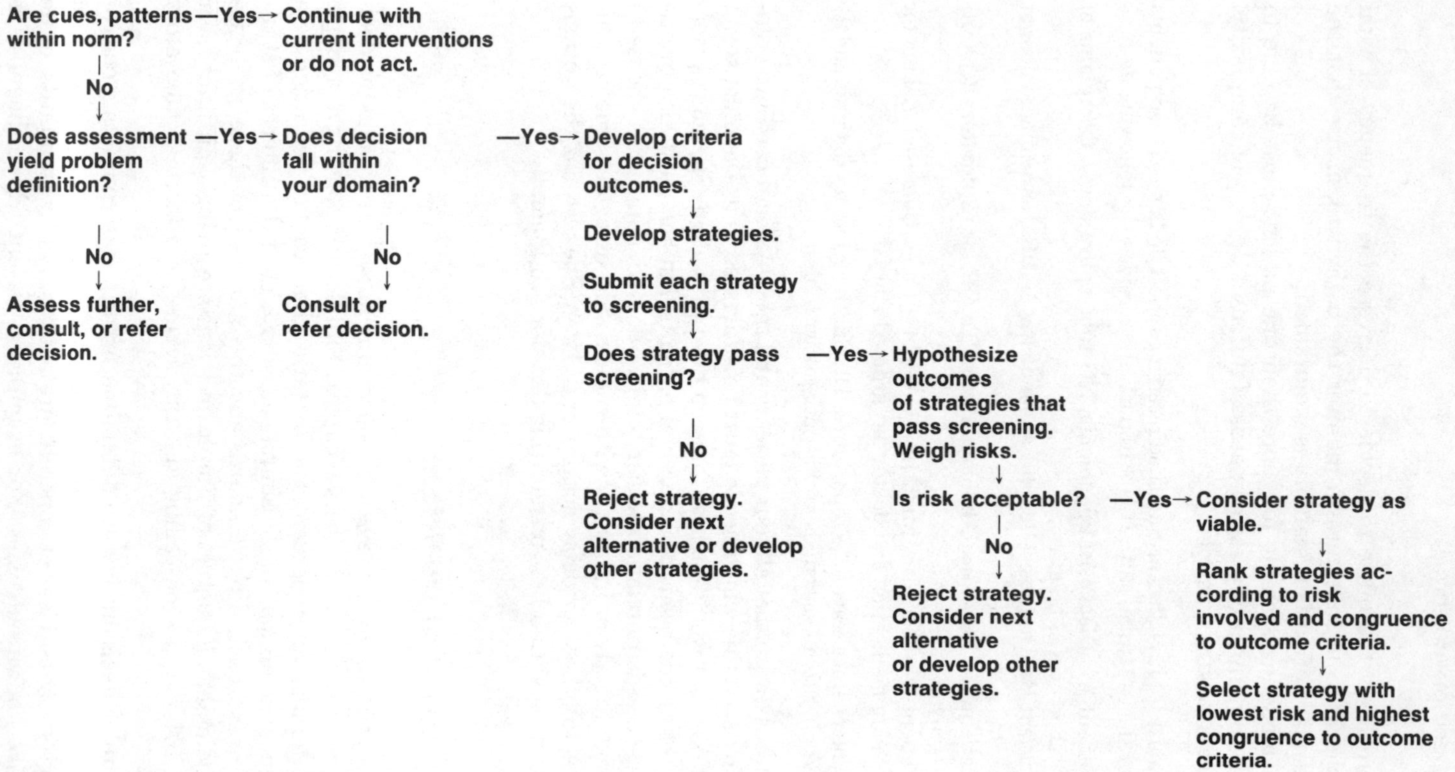

Are cues, patterns —Yes→ Continue with
within norm? current interventions
│ or do not act.
No
↓

Does assessment —Yes→ Does decision —Yes→ Develop criteria
yield problem fall within for decision
definition? your domain? outcomes.
│ │ ↓
No No Develop strategies.
↓ ↓ ↓
Assess further, Consult or Submit each strategy
consult, or refer refer decision. to screening.
decision. ↓
Does strategy pass —Yes→ Hypothesize
screening? outcomes
│ of strategies that
No pass screening.
↓ Weigh risks.
Reject strategy. ↓
Consider next Is risk acceptable? —Yes→ Consider strategy as
alternative or develop │ viable.
other strategies. No ↓
↓ Rank strategies ac-
Reject strategy. cording to risk
Consider next involved and congruence
alternative to outcome criteria.
or develop other ↓
strategies. Select strategy with
lowest risk and highest
congruence to outcome
criteria.

Figure 5-1 Diagram of the decision-making process.

83

standard leads the nurse to decide to decrease the frequency of vital signs checks. She continues to monitor the patient to ensure that the first standard of patient stability is maintained.

The nurse accountable for more than one patient must be able to prioritize a number of pressing needs of different degrees of complexity, as in the following example:

> Janice C., R.N., has just finished receiving report on her assigned patients for the 3–11 p.m. shift. It is 3:10 p.m. She received the following data.
>
> Patient A—Diagnosis: Pneumonia. NG tube not draining. Complains of shortness of breath.
>
> Patient B—Diagnosis: Possible appendicitis. In OR. Returning to floor at 3:30 p.m.
>
> Patient C—Diagnosis: Abdominal pain. To OR for exploratory laparotomy at 3:30 p.m
>
> Patient D—Diagnosis: Metastatic CA. Chest tubes. Confused. Asking for pain medication and doctor has ordered stat lab.
>
> When Janice leaves the report area, Dr. Smith arrives on the unit and asks her to make rounds on his patients with him.

Janice is aware that all four patients and the physician need intervention. To determine which needs must be addressed first, she must select the actions that would be best for each need presented. She must prioritize meeting the needs of individual patients, but she must also prioritize those needs in relation to her total work load. Janice can choose to intervene directly or indirectly with some needs, delegate some responsibilities to others, or delay actions until later. She also has the options of consulting with others or referring decisions to them.

Complexity of Decisions

By now you can see that even as a beginning nurse you are making decisions, some simple and others complex. Simple decisions have a single cue or familiar or congruent cue patterns that lead to definition of a problem. The domain of the simple decision is clear. Its choices of strategies are established by standards and the outcomes of these strategies are predictable. Examples of simple decisions are giving aspirin for fever above 101 degrees or calling the physician for abnormal laboratory results.

Complex decisions involve unfamiliar, multiple, or conflicting cues or cue patterns that do not present definable problems. The choices of strategies are not clear or concrete, are not covered by standards, or do not have known outcomes. For example, a patient whose diagnosis is unknown, who is febrile and complaining of pain may present the need for a more complex decision than the patient who has a urinary tract infection and expresses the same symptoms. Risk factors are greater in complex decisions because the outcome may alleviate one set of cues while aggravating another set. Weighing the risks of possible outcomes is particularly important in complex situations.

The nurse's ability to identify the degree of a decision's complexity will influence her ability to select the appropriate strategy. Knowledge base and experience can influence the perception of the complexity of the decision. For the proficient clinician, some complex decisions have become simple. Her decision making has become almost automatic.

However, a situation that appears simple to a new nurse may be considered complex by a more experienced nurse. The opposite situation of decisions appearing more complex to the beginning nurse and simple to the experienced nurse would be expected. Frequently, that will be the case due to the experienced nurse's ability to assess numerous cues simultaneously. However, having the ability to predict the impact of a decision in terms of the whole picture can change the assessment, the strategies considered and, consequently, the action taken. The beginning nurse can be very alarmed to realize that decisions she thought were simple and clear-cut are actually very complex. She can see that the outcome of the decision could have great impact on the entire organization.

The environment also affects the perception of complexity. If the experienced nurse moves into management or another clinical specialty, she may be less proficient in making decisions. Going back to the structured process may help her see situations more clearly and make more orderly decisions.

New situations present different levels of decision making. You must be conscious of the situation and the environment, and be willing to use structure and draw upon knowledge, theories, and experience, rather than make decisions automatically.

Use of Process in Other Decision-Making Situations

Until now, the decision-making process has been related primarily to patient care. However, the same process applies in other situations. For example, you may be involved in making a decision to initiate a new nursing procedure.

Assessment is done during committee meetings, personal interactions, and observation of staff performance. Once your assessment has led you to define the problem, you will plan your actions by setting criteria for outcomes and discerning who holds responsibility for making the decision. If the responsibility is not yours, you will refer the decision to someone else. If the responsibility is yours or yours and that of others, you will develop strategies for resolving the problem and then hypothesize their outcomes. Based on their risks, you will choose a strategy. Using resources at hand or negotiating for others, you will implement your decision and evaluate its outcomes.

Summary

This step-by-step approach to decision making may seem time consuming at first glance. However, by following this process, you should be able to make sound, rational, justifiable, and effective decisions. By repeatedly applying the process, you will integrate it into your nursing practice and can, with time, become a proficient decision maker.

Bibliography

Aspinall MJ, Tanner CA: Decision Making for Patient Care: Applying the Nursing Process. New York, Appleton-Century-Crofts, 1981

Bailey JT, Claus KE: Decision Making in Nursing: Tools for Change. St. Louis, CV Mosby, 1975

Benner P: From Novice to Expert. Menlo Park, CA, Addison-Wesley, 1984

Carnevali DL, Mitchell PH, Woods NF, Tanner CA: Diagnostic Reasoning in Nursing. Philadelphia, JB Lippincott, 1984

Drucker PF: The Effective Executive. New York, Harper & Row, 1967

Drucker PF: The Practice of Management. New York, Harper & Row, 1954

Ford JAG, Trygstad-Durland LN, Nelms BC: Applied Decision Making for Nurses. St. Louis, CV Mosby, 1979

Gillies DA: Nursing Management: A Systems Approach. Philadelphia, WB Saunders, 1982

Gordon M: Nursing Diagnosis: Process and Application. New York, McGraw-Hill, 1982

Rudizitis I: The Art of Effective Decision Making. New York, Research Institute of America, 1983

Stevens, BJ: The Nurse as Executive, 2nd ed. Wakefield, MA, Nursing Resources, 1980

Chapter 6

Conflict management and change

SUSAN C. ROE

During the last decade, recent explosions of technology, development of multiple avenues for delivering health-care services, the urgency to contain spiralling costs and, most recently, the prospective payment system, have brought about a health-care environment that can be characterized as turbulent. The components of this turbulence—conflict and change—have always been a consideration in organizational life.

The scope and intensity of conflict and change in today's health-care organizations have challenged all health care professionals to reevaluate the roles they play and the methods and processes used for the financing and delivery of care. This challenge has resulted in both positive and negative outcomes.

Some health-care organizations have been able to expand their marketability and services; others have become vulnerable and foundered. Organizations with difficulties often find that a key contributor to their dilemma is disgruntled employees who feel alienated from organizational objectives. This greatly affects their ability to deliver patient care.

The health-care organizations that seem to fare well are the ones in which a commitment to the organization's mission and resources are made by both the organization and its workers. In these organizations, a positive work climate seems to foster success in the marketplace and promotes effective delivery of quality patient care.

Nurses can only profit when they work toward building a positive work climate. Such a climate is built through the establishment of cohesive work relationships and the effective management of conflict and change.

This chapter includes the key components needed to build a positive work climate and will enable you to

1. Describe the five components for building a positive work climate.
2. Outline two strategies for establishing rapport.
3. Discuss "power balancing" as a means of developing collegial relationships.
4. Identify three ingredients for becoming a team player.
5. Summarize the conflict management process.
6 Compare and contrast the methods of conflict resolution.
7. List the guidelines necessary to participatively implement change.

Building a Positive Work Climate

Building a positive work climate in any organization can be a difficult but worthwhile task. There is really no mystery regarding the difficulty of this task. Gathering a large and diverse group of people and giving each person a specific role so that each may harmoniously achieve some prescribed objective is as difficult as attempting to climb Mount Everest. However, when combined with thoughtful planning, necessary resources and skills, and concentrated energy and commitment this objective is surely attainable.

For many, reaching the top of the mountain results in the satisfaction of using one's individual and team-work skills to their fullest. In addition, the excitement of experiencing the view from the top cannot be minimized. Payoffs resulting from helping to build a positive work climate are similar.

Attainment of greater job satisfaction can occur through the full utilization of one's knowledge and skills in patient care and team assignments. Furthermore, the excitement of experiencing the potential of a fully functioning team and organization can be truly breathtaking.

Development of a positive work climate requires consideration of five key components: the establishment of rapport; the development of collegial relationships; teamwork; the management of conflict, and dealing with change. Each component interacts with the others. The skills and knowledge gained from exercising each successive component build a framework for the next. The first component, the establishment of rapport, allows for a growth-enhancing environment between oneself and one's colleagues. Such an environment promotes the development of collegial relationships. This is the second component.

Collegial relationships tend to maximize collaboration and teamwork—the third component. As in all work groups, conflict (informational, perceptual, emotional, or value differences) can occur. An understanding of conflict and how to bring differences to productive resolution constitutes the fourth component.

Dealing with change, the fifth component, is a vital skill for nurses working in health-care organizations. When the rate of change is rapid, both workers and organizations tend to become rigid and cling to practices that may be familiar but nonproductive. Building a positive work climate, where trust and participation are hallmarks and where conflict and changes are seen as productive, can produce a dynamic and flexible organization. As a result, change allows for growth, not stagnation.

Integrating the five components of a positive work climate into one's nursing practice can be accomplished by understanding and applying the theories, concepts, and techniques discussed in the remainder of this chapter.

Managing Work Relationships

ESTABLISHING RAPPORT

To be successful in today's health-care environment requires that nurses demonstrate excellence in their clinical skills. However, clinical skills alone are not enough. As high technology increases in health care, there seems to be a need for a counterbalancing or compensatory reaction on the part of humans. This response is known as "high touch" (Naisbitt, 1984).

High touch means that nurses must have expertise in and an understanding of what it takes to establish positive relationships with others in the work setting. These relationships are equally as important as the finetuning of clinical skills. The development of positive relationships among fellow nurses, patients and their families, physicians, as well as other health-care personnel is an essential ingredient for nurses who want to thrive, rather than just survive, in health-care organizations.

Positive relationships include communication patterns between and among persons that are built on trust, clarity, common goal orientations, and collaboration. The basis for these positive relationships is rapport. When similarities, rather than differences, are emphasized, rapport is more easily established (Richardson and Margulis, 1981). Therefore, rapport in nursing settings is established by setting a tone that is mutually growth producing. Rapport is further established when nurses treat each other as allies and maintain a common goal of enhancing each other's practice.

Setting a positive tone in a health-care environment requires a work philosophy that focuses on what *can* be done, rather than on what *cannot* be done. For example, talking about what was accomplished during the shift or workday allows nurses and their colleagues to feel the day was productive. Sometimes just getting through the day is accomplishment enough.

A positive tone also means that the underlying perceptual base for communicating is a positive one. The nurse who is able to set a positive tone sees the world as "half-full" not "half-empty." Assessment of situations and the words that are used focuses on strengths. While not all situations are positive, those areas that are perceived as weaknesses can be seen as learning opportunities.

Giving positive feedback or compliments to others can be used to reinforce strengths. When nurses note another's strength, that individual tends to repeat the positive behavior or action. In addition, compliment giving can promote positive feelings about one's work, work skills, and others in the work environment. Giving feedback provides an opportunity for self-growth through the assessment of another's skills. In addition, "compliments beget compliments."

Despite the potential growth producing aspects of giving feedback to others, most "typical" responses to compliments tend to negate compliment giving. More often than not, when positive feedback is given, recipients tend to become embarrassed and respond by negating the compliment. Unfortunately, this kind of embarrassed response indicates to compliment givers that they are not very effective evaluators. As a result, few compliments are given. In fact, in some work environments, there are very few compliments given at all.

To ensure a positive tone that promotes rapport, use the following guidelines for giving and receiving positive feedback:

1. Give positive feedback on genuine characteristics, qualities, or behaviors. Giving a compliment just for the sake of giving compliments can be seen as manipulative and suspicious.

2. Be specific about what is shared. Specificity serves two purposes. First, it offers feedback that is focused on the person to whom it is being given. Second, if it is feedback about specific skills, it pro-

vides the reinforcing mechanism necessary for repeated performance. An example of specific feedback might be:

"I was most impressed by the way you were able to handle Mrs. Lane's son. Your willingness and ability to listen to his complaints sure helped zero in on his concerns about his mother."

3. Use "I" statements when giving positive feedback. Since the assessment is made by the compliment giver, the message must have the appropriate frame of reference.

4. When receiving positive feedback, simply say, "thank you." This response says to compliment givers that their evaluation is acknowledged.

5. Allow the richness of the compliment to penetrate. Positive feedback is a means of renewing energy. Enjoy it!

6. Encouraging further compliments can be accomplished by adding to the "thank you," "I appreciate that you shared that with me."

The selection of words is not enough for setting tone. Nonverbal communication must align with the words that are used. Positive words can only be perceived as positive when the nurse's body language conveys the same message. In fact, it has been found that if there is an inconsistency between verbal and nonverbal communication, the nonverbal communication (that is, facial and vocal expressions) will have a far greater influence on the message than the words themselves (Mehrabian, 1971). Therefore, if nurses want to convey that they are willing to listen and be open to what another has to say, they must not only express themselves verbally but they must also express a willingness to listen through direct eye contact and "open" body gestures (arms to sides; not folded across the chest).

A positive tone in the workplace is contagious. Concerted energy toward establishing rapport can influence the members of an entire work unit. Just one nurse's efforts can encourage others to look at work as a meaningful challenge where strengths are identified and shared, and where there is clarity in and congruence between words, expressions, and gestures. This kind of positive environment builds a foundation for the development of collegial relationships.

DEVELOPING COLLEGIAL RELATIONSHIPS

Nurses who collaborate as colleagues "come to value and respect their peers who share a mutual interest in providing quality health care" (Shea and Clark, 1979). This can only develop when a nurse is willing to reach out to another coworker. Moreover, collegial relationships are based on appropriate use of power sources. When two persons attempt

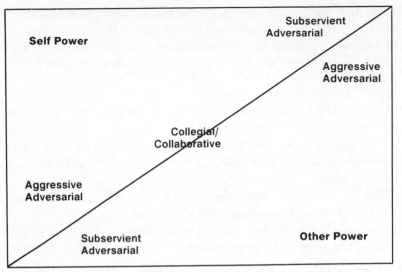

Figure 6-1   Model for developing collegial relationships in nursing.

to develop a relationship, each party exerts some form of influence on that relationship. When one person or the other has more power sources (formal authority, expert power, or information) and uses it to the detriment of the other person, then a subservient or aggressive adversarial relationship can develop.

Whether subservient or aggressive, relationships depend on the nature of the power sources and how power is used in the situation. It is only when there is a "power balance" among the two parties (a willingness to share power resources or to collaborate), that a collegial relationship can occur. (Figure 6-1).

> For example, suppose an experienced floor nurse chooses not to help a nurse newly assigned to the unit. The experienced nurse decides that, since there was never any help offered to her, she will not offer help to the newcomer.

It will not take long before an adversarial relationship develops. In this case, the experienced nurse has a great deal of power (information and expertise) and the new nurse has very little. An imbalance exists. Only when the experienced nurse shares information and expertise will the power between the two nurses be balanced. As a result, a collegial relationship can be established.

The process of "power balancing" incorporates the interactional components of setting a positive tone. It also requires that nurses develop clear communication patterns, communication skills, and set personal goals for working as team players.

BECOMING A TEAM PLAYER

The development of a team and teamwork does not happen just because a group of individuals happens to work together. There are certain factors that determine whether work groups—be they staff members at a meeting or a team working on an assignment—can be considered a team or merely a collection of individuals.

Members of a team choose to be team players. They work "together" because they are willing to assist each other and operate under a set of common rules. Team players fully participate in work planning and problem solving and positively confront conflict.

Work groups are composed of human beings, and therefore, can be considered "organic." To function fully as a team, they must mature. In order that any work group may become a team, nurses must be conscious of how groups function.

There are two sets of functions that operate interactively within a group at all times. One set of functions focuses on the tasks of the group, that is, the actual work being done by the group. The other set of functions deals with the personal relations among group members and serves to maintain the group process while tasks are being performed. These functions include such activities as encouraging others to speak or making sure everyone has the necessary information (Langford, 1981). While the leader of the work group has responsibility for these functions, so do the members of the group.

To reach optimal levels of team development, groups must pass through several stages of development. Each developmental stage integrates specific task functions with personal relations processes. For instance, when groups first form, group members often feel dependent on others for information. As a result, to reach the next stage of development, orientation must occur. In a similar fashion, each stage of development is illustrated by a type of personal relation and the task function necessary for movement to the next stage. Optimum team development is characterized by interdependence and mutual problem solving (see Figure 6-2).

While reaching optimum team development is a goal, it is not always achievable. As new members (such as new employees) are introduced into the work group, the dynamics of the group may change and the group may regress to an earlier stage of development. However, effectively functioning work groups continually reach for optimal team devel-

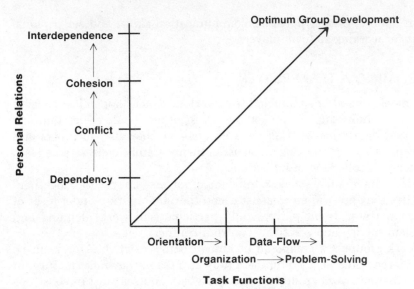

Figure 6-2   *Stages of group development. (Reprinted from Pfeiffer JW, Jones JE (eds): A Handbook of Structured Experiences for Human Relations Training, Vol. 2. San Diego, University Associates, Inc., 1974. Used with permission)*

opment (teamwork). The ability of a work group to be successful in becoming a team is contingent upon its members becoming team players, no matter what the stage of development. Nurses who are team players have

1. A clear understanding of and commitment to the goals of the work unit, that is, delivering quality patient care however that may be defined in the organization
2. Access to the knowledge, skills and expertise of fellow colleagues, such as sharing patient information informally or in a staff meeting
3. A willingness to trust others
4. A commitment to clearly and directly communicating work group problems

Optimum levels of teamwork occur when team members are flexible and are sensitive to the needs and feelings of others. Involvement and creativity are maximized through participation. In a service industry such as health care, organization goals must always be at the forefront. A strong sense of belonging to a team encourages the attainment of those goals.

It is not easy to be a team player since there are so many different individuals to deal with on a daily basis. As a result, an understanding of conflict and how to effectively deal with differences among people is helpful.

MANAGING CONFLICT

Anytime two persons come together, there is a potential for conflict. The potential is there because each individual has his own unique way of perceiving or "seeing" situations and "understanding" information. As a result, when perceptions and understanding of situations or information differ, conflict occurs. Therefore, conflict may be defined very simply and directly. Conflict represents "differences" between and among individuals or groups. There can be *interpersonal* conflict (between individuals or groups) or *intrapersonal* conflict (internal to an individual, such as a nurse having difficulty making a choice between taking one job or another).

Conflict within the work setting is a natural phenomenon and can be expected. If no conflict occurred, there would be complete agreement at all times. Under these "no conflict circumstances," persons would think alike, much like robots. Not only would the work environment be dull and boring, but no progress would be made. Creativity would not exist.

While conflict occurs as a normal part of work, the goal in conflict management is to intervene quickly. Conflict only grows in intensity when ignored. Therefore, conflict can be effectively managed by confronting it positively.

Confrontation can be an exciting challenge and the potential outcomes are well worth the investment. When conflict is handled well, a great deal of learning takes place. Greater understanding regarding different interactions can occur. Communication between persons increases as relationships grow. However, liking a person better is not the intended outcome. Being able to work together more effectively is the goal. Other positive outcomes of conflict include the generation of new ideas and the solutions to difficult problems.

In today's health-care environment, conflict abounds. Involved individuals and groups have their own opinions about how to handle the many challenges that lie ahead as a "new" health-care system emerges. As a result, there exists a variety of conflicts.

There are conflicts between health-care organizations and society as persons ask for health services in particular quantities and at a level of quality that varies from what can be delivered. Changing demographics and limited finances have stimulated professional groups to vie for the consumer's attention. Conflicts are occurring between the private and public sectors as federal and state governments attempt to determine what their appropriate role is in financing and delivering health care.

As resources have become scarcer, health care organizations are encountering increased internal conflicts, where personnel and/or work units compete for their "fair share." Finally, with an environment laden with conflict and stress, relationships and interactions among colleagues are potentially more labile. It has never been as important as now for nurses to become comfortable managing conflict situations.

Managing conflict is much like assessing and intervening when there is a patient problem. There are various causal factors that need to be identified, and this can be done by identifying the subject matter of the differences that have caused conflict. For instance, there may be conflict because of given information or set of facts, emotions, perceptions about a situation that occurred, or the values held by other nurses. The causal factor should first be identified. In conflict, knowing the etiology helps determine the ease with which the conflict can be resolved. It is much easier to deal with differences in information than to come to terms with differing values system, such as the ethics related to the "right to die."

Embedded within conflict management are several personal emotional barriers. A key barrier is exactly what an individual has learned about conflict. Notions of conflict develop from the messages sent over time by parents and significant others. Suppose a child learns that conflict is negative and should be avoided. When this child becomes an adult and encounters conflict, a definitive pattern of avoidance behaviors may be seen. Likewise, children can also learn that conflict is harmful and defenses should be drawn to guard against any potential threats. This message may lead to an aggressive response to conflict.

Learning about conflict can also be differentiated by gender. Many women were socialized into believing that they were not suited to the vagaries of conflict. Being angry was not considered an acceptable response and when differences occurred, women were supposed to either avoid or accommodate. Learning this message can cause women to feel fearful, powerless, and immobilized when confronted with conflict situations.

Today, gender socialization and parental messages about conflict are changing. Children are being taught that outcomes of conflict can be positive. Nonetheless, the remnants of the past still influence a great segment of the population.

The frustration and anger associated with conflict is another major barrier. Anger occurs as a result of a perceived threat. A threat may occur when a nurse "puts down" another by criticizing patient-care skills. When that threatening event occurs, assumptions are made about the intensity of the threat. The assumptions help determine how much power one has to ward off the threat. If the threat is not perceived as dangerous or if one feels powerful enough to confront the threat posi-

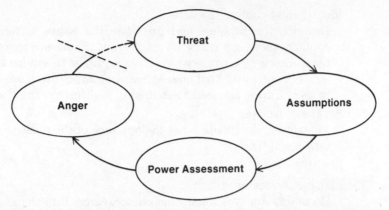

Figure 6-3   The anger cycle. (Illustration by John E. Jones and Anthony G. Banet, Jr. Reprinted from Pfeiffer JW, Jones JE (eds): The 1976 Annual Handbook for Group Facilitators. San Diego, University Associates, Inc., 1976. Used with permission)

tively, then anger does not ensue. However, if the reverse is true, and the threat is perceived as dangerous or a feeling of powerlessness emerges, then anger erupts as a means of protection (Kelley, 1979). This process is circular and can intensify as conflict situations repeat themselves (Figure 6-3).

While a usual response to conflict, anger becomes a barrier to its management since it is difficult to problem solve rationally when there are intense emotions. Dealing with the emotional barriers of conflict is one of the most difficult parts of conflict management.

Conflict management encompasses a problem assessment and intervention process utilizing the technique of positive confrontation. The rationale and logic of this step-by-step process enable the nurse to control the influence of emotional aspects of conflict. The steps of this process include:

Assess:

1. Analyze the conflict situation:
    Identify the type of conflict to determine the necessary time investment.
    Review the facts and validate any assumptions through further investigation.
    Examine who is involved in the conflict and the role they play.
    Determine to what degrees the situation can be changed.
    Become aware of personal messages that are blocking the ability to act. Realize that the other individuals involved may be dealing with similar messages.

2. Identify and confine the issue:
    Describe the problem and prioritize the issues. Oftentimes in conflict, there are many issues present. Some are more critical than others. Determine which issue is crucial to solving the problem and start with that one. Attempting to resolve more than one issue at a time can lead to confusion and further frustration.
3. Set the objective:
    Visualize and describe what the outcome of the positive confrontation will be.

    Identify:
4. Manage the feelings:
    Becoming angry is a personal choice. Entry into the anger cycle can be circumvented by identifying what personally triggers anger. Each person has a unique response pattern related to certain words, actions, and expressions. Whatever the situation, should that work, action, or expression be used by another individual, the anger response will quickly take hold. For example, for some persons, an anger trigger response results from a particular tone of voice that sounds condescending to them. If a person is aware of the behaviors that stimulate anger, then the choice to be angry is truly a choice.
    Check the reality of assumptions that are made in the anger cycle. Assumptions lead to the assessment of power. The more factual the assumptions, the stronger the power assessment. The intent is to feel as powerful as possible. The equation is direct. As powerfulness increases the likelihood of becoming angry decreases.

    Intervene:
5. Enter the conflict believing that there will be a positive outcome.
6. Select the appropriate method for resolving the conflict:
    Each situation often requires a different method for bringing conflict to resolution. Selection of a method is dependent upon desired outcomes. Furthermore, each method requires a different set of skills (Table 6-1).

The methods often selected for conflict resolution are either compromise or collaboration. These methods assume that the nurse has decided to approach the conflict positively, utilizing a problem-solving framework.

The major differences between compromise and collaboration lie in their intended outcomes and the time it takes to reach those outcomes. Of these two methods, collaboration can be considered more growth enhancing.

Table 6-1 Methods for Resolving Conflict

METHOD	RESULTS	APPROPRIATE	INAPPROPRIATE	SKILLS REQUIRED
Denial or withdrawal	Person tries to solve problem by denying its existence; results in win-lose	When issue is relatively unimportant; when issue is raised at inopportune time	When issue is important; when it will not disappear, but will build to greater complexity	Judgment of what is needed in the situation
Suppression or smoothing over	Differences are played down; results in win-lose	Same as above; also when preservation of relationship is more important than issue	When evasion of issue will disrupt relationship; when others are ready and willing to deal with issue	Empathy
Power or dominance	Authority, position, majority rule, or a persuasive minority settles the conflict; results in win-lose	When authority is granted by one's position; also when group has agreed on method of decision-making	When those without power have no means to express their needs and ideas, especially if this lack of opportunity has the potential of future disruption	Decision making; running effective meetings
Compromise or negotiation	Each party gives up something in order to meet midway; results in some loss of each side's position	When both sides have enough leeway to give; when resources are limited; when win-lose stance is undesirable	When original position is inflated or unrealistic; when solution must be watered down to be acceptable; when commitment by both parties is doubtful	Attentive listening and paraphrasing; problem solving
Collaboration	Individual abilities and expertise are recognized; each person's position is clear, but emphasis is on group solution; results in win-win	When time is available to complete process; when parties are committed to and trained in use of process	When time is limited; when parties lack training in or commitment to collaborative efforts	Attentive listening and paraphrasing; problem solving

(Hart LB: Moving Up! Women and Leadership. Lyons, CO. Leadership Dynamics, P.O Box 320. Reprinted with permission)

In collaboration, the goal is to have both parties win; no one is asked to give up anything. The problem-solving process continues until each party is satisfied with the resolution. Having both parties win is certainly a goal worth striving for but it is sometimes difficult to reach. Time, commitment, and expertise in the skills of problem assessment, identification, and intervention are essential. On the other hand, compromise takes less time. The process of problem assessment, identification and intervention takes less time because the goal for resolution is different. In compromise, both parties are willing to give something up. (Hart, 1983; Bolton, 1979).

While the outcomes of compromise and collaboration differ, their approach to conflict resolution is similar. The centerpiece of both compromise and collaboration is mutual respect. Listening skills are also essential. All the facts, assumptions, and feelings must be "heard."

Positive confrontation is a technique that can be used to verbalize facts, assumptions, and feelings. This technique offers a nondefensive, rational approach. Therefore nurses can effectively communicate their perception of the other person's behavior, their feelings about that behavior, and the effect the behavior had on them. This three-part assertive script is planned ahead of time and is both verbally and nonverbally expressed as clearly and succinctly as possible. Communicating the script effectively requires that all three parts are shared in the following pattern (Bolton, 1979):

WHEN YOU . . . . . . (State the behavior in descriptive terms).
I FEEL . . . . (Disclose feelings).
BECAUSE . . . . . . (Talk about the consequences of the behavior).

Once the script is shared, the next step is listening to and dealing with the response. This phase of conflict resolution can be considered negotiation.

Negotiation is a communication process in which a mutual decision is made (Fisher and Ury, 1981). If the decision is to move toward a win-win strategy, then collaboration is the method of choice. If concessions will be made by both, then a compromise will be reached. In any case, Nierenberg (1981) asserts that a basic ingredient in negotiation is preparation. The nurse must be clear about the desired outcomes and be sensitive to what is happening during the entire resolution process. In addition, the nurse should decide if, as part of the resolution, she is going to ask for a change in behavior.

There is an underlying assumption regarding a request for a change in behavior. The nurse must feel that she has a right to ask another to modify her behavior. The foundation for the request emerges from the impact that behavior has on the nurse's activities. The request must outline the specific change in behavior and be communicated as an "I" statement. For instance, "I am asking that the next time we work together you also let me know when you are going to take a break. Would you be willing to do that?" In addition to the request, consequences for the change should be described. Positive consequences resulting from the change should also be identified (Bower and Bower, 1976). Discussion should continue until a resolution is reached.

The following is an example of how a nurse can manage a conflict situation:

Assume that two nurses were in conflict because one nurse continually asked the other to do "little favors" for her. These "little favors," such as checking her patient's IV, were part of that nurse's patient-care assignment. The "little favors" never seemed to be just "little." The favors often took more time than calculated and sometimes caused the nurse performing the favor to fall behind in her own assignments. When she did fall behind and asked for help, she was told by the other nurse that she (the other nurse) "didn't have time." At first, the nurse being asked to do the favors did not mind because she felt that it was part of being a team player. After the requests became a continual pattern, the nurse started to become increasingly angry. The relationship between the two nurses deteriorated quickly. Intervention was necessary.

After problem assessment and identification, the intervention chosen was positive confrontation. The hope was that collaboration could be the method employed. The positive confrontation the nurse used follows:

> *When you* continually ask me to do your "little favors" and then don't offer to help me when I get behind,
>
> *I feel* angry
>
> *Because* the "little favors" take time away from the care I need to give the patients assigned to me and I fall behind.

The next step would be to cope with the other nurse's response. Negotiating a resolution could then be accomplished by both nurses listening to each other and focusing on an acceptable outcome. It is important that no assumptions be made regarding motives, intent, or reasons why the nurse keeps asking for favors. If it is assumed that the nurse is lazy, incompetent, or doing this "on purpose," resolution will be difficult or even impossible. A descriptive, rational approach is imperative.

In this situation, a request for a change in behavior might be appropriate. Depending on the course of the resolution process, one request might be:

> I am willing to help you as long as I am also able to finish my assignments. I am requesting that, if I am willing to help you and then if I ask you for

help, you will reciprocate. If you are willing to do this, the positive consequence will be that both of our patient assignments will be completed.

Should one nurse not comply with the request, the next step for the other nurse would be to identify the consequences for the noncompliance. Unfortunately, the consequence might be that requests for help in the future would be carefully scrutinized.

Managing conflict can be an exciting challenge when seen as a way of improving communications and promoting growth. Communication and growth are essential as nurses attempt to direct the system of health care toward a positive future.

DEALING WITH CHANGE

"Change is the process by which the future invades our lives" (Toffler, 1970). This statement has never been as true as in health care today. The rate of change is so quick that often there is little time to respond. But respond we must!

Mauksch and Miller (1981) conceptualized change on two levels. The first level, *macroscopic,* is change that affects the health-care universe. An example of a macroscopic change would be the impact of diagnosis related groups (DRG's) on health-care organizations all over the country.

Microscopic change, the second level, has only a small influence on the universe of health care. Change that might occur within one region, health-care organization, or part of an organization would represent a microscopic change. A microscopic change can range from broad to narrow in focus. Examples could range from the formation of a statewide nurses' political action committee, on the one hand, to the introduction of a new form into one department of a health-care organization.

Organizations tend to have their own unique response to change. This response is often predicated on the organization's style of management. Some organizations assume a reactive posture toward change, thus allowing both external and internal changes to control the organization. Others are proactive and attempt to respond to change by carefully planning for it.

When change is unplanned, there is great potential for negative outcomes because there are limited opportunities for involvement in planning for or implementing the change. On the other hand, if it is possible to plan for change, the outcomes can be worth the investment. This is especially important because, even when change has potential for positive outcomes, individuals tend to resist it.

Resistance occurs because many persons, especially in the work setting, like the comfort of routine. They are secure when things are status quo. By its very nature, change connotes some degree of risk and may require persons to try out or learn something new. As a result, change may be perceived as a frightening event.

For some, resistance results from personal attitudes toward change, fear of the unknown, fear of the change itself, or myths or assumptions about the outcomes of a particular change (Kossen, 1978).

Information giving is a powerful strategy for combating resistance. When change occurs and limited information is given, the response from some health-care personnel is oftentimes fear. When information can be shared, faulty assumptions are less likely and, as a result, rumors can be curbed. Coping with unplanned change can be difficult. A positive work climate encourages the flexibility and collegiality needed to maintain personal and professional productivity.

Planned change can occur at all levels of an organization. Sometimes change is directional: initiated from the top down or from the bottom up. For instance, a top-down change might be a new policy. Bottom-up change might come from a suggestion made by a nurse on a work unit or from a problem-solving group such as a quality circle.

When change is planned, the nurse can play a very important role as change agent. To achieve the desired response, it is helpful to have support from top administration and to include all persons involved in the change. There are several guidelines that are helpful when implementing change participatively (Kron, 1981; Douglass and Bevis, 1974):

1. Identify practical and realistic goals.
2. Set priorities.
3. Reduce any surprises by keeping everyone informed.
4. Try to get everyone to agree on the change.
5. Set up a process among those involved in the change that includes such norms as willingness to listen to each other's contributions and making conflict acceptable so that all emerging issues can be handled.
6. Allow for modification at any point during the implementation of the change.
7. Keep the group on the target. Failures can then be minimized and salvaged.

Nurses can have a powerful influence in their organizations as they respond positively to change by acting as information links in their health-care setting. By their example, nurses can be helpful change agents as they initiate and participate in the change process.

Summary

Working in health-care organizations can be an exciting challenge for all nurses. Establishing rapport by acquiring a positive work philosophy and focusing on the strengths of one's colleagues, sets a tone for the sharing of power sources. The sharing of power sources or "power balancing" is critical to the development of collegial relationships.

The primary goal of health-care organizations is the delivery of a set standard of patient care. Understanding and being committed to this goal is essential to teamwork. A sensitivity to another's needs and feelings, the sharing of skills and knowledge, and full participation in team activities are just a few of the ingredients that help make a nurse a team player.

One benefit of developing a positive climate is the enhancement of relationships with others. A great deal of learning comes from managing the differences between and among individuals. Conflict management provides an opportunity for nurses to sharpen their problem assessment and intervention skills. Positively confronting a situation in order to bring conflict to resolution requires abilities in overcoming personal emotional barriers, using a logical process to assess problems, and selecting the appropriate method for conflict intervention. Methods such as compromise and collaboration suggest that the resolution of conflict should be based on respect and mutual problem solving.

What the future holds in store for health care will be determined by what is done today. By responding to the many changes ahead, both planned and unplanned, nurses will become indispensable transmitters of information. Nurses must also assume a leadership role in advocating a participatory approach to planning for and implementing change. Identifying realistic goals, setting priorities, encouraging agreement and involvement, and maintaining the desired direction will assure a smooth and steady transition to the future.

A positive work climate is the foundation for a productive and growth-oriented work environment. In such an environment, nurses will have unlimited opportunities to use their creative leadership skills!

Bibliography

Bolton R: People Skills, Englewood Cliffs, NJ, Prentice-Hall, 1979
Bower SA, Bower GH: Asserting Yourself: Practical Guide for Practical Change. Reading, MA, Addison-Wesley, 1976

Douglass LM, Bevis EO: Nursing Leadership in Action: Principles and Application to Staff Situations. St Louis, CV Mosby, 1974

Fisher R, Ury W: Getting to Yes. Negotiating Agreement Without Giving In. Boston, Houghton Mifflin, 1981

Hart LB: Moving Up! Women and Leadership. Lyons, CO, Leadership Dynamics, 1983

Kelley C: Assertion Training: A Facilitator's Guide. La Jolla, University Associates, 1979

Kossen S: The Human Side of Organizations. New York, Harper & Row, 1978

Kron T: The Management of Patient Care. Philadelphia, WB Saunders, 1981

Langford, TL: Managing and Being Managed. Englewood Cliffs, NJ, Prentice-Hall, 1981

Mauksch IG, Miller MH: Implementing Change in Nursing. St. Louis, CV Mosby, 1981

Mehrabian A: Silent Messages. Belmont, CA, Wadsworth Publishing, 1971

Naisbitt J: Megatrends. New York, Warner Books, 1984

Nierenberg GI: The Art of Negotiating. New York, Simon & Schuster, 1981

Richardson J, Margulis J: The Magic of Rapport. San Francisco, Harbor Publishing, 1981

Shea CA, Clark CC: Considerations in developing alternatives: Autonomy and collaboration. In Clark CC, Shea CA (eds): Management in Nursing. New York, McGraw-Hill, 1979

Toffler A: Future Shock. New York, Random House, 1970

Chapter 7

Making the most of expertise

NANCY R. KRUGER

Today's health care climate demands that all care-givers maximize the use of their resources. Among the types of resources available are diagnostic tests, specialized facilities, and persons with specialized talents and technical skills. Each needs to be managed effectively in order to assure full productivity. One of the resources often overlooked is the effective management of expertise.

According to the dictionary, *expertise* is a specialized skill or technical knowledge applied for some use. In this chapter the discussion will focus on using expertise that is available to newly graduated professional nurses.

This chapter will enable you to

1. Identify components of job descriptions that define areas of worker responsibilities.
2. Identify principles of time management.
3. Identify components for the development and utilization of self and others.
4. Identify the importance of a positive self concept in the successful utilization of experts available for consultation.

Using available expertise is more than notifying the appropriate expert, requesting assistance, and then expecting the problem to be solved to everyone's satisfaction. It begins with insight into one's own self-concept, identification of personal strengths and weaknesses, and an understanding of the defined job expectations.

Superimposed upon this foundation is the effective use of good resource management skills. These skills include the application of time management concepts, proper identifications of work that must be accomplished, acceptance of direction from supervisory personnel, appropriate delegation of jobs to optimize one's own talents as well as those of colleagues, and a minimization of conflict over turf issues.

For the new nurse, an understanding of the job expectations is fundamental. The job description serves as the explicit and implicit guide to behavior and performance expectations. Supervisory personnel rely on this framework for optimizing staff talents. Colleagues depend on each other to act within the defined guidelines, to prevent duplication of effort, and to capitalize on the inherent expertise built into each job. The job description serves as a useful structure for building and using expertise.

Job Descriptions as a Reference for Optimizing Staff Talents

Ordinarily, obtaining the most efficient productivity from staff members by optimizing staff talent is the responsibility of the head nurse. Often the head nurse has had significant input into the development of the staff member job description. Consequently, when a particular problem arises, the head nurse is able to identify quickly and then assign the staff member best equipped to handle the situation. However, the staff nurse who knows the special talents, expectations, and responsibilities of various members of the staff, including her own, will be able to initiate care quickly and effectively rather than wait for a series of contacts to be made in order to obtain the resource to solve the problem.

In reviewing a job description, certain standard elements are necessary: a summary of your duties and responsibilities; to whom you report;

whom you supervise; what the minimum qualifications are for the work, and what the working conditions will be.

Most institutions have a form such as the one illustrated on this and the following page, that is used for all jobs. The content of the form changes, depending upon the position. Usually the title of the position is stated followed by the department in which the position is located. Next, a statement appears describing reporting responsibilities. If the employee is expected to supervise any personnel a separate area will designate those positions. Occasionally a job code and a grade are involved;

POSITION DESCRIPTION

TITLE: Clinical Nurse	DEPARTMENT: Nursing Service		F.L.S.A STATUS:
REPORTS TO: Head Nurse	GRADE 14	POSITION CODE 1406	__X__ Non-Exempt

POSITIONS SUPERVISED:
Staff Registered Nurses' Ward Clerks and Nursing Assistants

Exempt
_____ Administrative
_____ Executive
_____ Professional

PRIMARY FUNCTION:
Responsible for Clinical management of patient care on the unit.

PRINCIPAL DUTIES AND RESPONSIBILITIES:

1. Assist the staff nurses' with nursing process by making daily clinical rounds and reviewing the patient care and patient documentation with the staff nurse.

2. Review patient care plans and update daily with the staff nurses.

3. Holding patient care conferences at least monthly with the staff nurses to establish clinical care practices and review of these practices. Encourage staff to participate in the area.

4. Review, revise and develop written care plans protocols through nursing Standards Committee.

5. Participate in the evaluation of these protocols and the staffs ability to implement these protocols. Implement all policies and procedures with staff.

6. Participate and coordinate with the Head Nurse and Assistant Director for Education al Programs in the orientation of new staff.

7. Provide assistance to the staff for the Discharge Planning Process—utilizing the patient, family, Utilization Coordinator and Social Service Department.

8. Coordinate with the Nursing Quality Care Committee and follow-up recommendations from the committee.

POSITION DESCRIPTION (*CONTINUED*)

QUALIFICATIONS:

Education: Registered Nurse—Pennsylvania—BSN

Experience: One year-Med/Surg. 6 months ophthalmic—demonstrated ability in all
     steps of Nursing Process.

Certification/Licensure: Current licensure in Pennsylvania

WORKING CONDITIONS: Lifts weights over 25 pounds, repeated bending, squatting, stooping, Pushing and pulling movements. Prolonged walking and standing. Exposed to infections occasionally, cuts when handing instruments and hazardous gases in anesthetized areas. Exposed to electrical and radiant energy hazards.

DESCRIBED BY:	DATE:	APPROVED BY:	DATE:

Position Title	Department	Subdivision	Work Area
Clinical Nurse	Nursing Service		Patient Care Floor Operating Room

---

  9. Self continuing education. Attend a minimum of two "outside," and eight inhouse conferences/year.

10. Monthly rotations on evenings nights as needed.

11. Provides staffing relief as needed.

12. Additional functions as assigned by the Assistant Director for Patient Services.

---

this is usually for comparative purposes with other similar positions and responsibilities. A statement of the primary function is made and may be followed by the summary of duties or the principal duties and responsibilities.

Qualifications including the minimum required education, required experience, and required certification and/or licensure should be stated. Within this section, one may note that certain things are preferred. When applying for a job these requirements may give you a clue as to the level of person being sought. If you have this additional prerequisite you may have a better chance of obtaining the position. For example, if the position requires a diploma but a B.S.N. is preferred your chances are much better if you possess a B.S.N..

Finally, and certainly one of the most important elements, are the working conditions. This section includes a statement about the hours of work, exposure to various hazards and stresses as well as physical requirements for lifting and reaching. Occasionally, there may be some ambiguous statements within a job description that may cause some confusion. It is essential that the published job description is also the way in which the practice is carried out on the work unit. Any discrepancies need to be clarified with actual expectations clearly defined.

Once a clear idea of the job description is understood and some proficiency in practice is gained, learning the performance expectations of other staff members will help identify appropriate resources. This type of investigation will also pinpoint areas of redundancy, that is, areas where more than one type of staff member may be available to perform a task, structure a program, or give information to patients.

A careful analysis of various jobs may suggest responsibility for the same activity. Administration of medications is one such example. Not only may all R.N.s have this duty as part of their job descriptions but L.P.N.s may be required to administer medications and have it so defined in their job description. Who then, you might ask, administers medication? The answer: it depends. It depends on the situation and the institutional policies that affect where the responsibility resides. In some situations the R.N. may delegate this activity to the L.P.N.

Frequently during the orientation period, questions of shared responsibility are discussed. The new nurse may be instructed to contact certain staff members for advice in specific matters. These designated expert staff members may include more experienced staff, inservice instructors, supervisors, or clinical specialists.

As one begins practice, knowing the job expectations of fellow staff members permits the nurse to delegate tasks to appropriate others as well as request their assistance. Since the initial task of the new practitioner is to gain proficiency in basic nursing assessment, planning, and treatment skills obtaining assistance from more experienced staff is one method of developing the skill of using experts for specific purposes.

Knowing the job description of other staff members permits the nurse to delegate tasks to others as well as to foster the request for help. Although the new nurse is often the person to whom tasks are delegated, certain instances arise where the nurse properly delegates to others. A patient may require transportation off the floor for diagnostic studies. Instead of accompanying the patient, the nurse might direct the patient escort or a member of the nursing auxiliary staff to transport the patient.

Each of us has varying levels of technical skills. Identifying particular personal skills allows us to capitalize quickly on our own expertise. Using personal expertise is often more efficient since it does not require additional time to make appropriate arrangements with others. Consequently, care may more often be delivered at the mutual convenience of the nurse and patient.

Certain types of experts are particularly valuable to the new nurse. These include persons with experience in comfortably moving patients on and off bedpans, transferring patients out of bed to chairs, wheelchairs, and stretchers, or undressing an unconscious patient quickly and without damaging the patient's clothing.

There are numerous members of the staff with particular talents either by personal ability as an individual who speaks a foreign language or expected talents by virtue of various roles. They may include nurses' aides, L.P.N.s, ward clerks, unit managers, other staff nurses, clinical specialist technicians, staff from various departments (such as home care, discharge planning) and pharmacists. Others include I.V. therapists, dietitians, lab technicians, diagnostic department members, nurse practitioners, physicians, and purchasing agents. While this list is not exhaustive, it provides at least some of the areas that interface with patient care activities.

Since the need to establish a working relationship with other departments is crucial in order to assure successful patient care, the nurse would be wise to recognize and understand the concept of mutual dependence.[1] The concept of mutual dependence recognizes the fallibility of two human beings but also the need for accomplished persons to rely upon and trust each other. It is therefore reasonable to recognize not only one's own talents but also the talents of others. Furthermore, it is essential to acknowledge explicitly the help received from a colleague or subordinate.

Head nurses and supervisors do not have infinite wisdom and knowledge. Occasionally, an improper assignment may be made—improper because the nurse in question has neither the experience nor the expertise to perform the assigned task. The new nurse who understands personal talents and those of her coworkers, who accepts direction graciously and tactfully delegates or redirects problems to appropriate staff members will develop into a positive health-care team member.

Perhaps the most difficult issue for the new nurse to resolve while learning to make the most of expertise is the turf problem: dealing with overlapping responsibilities. Several members of the staff are likely to view themselves as experts in the same area. Each person has a particular way of approaching the problem. Although differences may not appear significant on the surface, to the competing groups these differences may seem like a chasm.

For example, preoperative education may pose some turf problems. On one hand the patient's nurse is often expected to provide preoperative education. The content usually includes a description of the sequence of events expected to take place on the day of surgery, the anatomy involved, postoperative diet and exercise, and expectations about pain and how it will be managed. On the other hand similar information may be given to the patient by a clinical specialist with expertise in the problem at hand.

When the same information is somewhat different when presented by the staff nurse and by the clinical specialist, and where the patient asks questions that suggest a misunderstanding, one nurse may feel the second nurse acted in an inappropriate manner. At the very least there might be angry feelings between the two nurses. Unfortunately, patients may become aware of the differences of opinion. As a result, the patient may become further confused and lose trust in the nurses' capability to provide care.

In order to prevent or diminish turf problems, it is essential to discuss potential areas of disagreement with the charge nurse and then to share those concerns with the consulted "expert." As part of the investigative process, the nurse should routinely ask the unit leader if there is likely to be any difficulties with other team members if a problem is approached in a certain way. Other references available to assist in this process are policy manuals, nursing practice or nursing standards, as well as the clinical literature.

Aside from turf issues, other problems likely to be encountered are perceptions about what kind of person the new staff member is. Will this new person fit in with the group? Is the nurse a safe practitioner? Accusations such as "brown nosing," trying to make colleagues look bad because of conscientiousness and thorough practice, or being accused of taking too much time are frequent criticisms of the new nurse. These circumstances may lead to conflict. However, if one is prepared to state the reasons, including admitting when certain actions have created additional problems, then it is likely that hostility may partially be defused.

Finally, in optimizing staff talents, the flow of information needs to be timely and correct. There are several types of information pertinent to patient care and the management of the patient care unit. The flow pattern will be different depending upon the organizational structure of the institution. In some facilities the staff nurse must ask an assistant head nurse to make phone calls to physicians to clarify orders. Other settings foster a more independent practice and the staff nurse is expected to direct all of the care without seeking permission to carry out a particular plan. Instead the nurse is expected to keep colleagues and supervisors informed about patient progress and solicit advice when needed.

In the first instance the information flows from the nurse to an assistant head nurse and higher if necessary. Answers are returned through the same centralized structure. In the second case, information is more decentralized and direct. It flows from the physician to the direct care-giver and returns directly to the physician.

As another example, the nurse requires certain supplies in order to change a dressing. Here the nurse may be able to delegate the responsibility to a ward clerk simply by asking the clerk to order the supplies when she "takes off the physician orders." When the supplies arrive on the unit, the clerk notifies the nurse. The dressing change is made. The nurse documents the condition of the wound in the medical record and reports orally any pertinent information to colleagues and physicians. The information flow pattern is from the chart to the nurse and ward clerk. Each acts in a specified manner because of the pattern and the expectation of what each is to do with the written instructions (information). Similarly, the return activity is based on the receipt of information. The dressing is changed when the nurse is told the supplies have arrived. In another setting the nurse may be expected to act entirely differently because the flow of information excludes the ward clerk, leaving the nurse to make all of the arrangements.

It is also important to be aware of the existence of the informal information structure. Critical information about a patient's condition may reach the nurse too late. A nurses' aide, for example, may have overheard a patient and physician talking about a change in treatment. When the aide fails to notify the nurse of the conversation, a previous treatment may be delivered to the patient with serious consequences. By developing a good working relationship with a subordinate, the nurse would have been made aware of the change. In ignoring the importance of these employees and/or projecting such as impression, the nurse may prompt the aide consciously to withhold the information and thus make the nurse appear incompetent.

Clinical information needs to be relayed to the rest of the nursing staff, particularly changes in orders, test results, and patient responses to medical and nursing interventions. Naturally, critical value changes need to be reported (falling vital signs or abnormal laboratory values). When you are unsure of the implications of certain data, report it to your supervisor. The method of reporting may be written as well as oral. Above all, be clear about the handling of such information—to whom it must go, in what form, when follow-up is required, and how urgent notification needs to be made.

Other types of information are administrative questions. For example, equipment that malfunctions, or a failure by the laundry to provide an adequate supply of linen both need the attention of other departments. Knowing the proper channels to report problems may mean the difference between solving the problem or being plagued by their continuation.

Understanding the nature of the job, the expectations of colleagues and coworkers, along with turf issues and the direction of information flow is essential so that the new nurse may make the transition from student to professional. As these elements of knowledge are incorporated into daily practice, the nurse is able to concentrate on a more effective use of time.

Time Management

Although a staff nurse's time may seem highly regulated by factors outside her control, principles of time management may nevertheless be applied to enhance planning and execution of the job. These principals are outlined below. There are only 24 hours available in the day. It is not possible to create more time but time may be effectively managed for more efficient and productive outcomes.

Prioritization of work is a method of ranking work in order of preference. It begins with problem identification of those areas that may respond to nursing interventions. Three models for priority setting have been suggested. These include the problem-oriented model, the process-oriented model, and the outcome-oriented model.[2]

The problem-oriented approach tends to focus priority-setting on the severity of illness. Housing of critically ill patients or increasing staff may be a response to such an approach.

The process-oriented approach tends to focus on the types of interventions that might be most successful. The outcome-oriented approach

PRINCIPLES OF TIME MANAGEMENT

1. Prioritization of work
2. Plan work
3. Break difficult tasks into their smallest parts
4. Set deadline for achievement of smallest parts and the overall project
5. Group activities into logical sequences
6. Organize supplies and tasks
7. Control the environment to minimize interruptions
8. Use telephones to your advantage
9. Participate in meetings by adhering to the main topic

tends to set priorities along economic lines so that discharge planning might receive very high priority for patient care.

While each of these models seems very simple, there are numerous factors that often come together to prevent the implementation of a single system. Variables that have a significant impact are the employing institution and its policies, persons who work in the institutions, and the patients themselves.

Each constituency has its own goals. Dilemmas occur in priority-setting when the needs of the interacting variables are not congruent. When a consistent method for priority-setting is adopted and then applied to the practice-setting on a consistent basis, the opportunities for problem resolution are increased.

The new staff nurse will most likely encounter difficulty in priority-setting at two levels. The first level is that of the patient-nurse. The second level is the nurse-institution level. Through the assessment process, patients help the nurse define their needs, establish interventions, and implement the plan of care. This is where individualized priority-setting between patients and nurses occurs.

Since all patients assigned to a particular nurse may not receive care simultaneously, the nurse must determine the order in which patients will receive care. By necessity some care needs will be delayed in preference to more pressing needs of other patients. One method of ordering patient needs is to apply Maslow's theory to the situation. Maslow's theory, a hierarchy of needs (displayed elsewhere on this page), states that human needs—physiology, safety, love, self-esteem, and self-actualization—are arranged in an order to preponderance.[3] Though all people

Maslow's Hierarchy of Needs

Self-
Actualization

Self-
Esteem

Love

Safety

Physiology

strive for satisfaction of love, self-esteem and self-actualization, when more basic requirements such as physical health and safety are threatened these must receive first attention. Hence, if a patient has a cardiac arrest, this condition must be attended to in preference to the patient who is giving a return demonstration for medication knowledge. This example represents the difference in the physiological integrity of a patient and that of safety/self-esteem.

The second level of priority setting is nurse-institution needs. At this level general schedules that govern the typical day at the institution provide restrictions to priority setting for individual patients. In this area there are activities that must be done, should be done, and are nice to do.[2] Within this schema, nurses would order their activities to prevent or respond to emergencies, follow medical and nursing orders, promote progress toward the therapeutic good, and plan or initiate progress toward new goals.

Beyond general schedules and individual patient needs, priorities may be modified still further by staff needs such as conferences, staff meetings, and change-of-shift reports. In addition, the organization of the nursing staff into team nursing, primary nursing, or functional nursing may determine the priorities of an individual nurse's practice. The nurse may be the medication nurse for example. All patients would receive their medication in a designated order while another nurse may give treatments.

Priorities, then, may be set by order of importance for patient needs within the confines of predetermined institutional policies, staff assignment practices, and staff institutional obligations.

After the work has been prioritized, it should be planned. While taking some time, planning will allow the nurse to work smarter, economizing in time and energy. Otherwise the nurse may find the work may be accomplished only by working faster and longer. The need to work faster and longer because of poor planning often leads to poor judgment and mistakes. The result is the requirement to perform the task a second time, using additional time and resources.

Lack of planning may interfere with work priorities to such an extent that chaos will exist. Planning to work smarter also means identifying other persons on the health-care team who are in a position to assist in completing certain tasks. Self-discipline through the planning process is crucial if successful implementation is to be achieved.

The next step in time management is to survey the work at hand and to select difficult tasks and tasks that you may find distasteful. Teaching a patient how to perform a colostomy irrigation, for example, may be difficult and time consuming. By breaking down these tasks into their smallest possible parts with deadlines established for each segment, a sense of achievement for each completed portion may serve as a stimulus to continue onward as successful accomplishments have already been attained. "To do lists" are helpful tools in this process.[4] A sense of satisfaction is felt as one is able to cross off items on the list leaving fewer and fewer things to accomplish.

In conjunction with this technique, giving yourself and the patient a little reward at each step or at each group of steps along the way may act as further incentive to complete an activity. The nurse may reward herself with a coffee break at the end of the session while the patient may watch a favorite TV show.

Another time-management technique is to group activities into a logical sequence. For instance, if a patient is to have a colostomy irrigation with instruction and the patient's bed linens need changing it would seem appropriate to change the linens after the irrigation has been completed. This may mean that, rather than following the institutional routine of changing all of the patient's linen by 9 a.m., a particular patient may not have his linen changed until 11 a.m. following the warm soaks for phlebitis.

Other similar problems of grouping and sequencing activities may revolve around a group of patients. For example, several patients may need to leave a nursing unit for diagnostic tests or surgical procedures. All of these patients may need to have modified hygiene care in order to meet their appointments. These patients would receive care first, leaving the remaining patients to "sleep in." The needs of patients who "sleep in" would be delayed until later in the day.

Organization of supplies and tasks is important when activities are grouped together. Organizing items prevents multiple interruptions during a procedure in order to collect things that were forgotten. When this occurs the nurse may be perceived as being incompetent to care for the patient.

Once priorities are set, the work planned and organized, the nurse is ready to act. One additional precaution should be considered before the care is actually delivered. That precaution is environmental control to avoid unnecessary interruptions. Care should be taken to assure privacy, to be certain there is sufficient light, and to be sure it is quiet. In most instances, it is also important to have the patient's attention. This is best achieved when the environment is controlled and when the patient believes the nurse is interested only in him.

Some relatively simple measures that may be taken to assure privacy include letting your coworkers know where you are, what you are attempting to accomplish, and how long you expect to be involved in the activity. Closing the patient's door and drawing the curtain around the bed for screening are additional steps that might be taken. When an activity involves some explanation, sitting alongside the patient's bed rather than standing projects not only interest but also tends to make the patient believe the nurse has spent more time with him than if the nurse were to stand and conduct the same counseling session.

Time management should also be applied to the use of the telephone. The telephone may be viewed as a tool of enormous assistance or as a device of interruptions. Calls should be grouped together so that all information that might best be transmitted by phone is done at once. Socializing by phone should be kept to a minimum. Consideration of frequent interruptions of the party you are calling should also be given some thought.

One area frequently called is the clinical laboratory. Results of blood tests used to guide therapy must often be obtained quickly. However, when technicians are frequently called for test results, they are unable to perform the tests. By grouping information needs together, one phone call for all of the patients would be more efficient for both the nurse and the laboratory technician.

It is also essential for the nurse to have some idea of the turn-around time for the test. A call should not be made 15 minutes after the blood has been drawn if it takes 15 minutes to get to the lab and then another hour to run the test. If your hospital has a functioning computerized laboratory transmission results program, calling the laboratory will not enable you to obtain results any faster. Results will only become available as the computerized machines print out the results.

One additional consideration is to be aware of the actual urgency of need for the test results. What harm or alteration in treatment might one expect when this knowledge is available? Will the nurse's priorities of care be materially affected? If so, what preparations would be appropriate, pending those results?

Finally, meetings are a regular part of any staff nurse's working day. Whether the meeting is the report at the change of shift, a staff meeting with the head nurse, or a patient care conference, judicious use of time to accomplish the meeting's purpose is essential. During these meetings, valuable information is often mentioned that assists the nurse in identifying potential expert resources. Asking appropriate questions and adhering strictly to the main purpose of the meeting save time while also helping to collect accurate information.

Deterrents to Proper Time Management

Time has a way of passing very quickly. When time is not used effectively, work is not completed. One of the biggest problems is procrastination. All of us at some time will delay completing a task because we become involved in other activities. The task might simply be delayed because it is unpleasant or we have had little or no experience with the procedure and therefore put it off.

The obvious result of procrastination is that activity must still be completed and often under less than ideal conditions. The patient may not only suffer physically because of pain, but healing may be delayed, as in the case of a large, foul-smelling dressing not changed in a timely manner. Patients also sense avoidance on the part of the nurse who does not want to deal with difficult problems. Sometimes this feeling is adopted by the patient and he may avoid learning how to provide for himself.

As you might expect, procrastination may also occur under the guise of need for more information before a decision can be made. At this point it is necessary to determine whether or not additional information (and what type of information) will contribute to the ultimate outcome. In these situations it is better to understand or acknowledge that you cannot always make decisions with all of the possible facts known. Foregoing the decision may result in an outcome more detrimental to the patient.

Avoiding procrastination may be accomplished in at least two ways. One is to do the unpleasant task first, breaking it down into manageable parts, and second, to identify what is unpleasant about the task. In identifying what is unpleasant you may be able to obtain support from other staff members or find reference material that will make the job easier to complete. When it is a task with which you are unfamiliar, additional practice may make the task easier and less unpleasant because a certain amount of proficiency is achieved.

Finally, one might promise oneself a reward for good management when a task that is unpleasant is completed sooner than foreseen. The project focus may then be viewed with a far better attitude because a reward will follow hard work.

A second major deterrent to proper time management are unplanned interruptions. These may be related to family concerns and complaints, physician demands, patient emergencies, or institutional emergencies. In each instance, it is essential to identify the specific problem as quickly as possible, determine the resources available to meet the need, volunteer to assume responsibility for areas in which you are proficient, and cooperate in reestablishing an equilibrium in the system as quickly as possible.

By learning to utilize time effectively through prioritizing and planning, a good foundation will be laid to advance personal expertise in practice, as well as to identify and use available resources.

Utilizing Expertise of Self and Others

Once talent and expertise have been identified in certain team members, the next step in the process is to use these talents appropriately. Creating the proper match between patient requirements and the available resources begins with identifying patient needs and staff talents.

This process forces strengths, weaknesses, and personal style to be placed in the equation for a proper match. When resources are limited, the decision is easy: either the resource is used or it is not.

If no particular expert is available, then the nurse has an opportunity to create a certain amount of expertise within herself. Utilizing oneself, particularly in areas of interest or previously identified competence, fosters the development of more accomplished practice.

At some time, the nurse will need to do something in an area where knowledge and skill are particularly weak. In these cases, it might be helpful to notify or acknowledge both to one's colleagues and head nurse that you are not proficient and that some extended time may be required to complete the task.

With patient needs and staff assigned or consulted, suggestions and recommendations are made. Each recommendation must be evaluated. Among the things that need to be considered for each suggestion before implementation are: how long it will take; how many sessions will be required and with what frequency; whether other persons will need to be in attendance (family, friends, staff); how much it will cost; whether outside resources need be obtained; how complex the process; what supplies are required and finally, but perhaps most important of all, does the proposal really fit the patient and the situation.

When these questions are answered realistically, consideration for the implementation process can begin. Will the identified expert (nurse's aide, therapist) perform the task in its entirety or will the nurse share some responsibility? If responsibility is to be shared, what portion will be delegated and what portion will be retained by the nurse?

Following evaluation of the recommendations, the amount of time for completion should be determined. When determining time, it is always prudent to allow some additional time for interruptions and delays. As with most care interactions, providing the patient with courteous and complete attention is worth any additional time required. Conversely, the need to complete a task quickly is not an excuse for rudeness.

Defining the time frame for a patient-care activity within the unit schedule is affected by the activity completion time. An activity that might take an hour to complete should not be started 15 minutes before the change of shift. To accommodate a lengthy procedure, some activities may need to be changed from the morning to the evening. Often cited is the complete bed bath. This has traditionally been performed in the morning. Under certain conditions, there is no reason this could not be done at night. However, the amount of freedom in altering implementation may be either guided, restricted significantly, or highly unstructured, depending upon the rules of the unit where you work.

Utilization of expertise is also influenced by the level of interpersonal skills. For example, working relationships are enhanced when you like the individuals with whom you work. Certainly experts may be used effectively when persons are not close friends; they do not have to "like" one another in order for a task to be completed. However, when coworkers genuinely like each other, tasks are more likely to be completed in a positive manner. The atmosphere within the organization is enhanced.

Working relationships in which persons like each other also bespeaks an understanding of mutual expectations. Specified paths of information transmission are likely to occur so that persons who require the information receive it in a timely manner and the information is likely to be accurate.

The new nurse will come to trust those more experienced coworkers when she learns that these colleagues want to help her succeed. Even when disagreement or conflict arises, an honest evaluation of a mistake is highly worthwhile. Being dependable and honest under these circumstances establishes one's credibility.

When the nurse demonstrates an ability to use time wisely and resources appropriately, personal value is enhanced. This practice is obviously necessary if the nurse expects to receive recognition for excellent care and good management skills.

Once this type of credibility is established and interest is shown, the nurse may be considered for promotion. Certainly without the development of good time and resource management, both clinical proficiency and management skills will not mature and this is to the detriment of future patients.

Positive Self-Concept as a Tool for Success

Making the most of expertise, whether it is personal expertise or the expertise of another individual, entails a positive self-concept. A positive self-concept is essential so that the nurse can feel comfortable with the decision to delegate a job to another person, request assistance at the risk of appearing less competent, or assume responsibility in situations that may be unfamiliar.

Self-concept—how we see ourselves—acts as a filter for how we see, hear, and perceive *everything*. It influences what we say and how we say it. Our actions in part are a result of our self-concept and therefore influence how others view us.[5]

Development of the self-concept occurs over time and emerges from the individual's social interaction.[6] However, self-image does not simply mature to a certain point and then stop changing. The new professional nurse arrives in the clinical setting with fixed feelings about herself, feelings that have been shaped through childhood and formal education. As the nurse progresses through the orientation program, new knowledge and skills are learned that modify behavior. With each alteration in behavior comes a change in self-concept.

Gradually the role of a professional nurse is assumed during this formative period. With positive feedback for the successful application of newly acquired skills in the clinical setting, self-concept is enhanced. Growth and maturity during this time continue to occur, particularly when the nurse engages in some introspection about what skills she possesses and what skills need improvement.

Part of the process of developing a positive self-image is the establishment of a certain congruency between how we see ourselves and how others see us. If one believes one is capable of performing certain activities while it is evident to others that this is not the case, then the recognition sought will not be forthcoming. Patients' positive responses will decrease. Only a realistic assessment, a willingness to engage in an honest evaluation, enables the nurse to take corrective action that will enhance performance.

Beyond a realistic appraisal of whom we are, another difficulty with self-concept is that all of us are engaged in playing different "roles." Sometimes we may be friends, at other times we may be mothers or fathers, and still other times we are nurses. Conflict arises within ourselves when we are expected to act within a certain role but find ourselves in a situation that calls for us to play a second role. For example, the nurse may be working on a unit and an acquaintance appears for some conversation. The nurse switches "roles" to that of a friend and is no longer acting as a professional nurse. Reactions by coworkers and patients who observe this change in behavior in the work place may indicate disapproval toward the nurse. Later, when again acting in the nursing role, the nurse may receive some negative feedback because her role change was considered inappropriate in the work place.

It is essential to the development of the nursing role to incorporate the notion in the self-concept that one is a "nurse." That role definition is most successfully integrated by the new nurse when the nurse's idea and the patient's idea of what a nurse is and what she does coincide. One of the most frequent causes of nurses leaving the nursing profession is a result of the disparity between these two concepts.[6] If this is recognized, patients may be educated by the nurse as to what they should expect in terms of care and how it will be delivered. The nurse also needs to evaluate patients' expectations of a nurse. Nurses may need to incorporate some of the patient values into their nursing roles in order to achieve professional success and personal satisfaction.

Successful integration into the health-care system as a professional nurse depends upon a positive self-image. With a realistic appraisal of strengths and weaknesses and the courage to use constructive criticism for that development, the nurse will attain a strong self-concept.

Summary

New nurses need to be able to manage expertise, be it their own or those of others. This is achieved by identifying patient needs, prioritizing the work, delegating where appropriate, and asking for assistance when required. By knowing the job expectations, stated and implied, as well as the expectations of others, the nurse will be better able to use expertise in an appropriate manner without infringing on the territory of other workers. Finally, a positive self-concept will translate into a belief by patients and colleagues that this individual is an asset to the agency and patients in contributing to a positive health outcome.

References

1. Gabarro J, Kotter J: In Collins E (ed): Executive Success: Making It in Management, pp 333–344. New York, John Wiley & Sons, 1983
2. Feldman E, Monicken L, Crowley M: The systems approach to prioritizing. Nurs Admin Q7 (2): 57–62, 1983
3. Hampton D, Summer C, Weber R: Organizational Behavior and the Practice of Management, 3rd ed. Glenview, IL, Scott, Foresman, 1978
4. McNiff M: Getting organized—at last. RN: 1984 June, 23–24
5. Brouwer P: The power to see ourselves. In Collins E (ed): Executive Success: Making It in Management, pp 15–28. New York, John Wiley & Sons, 1983
6. George T: Development of the self-concept of nurse in nursing students. Res Nurs Health 5: 191–197, 1982

Bibliography

Barros A: Time management: Learn to work smarter, not longer. MLO: 1983 August, 107–111

Burke R: Personality, self-image and situational characteristics of effective helpers in work settings. J Psychol 112: 213–220, 1982

MacStavic RE: Setting priorities in health planning; what does it mean? Inquiry 15: 20–24, 1978

Murray M: Role conflict and intention to leave nursing. J Adv Nurs 8: 29–31, 1983

Chapter 8

Financial management

NANNETTE L. GODDARD

In the educational process of the nursing profession much time is spent familiarizing the student with the clinical functions and departments of the health-care institution. As the on-the-spot clinician who oversees the total needs of the patient, the staff nurse interacts most frequently with other clinically-focused hospital employees who work in laboratory, central supply, pharmacy, radiology, other diagnostic/treatment departments, and the other nursing units. There is little call for the individual nursing care-giver to be involved with the personnel of the business office or financial planning department on a day-to-day basis. Yet the pivotal role of the staff nurse and the contribution of that care-giver are vital to the financial picture of the institution.

This chapter will explain the general trends that relate to health-care costs, hospital financing, and the functioning of the nursing unit. The link between staff nurse practice or behavior and the financial implications of clinical work patterns will be established. Some specific strategies for developing fiscal awareness and responsibility will be introduced, along with ideas that the staff nurse might implement to improve the productivity and job satisfaction of the entire unit staff.

This chapter will enable you to

1. Explain the general trends related to financial issues in nursing.
2. Describe the link between clinical nursing practice and the unit financial function.
3. State strategies for assuming accountability for cost-effective nursing practice.
4. Discuss ideas for improving clinical productivity.

Health Care Costs and Issues

The nurse manager or administrator may function as an intermediary between the payroll department and the staff in matters regarding wages and paychecks. The staff member may have to interface with the admitting and business office if the staff nurse (or a family member) becomes ill, is hospitalized or treated in the institution, and therefore becomes involved as a consumer of health-care services, rather than as a provider, for a brief period of time. Typically, however, it is the nurse manager or assistant head nurse who is asked to be more responsible for the business communications representing the nursing unit's staffing and budgetary needs.

HOSPITALS ARE BUSINESSES, TOO

The trend in many health care centers around the country is to consider the unit nurse-manager position as a department head position, requiring a combination of clinical expertise and business management skills. With the changes in governmental regulation and reimbursement methodology that have occurred recently, hospitals have had to place more emphasis on evaluating each phase of their operation. Each manager has been required to gain new skills relating to financial analysis and productivity monitoring; costs need to be reduced, and practice patterns need to be streamlined. Increasingly, it is becoming essential for each clinical practitioner to comprehend the economic pressures faced by hospitals and to understand that the institution must be run as a business, if its doors are to remain open.

"The hospital as a business" may be a difficult concept for some persons. In the United States, the population at large tends to regard access to health care as an inalienable right, not a privilege or luxury. Society has been oriented to expect that the appropriate amount of the best care will be provided to any individual, regardless of his ability to pay or the extent of his illness and injury. From the critically ill neonate to the multiorgan transplant candidate, past focus has been on the provision of the highest quality inpatient care—frequently to the exclusion of cost considerations.

The laws of the land have provided for most disabled, indigent, and/or elderly sectors of society to be served accordingly through the use of federal, state, or locally supported programs. Hospitals, therefore, have been perceived as benevolent organizations from which society expects excellent care and services.

It is easy to walk through the corridors of the modern hospital and be impressed with the array of equipment, supplies, and professionals who appear to be in abundance. It is easy to think that the hospital has much to give from its seemingly "limitless resources." It is more difficult to try to fathom the costs of such a mammoth operation and the size of the institution's bills—even for such basics as water, electricity, and waste disposal. When consideration is given to the amount of research and technological development involved in medical science and health care, the ultimate cost in time and dollars becomes staggering. Progress made over the last few decades, including the radically new surgical techniques, complex space-age equipment, new treatment modalities, and life-saving drugs, clearly underscores the need for reconciliation between the amounts that hospitals must charge in order to pay for these services and what our society, in turn, is willing to pay.

SOCIAL POLICY AND ECONOMIC DECISIONS

In the last 30 years, the nation's budget allocation for health-care expenditures has grown at an alarming rate and has developed into a major issue in the country's legislative bodies, where tax rates must ultimately be adjusted to fund much of the increase. Laws were passed that mandated or supported programs such as Health Systems agencies, Certificate of Need applications, Professional Standards Review organizations, and the expansion of Health Maintenance organizations—all in what now seems a vain attempt to curtail the rapid growth in spending. According to Carolyne K. Davis (July/August, 1983), past administrator of the Department of Health and Human Services Health Care Financing Administration (HCFA):

... public programs went from paying 25% of the nation's health bill in 1950 to 42% in 1980. When Medicare and Medicaid began paying claims in 1966, the total expenditures for that year were approximately $6 billion. In 1982, the programs spent more than this amount each month, giving HCFA the third largest budget in the federal government. For programs like Medicaid that use tax revenues, rapid growth in spending only exacerbates the federal deficit; for Medicare it means serious long-term problems for the trust funds. . . .

In addition to social programs for the needy, Americans have grown to expect that employee benefits packages would provide health insurance covering the payment of hospital bills. Many citizens lost track of how much their families' health care really cost because someone else was paying the bill. The relatively small deductible that was paid by the individual worker was much easier to swallow when the insurer or employer picked up the bulk of the payment required by the health-care institution. The insured employee did not actually see the money change hands and found it easy to ignore the specifics of how much each x-ray or blood test or room charge actually cost the employee benefit system.

In truth, the costs were skyrocketing so dramatically that the employers began to wonder if they could continue to pay the increased insurance premiums. Again, according to Davis:

As real per capita health care spending increased threefold from 1950 to 1980, direct patient payments decreased from 59% (1950) to 29% (1980). During the same period, private insurance payments for health care increased from 10% to 26% of the national health bill.

American industry was compelled to join forces with various governmental bodies, labor representatives, and community groups to investigate new innovations in health care that would serve to hold the line on costs to employers.

The detailed history and specifics of the Medicaid, Medicare, and other entitlement programs are beyond the scope of this text and have been well documented in other sources. The complete set of statistics related to the cost escalations in the public and private sector are also available in other publications that the reader may choose to explore. (See the reference list at the end of this chapter.)

The main purpose of the preceding paragraphs has been to point out that the increased participation of American industry and the recent upsurge of concern in governmental circles have sparked the overall direction of change in health care economic and social policy. Decisions are being made more in response to business issues related to running our country's health care institutions, and not to clinical concerns. The United States is experiencing the emergence of a revised health care system. Staff nurses must be aware of the new trends developing and of the hospital's necessity to concentrate on financial stability in order to survive.

The New Direction in Reimbursement

The new major trend in health care reimbursement policy was engineered by the Health Care Financing Administration during President Ronald Reagan's first term in office. Payments made to hospitals on behalf of Medicare recipients are no longer based on retrospectively reimbursing the hospital for its "allowable costs" relating to the specific services and number of days of care provided to each individual patient. By categorizing the patients into diagnostic related groups and assigning an expected flat rate dollar payment to each diagnostic related group, the government can dictate how much money the hospital will receive for a specific patient, regardless of how many services or days of care the hospital provides.

In addition, by analyzing the normal case mix of the numbers of patients in each diagnostic related group for which the hospital usually supplies care, the government may provide the institution with lump sum payments prospectively. Therefore, the hospital is supposed to receive a predetermined, fixed amount of money for its Medicare patients and must then attempt to provide care to those clients while not exceeding the budgetary allotment it has already received from the federal government.

Under the old cost-based reimbursement plan, hospitals paid little penalty for being inefficient and were, to some extent, rewarded for the amount of money they spent. This led to increasing the amount of services offered and prolonging the days of care provided. Now hospitals are trying to minimize the amount of services and days of care, in order to spend the least money possible and attempt to live within the dollars Medicare now promises up front. In this way, the government has built in significant incentives for efficiency. Predictions are that the major insurance companies will follow in the footsteps of Medicare and adapt a similar prospective pricing and payment system, thus allowing them to set flat fees for their coverage plans and supply some relief to the employers and individuals who pay for benefits.

The Shift Away From Acute Care

The health care industry has been forced to decrease its concentration on acute care, inpatient services and instead focus on developing alternative and cheaper methods of delivering care through outpatient, home care, ambulatory, rehabilitation, long-term care, and health maintenance services. In many respects, the only patients who remain hospitalized in the system are those who are the sickest and who cannot be treated in or transferred to other facilities. There may be fewer persons hospitalized less frequently for shorter lengths of stay, but their acuity levels and their needs for more intense medical and nursing care may be higher than the average hospital census of the past. Nurses who are employed in these acute-care settings will be continually challenged to gain additional skills in the organization and management of their case-loads of patients, as well as in the clinical performance of the nursing process.

The changes of the last several years have spawned a higher level of emphasis on hospital competition, strategic planning, and marketing of health-care services. Competing hospitals in a given community want to outdo each other by offering the highest quality of care for the lowest possible price. Competent and speedy services delivered in a caring atmosphere will be the marketing strategy that hospitals will attempt to use to attract the consumers and employing industries who represent large groups of consumers. If the acute-care setting sees fewer total inpatients, then the percentage of total market share attained by the individual institution will be a vital statistic tracked in the boardroom and the executive suite.

Rather than forecasting the doom-and-gloom shrinkage of the health-care field and eventual demise of many American hospitals, some prognosticators are suggesting quite the opposite. At the 1985 annual meeting of the American Organization of Nurse Executives, Leland Kaiser announced that the United States is likely to become the state-of-the-art health-care provider to the rest of the globe. His vision of a boom in the country's worldwide standing in health foretells the American hospital system becoming the "transplant, implant, and replant capital of the world" (Kaiser, 1985). There are parallels to be drawn between the former dominance of the American automotive industry and the future dominance of the country's production of health-care and related services. Indeed, many international contracts are already being negotiated between foreign governments and domestic hospitals or corporations.

Regardless of which trend becomes a more viable and prevalent option to all health-care centers, the business acumen, financial savvy, marketing ability, and negotiating skill of the administrator and the hospital staff member will be of even greater importance to the survival of the fittest institutions.

Minimizing Losses Related to Unit Functioning

The basic revenue/cost center of the nursing department is usually the individual nursing unit. The nursing unit normally houses groups of patients who have similar or complementary medical diagnoses, treatment plans, and needs for nursing care. The nursing revenue/cost center is the common denominator of the nursing budget; in most cases, the supplies, expenses, personnel time and dollars, and capital equipment requests are tracked and allocated according to the individual nursing unit.

As the staff attempts to render the best care possible in the amount of time available, the staff nurse is often chided to police cost containment carefully and to utilize the hospital resources wisely. The hospital worker may be asked to conserve water, use supplies sparingly, and turn off electricity when lights or pieces of equipment are not in use. These are all things any household consumer might do to minimize costs at home.

RISK MANAGEMENT AND INSURANCE COSTS

Most staff functioning in the hospital are taught to be concerned about the safety of the environment—for the sake of both staff and clients alike. Safety campaigns and posters caution about potential electrical hazards, water spills on the floor, improper disposal of contaminated needles, and the dangers of cumulative exposure to radiation. Any homeowner or licensed driver learns quickly about safety issues, the costs of accidents or repairs, and the advisability of insurance policies. Similarly, most businesses attempt to cover themselves with the correct types of insurance that will serve to protect them against most claims and losses.

The costs of insurance policies are usually determined based upon a calculation involving the historic average number and types of claims processed and the average expected dollar payments needed to pay the insured or beneficiary for any loss. An automobile driver who has a good driving record is, many times, eligible for discounted insurance rates based upon the demonstrated past history of an uneventful experience on the road and the likelihood of that pattern continuing. However, rates are set in the higher ranges for younger male drivers and for those who own higher-powered, sporty vehicles; the insurance industry has compiled detailed customer and claims surveys to document that these types of drivers have historically represented a higher risk and expense to the insuring company.

Given the high-risk nature and complex environment of the acute health care setting, it is not surprising that insurance rates and premiums represent costly items in the hospital budget. In addition to the normal business coverage for accidents, theft, and natural disasters, hospitals must insure themselves and their employees or representatives against malpractice and negligence claims. Currently, the United States is in the midst of an "insurance crisis" and liability coverage for many businesses and professionals is becoming more difficult to find and fund.

Clinical care-givers who may on occasion exercise poor judgments and be responsible for errors or omissions in care (or in the documentation of care) may inadvertently expose the patient to potential harm and the health care institution to costly lawsuits, damaging press coverage in the news media, and escalating insurance fees. The American society is a litigious one and the level of consumer activism is a potent force in the marketplace.

Physicians and nurses are guided by codes of ethics, standards of practice, hospital policies, published procedures, and recommendations from their professional bodies, not to mention government statutes and rulings from other regulatory agencies. The beginning practitioner in any clinical discipline has the responsibility of understanding the skill level expected by the employer and of knowing when to seek advice and counsel from more experienced colleagues. Validating an opinion or discussing a planned course of action with a supervisor or clinical specialist may turn out to be the best timesaving and moneysaving approach in the long run; every institution has its own unique methodologies of operation and recordkeeping that the novice nurse must learn. The staff nurse working on a nursing unit will function more cost-effectively over an entire career by initially establishing good practice habits, recording facts and assessments accurately, and safeguarding against errors and omissions in care.

ABSENTEEISM

Risk managers, administrative supervisors, and personnel representatives are vitally interested in the safety and security of the organization's employees. Employees who value their jobs and their health are motivated to follow appropriate procedures when operating equipment or working with critically ill and potentially contagious patient populations; it is a matter of protecting oneself from injury or physical complications. Benefit time for illness and workman's compensation coverage are normally available to support full time or regular part-time employees who may be injured while on duty. However, it is best for everyone to stay healthy and avoid having to utilize such sick time and injury coverage, so that staff members remain productive and on the job.

There are many direct and indirect costs that the institution may incur due to the absence of a regular employee. Direct costs include the outlay of funds to pay for the benefit days or workman's compensation and the additional payroll dollars (which may have to be paid at overtime wages) required to replace the individual who is absent. Like any other employer providing health care benefits, the hospital must pay its promised share of health insurance premiums or payments. Most health care centers also fund and staff some sort of employee health office that serves to monitor the health care needs of the organization's employees and certifies when sick or injured employees are restored to health and may therefore return to work.

The level of functioning of the nursing unit suffers when one of its regular staff is absent and that person is replaced with someone who may not know the unit's routine or its patients. The productivity of the staff may also be undermined if other members of the same unit are asked to work excessive amounts of overtime and then become mentally or physically strained by the additional workload. A vicious cycle of fatigue, more illness, and more overtime coverage can become a demoralizing work experience for a unit staff and an expensive drain on the institution. Eventually, the staff's stress may affect its ability to work at peak performance. Errors and omissions in care are more apt to occur under these circumstances.

In some settings, a nurse manager may feel compelled to take a full clinical assignment and thereby cover the temporary vacancy left by the staff nurse who is ill. This may be one possible solution to the immediate need for staff coverage but, if the head nurse performs this replacement function repeatedly, the management work of the unit may not be accomplished in a timely fashion. This, in turn, may cause the unit to function less cost-effectively over a period of time. If supply orders are not processed, the next round of time schedules left uncompleted, and other management planning functions ignored, the unit and its staff can suddenly find themselves lacking such basic supports and in need of immediate crisis management.

PRODUCTIVITY OF THE STAFF AS A UNIT

The individual staff nurse may spend many months and years refining skills and applying a wealth of knowledge in order to gain competence in professional nursing practice. However, the delivery of nursing care is almost exclusively a "group sport" (Zander, 1979) rather than an individual endeavor. The nursing unit staff is comprised of many individuals, with differing backgrounds in education and experience, who are expected to work together to further the institution's goals and meet the needs of its patients. Nurses must rely on each other to communicate, follow through, and to substitute for one another. Even in a primary nursing or primary care setting, clients may require nursing care at a time when the assigned principal care-giver is off duty or at lunch and another nurse may need to act on behalf of that patient. During a cardiac arrest or other emergency situation, a multidisciplinary group is often called upon to function in the rhythm of a well-rehearsed team.

From a financial viewpoint, the staff's ability to work well as a team and to provide competent care for a group of patients, while utilizing an appropriate amount of hospital resources, is commonly measured by determining the staff's productivity. The institution's resources include manpower, supplies, buildings, equipment, and other assets. Jelinek (1979) described some key terms:

> ... *production* is defined as the output of the hospital operation. The output measures, in order to be meaningful, must not only reflect the quantity produced by the hospital but also must reflect the quality of these outputs. *Productivity* is defined as the ratio of output to input. Thus, productivity relates the output to the resources being expended (input) to produce that output.

In the case of an inpatient nursing unit, the inputs are primarily staff hours, supplies, and equipment; the output is patient care, usually expressed in terms of hours or days of care delivered (sometimes adjusted for patient acuity levels as explained later in this chapter).

Quantity of care and quality of care must be considered in any discussion of productivity. The radiology department could set a world's record in speed of performing chest x-rays and complete more chest films per hour than ever before accomplished, but the films would be of no diagnostic assistance if their quality was so poor as to render them useless.

Efficiency and effectiveness are related, but by no means interchangeable, concepts. The classic hospital industrial engineering text by Smalley and Freeman (1966) explains the difference as follows: "Effectiveness is the degree of achievement of objectives, while efficiency [like productivity] is the relation between achievement of objectives and the consumption of resources." Edwardson (1985) explained effectiveness in health care by referencing the work of the Applied Management Sciences, Inc., Department of Health and Human Services publication on productivity and health:

> Effectiveness refers to the safety, appropriateness, and excellence of care. An acceptable output specifies the minimum level of patient outcome, patient satisfaction, and change in health status approved by decision makers. . . .

Therefore, in establishing its own productivity goals according to its projected workload and standards of care, an organization provides a criterion for measuring the actual versus the expected performance of the staff involved in the "production" of each department. The nursing unit staff that meets the institution's productivity goals will be using the expected level of resources to deliver the projected workload (days of care) within the budgeted dollars of that fiscal year. The unit staff that uses more than the recommended amount of supplies or more than the allocated level of staff, to deliver the projected amount of care, may be causing the institution to spend more resources/dollars than planned, thereby diminishing the productivity of the department. If the staff is highly efficient, delivers care effectively, and utilizes fewer resources than expected per day of care delivered, the department will exceed its productivity and quality objectives and may present a more positive financial picture.

Edwardson (1985) points out that a broader interpretation of productivity might include other output indicators—"such diverse intangibles as employee morale, job satisfaction, and client satisfaction." Long-term survival of health care organizations may—like any other competitive business—depend on achieving a certain level of productivity relative to their competitors. Skillful implementation of an objective productivity monitoring system is a key step in establishing and maintaining a high grade of productivity and other significant operational benefits. According to Kaye and Utenner (1985):

> All levels of management should be able to evaluate the results of their current policies and operational decisions in order to plan for future adjustments. The system should be able to prove its worth by: improving teamwork and morale; reducing absenteeism, turnover and tardiness; increasing real productivity and the quality of product produced; improving service to the customer; and improving profit margin.

The role of nursing and the expected accomplishments of the nursing staff are negotiated at the uppermost administrative level in the organization. Professional bodies and regulatory agencies may publish recommended standards of practice for use in health-care settings, but subtle nuances of interpretation, variations in leadership styles, and philosophical differences may cause one institution to function quite unlike another in the same community.

Part of the task of setting realistic productivity goals for the nursing unit staff may revolve around the geographic design of the work setting itself. Some nursing units are designed for better visibility of patients, efficient work flow, and less congested traffic patterns. Long corridors can mean more nursing staff footsteps to reach patients, supplies, charts, telephones, medications, computer support, and other personnel. The placement of patient rooms or care areas in relation to supply closets, utility rooms, medication stores, and even laundry shoots is a science and architectural art in itself.

Having the ancillary or support staff deliver the most frequently used items to the patient bedside may increase the productivity of the nursing staff by eliminating many of its unnecessary footsteps. Depending on the labor force employed by the organization and the priority with which patient needs are addressed, the amount and function of ancillary personnel may vary considerably.

The staff nurse is wise to evaluate the institution's performance expectations of the individual nurse and of the entire unit's nursing staff before joining an organization, in order to determine whether practice according to one's own philosophy and nursing standards is feasible.

Relating to Other Departments

Swenson, Wolfe, and Schroeder (1984) cited two studies that highlight the importance of effectively employing support services as a method of increasing the productivity of nursing personnel:

> A well-organized materials management department can cut an average of 1.5 nursing hours per patient day. That means, for a hospital with a daily census of 150 patients, a savings of 39.5 full-time equivalent personnel. With support service instead of nursing personnel performing logistics and transportation activities, potential salary savings can run $118,500 annually if the salary difference between the two personnel groups averages only $3000. . . .
>
> In a suburban hospital with an average daily census of 200 patients, 46 nursing service hours per day were devoted to transport: 26 in "unnecessary" patient transport and 20 in the transport of supplies, equipment and papers—clearly not nursing tasks, although necessary in providing patient care. About three-fourths of the trips, none requiring nursing participation, had been made by registered nurses, including head nurses and supervisors.

Support services personnel, ancillary staff, and other professionals are not on the payroll for the convenience or whim of the individual nurse staff member; neither are nurses on the payroll in order to "pick up the slack" or pitch in and substitute for other workers. Role definitions and departmental functions must be established according to licensure laws and standards of practice, as well as within the financial resources of the institution and the labor force available within a community.

If the general goals of all related departments within the health care setting are focused on the provision of care and services to the consumers who are patients within the system, the stage is set for cooperative relationships between the personnel of those departments, interacting on a daily basis. Employee understanding of the basic institutional mission and the overall importance of patient satisfaction may help each staff group to view its daily tasks more in terms related to "the needs of the patient or family" rather than "the needs of my department."

Beyond the global raison d'etre, the employee needs to understand the fit of each job within the structure of a department and the accepted intra- and interdepartmental communications required to accomplish that job. O'Sullivan (1985) described the alternatives:

> To perceive their roles accurately, to work together with interest and enthusiasm, team members must know what is expected of them, must feel free to clarify vague messages, to validate what they know, and must understand changes before they take place.... Miscommunication can engender indifference and smoldering hostilities which undermine quality patient care.

The solutions to care delivery problems involving other staff members (whether across departments or across tours of duty) are discovered and negotiated more easily when the patient is the center of everyone's attention and problem-solving abilities. Delays in care are costly to the institution and inconvenient, if not detrimental, to patients. If vital information in a written request for diagnostic testing has been omitted by a staff nurse, an employee in another department may be forced to postpone a scheduled test until the appropriate information is supplied. If the patient has not been prepared for a radiologic procedure according to the standard or prescribed protocol, a full 24 hours or more may be required before another appropriate opportunity for testing may be arranged.

Similarly, the nurse may be hampered in the performance of patient care responsibilities if medications are not ordered correctly, dispensed accurately, and delivered to the nursing unit on time. When appropriate non-nursing staff do not respond to patients' requests or needs within a reasonable amount of time, it is primarily the nursing staff that must deal with the patients' questions, anger, or resultant complications in physical status.

There will always be a potential for human error in a system such as health care that functions with so much human involvement. While human error and personality cannot be excluded from the workings of the organization, it can be recognized that the majority of care-delivery problems stem from flaws in the design of the specific delivery systems and in the work flow/communications across the departments within a system. Quality assurance programs may identify some issues related to patient care; it may take additional support from management engineers, internal auditors, and task forces of staff members themselves to attack and solve the nagging and repetitive problems that disrupt the smooth operations and communications within and across departments.

PRODUCTIVITY OF THE INDIVIDUAL NURSE

Even when the nursing unit staff's collective productivity appears to be meeting the department's goals, attention to the practice of the individual within that work group is vital. Patient care provided by the individual staff nurse is a relatively intangible product. The professional component of the job greatly complicates the measurement of the individual's productivity by standard industrial engineering techniques, such as time and motion study or work sampling. How does one account for the thinking involved in patient care? How does one attempt to measure the amount of assessment or re-evaluation performed at every contact with the patient?

Benner (1982) documented that the proficient and expert levels of practice are more difficult to explain and describe:

> The expert nurse, with her/his enormous background of experience, has an intuitive grasp of the situation and zeros in on the accurate region of the problem without wasteful consideration of a large range of unfruitful possible problem situations.
>
> It is very frustrating to try to capture verbal descriptions of expert performance because the expert operates from a deep understanding of the situation, much like the chess master who, when asked why he made a particularly masterful move, will say, "Because it felt right. It looked good."

The consideration of individual productivity must have its foundations in both the degree to which the individual approaches expert practice and the philosophy by which one practices the profession. If productivity is the ratio of output per unit of input, then one must have a sense of one's output—not only in relation to outcomes, but also in regard to appropriateness of function, actual versus potential achievement, feedback from peers, and one's own sense of individual accountability.

A more wide-ranging look at the output of the individual staff nurse may incorporate the nurse's contributions (or lack thereof) to the work environment and work systems. Is there active support of fellow nurses and other personnel in the workplace? Is the individual advancing ideas to improve the systems, ethics, and methodologies of care? Is the staff nurse participating politically within the institution in such a way as to promote its philosophy and the highest standards of care? Is there a willingness to work fairly and forthrightly within the system to help bring about changes that may be beneficial to everyone involved?

Streamlined charting systems, flow sheet documentation tools, generic care plans, computer support, group teaching/counseling, and packaged patient information programs are just some of the latest time-saving techniques being introduced around the country. These are all attempts to lead the individual staff nurse toward more efficient ways of meeting patient and family care needs (Sovie, 1985). The staff nurse must not only be willing to experiment with these and other changes in the practice setting, but must also be willing to learn quickly and well those lessons that foster personal growth and professional expertise.

SUPPLY COSTS AND
MATERIALS MANAGEMENT

The health-care institution stocks myriad supply items, medications, and pieces of equipment. Its storerooms house the bulk of these items, with mini-storage areas set up in appropriate work stations or major departments throughout the organization. Some supplies must be packaged together to provide the convenience of correct assembly for use in a particular procedure. Many supplies must be sterilized for use in areas such as the delivery room, operating room, postanesthesia recovery, emergency department, intensive care units, and other specialty areas (Peterson, 1985).

The availability and integrity of supply items is crucial to the delivery of patient care. The nurse must feel confident that medications have not reached their expiration dates, that equipment is in good working order, and that supplies have not been damaged or contaminated in storage.

In a 1985 survey of 450 hospital administrators, 82% of the respondents believed that better management of supply purchasing could help control costs (Jensen, 1985). A good materials management system may save money through standardization of products, purchasing products via group consortium arrangements, centralizing purchasing activities, and controlling inventories.

The staff nurse is involved in the handling of supplies and medications on a daily basis. As professionals with the most consistent and constant patient contact and as care-givers responsible for carrying out the bulk of the treatment plan, nurses serve as the final link between the patient and most supply items. The nurse who exercises appropriate judgment in assessing and intervening with patients will use supplies and administer medications in a cost-effective manner.

Determining what supplies to purchase and stock in the institution is an important step in the involvement of staff nurses. Many health-care settings have established ongoing, multidisciplinary committees to review the institution's supply needs. One such task force was formed at Providence Hospital, located in a suburb of Detroit:

> This Committee evaluates each product for its safety, quality and price. Effectiveness, storability [sic], availability, delivery time, educational support, service and repair, other hospital user experience, competitive product comparison, and independent company studies also influence the final decision. (Eusebio et al, 1985)

Once the purchasing decisions are made and the selected items arrive at the institution, the procedures for stocking and delivering the routine or requested items to patient-care areas are set in motion. Determining realistic numbers of items to be stored at certain standard or par levels on the nursing unit may be accomplished by surveying periodically what supplies are actually utilized and at what frequency. Backup procedures for attaining additional items or special requests must be designed to meet the emergency situation or the unusual fluctuations in workload. Stockpiling, overstocking, or hoarding supplies or medications may result in items becoming misplaced, damaged, or out-of-date. The costs of spoilage, obsolescence, and maintaining too much inventory must be minimized. Storing too many items in unsecured areas, where the general public may have access to them, can contribute to losses due to theft. Stealing by employees and others is estimated to cost the industry $3,000 per hospital bed per year (Wilkinson, 1986).

Recording the items used by individual patients during their hospital stays or visits is an extension of the exacting system of accounting that documents the costs and/or charges according to the care provided each patient. In addition, good documentation on the patient record helps to substantiate the appropriateness of care administered (based on the individual needs of the patient) and offers rationales regarding why certain supplies and medications were necessary. Inadequate nursing charting or recordkeeping can lead to lost charges, which will not appear on the patient's bill, or charges that will be disallowed by insurance companies or other third-party payers who perform audits of patients' hospital bills. Beyond the direct cost of the item that will not be reimbursed to the hospital, there are other indirect charges for handling, storing, dispensing, and packaging supplies and medications for which the institution will not be paid.

The Nursing Care Delivery System and the Required Human Resources

DECISIONS REGARDING MODALITY OF CARE

The choice of which nursing care delivery system (that is, functional care, team nursing, total patient care, or primary nursing) may be best for a particular health-care setting is based on many factors. The administrative staff may evaluate the success of previously utilized practice patterns and systems currently in use and in vogue in other community institutions. The executives may be forced to consider the available labor pool in the community and the institution's track record in recruitment and retention of qualified staff. Leadership styles and political factors may cause the institution's management team to choose a system that is not their ideal, but that is the only feasible alternative at the time.

Evaluation of various delivery systems is beyond the scope of this chapter and has been addressed in the nursing literature since Nightingale's time. Total patient care and primary nursing have received more attention recently as economic issues have spawned some concentration on the increased productivity, versatility, and accountability that can be expected from the professional and licenced staff. Spitzer describes the administrative direction established at Cedars-Sinai Medical Center in Los Angeles:

> As technology advances, length of stay decreases and patient acuity rises, the licensed staff is legally, morally, ethically and educationally better prepared to provide total patient care and increase productivity than an unlicensed employee....
>
> A nurse who does not have unlicensed staff to supervise almost automatically becomes 25% more productive.... Therefore, if a hospital has all licensed staff members, fewer people will be needed. Also, the total cost for this staff will be lower....
>
> You'll be paying less people more money, but the benefits will cost significantly less (Franz, 1984).

PLANNING FOR APPROPRIATE STAFFING

A host of other management decisions involved in staffing the nursing department must be addressed following the basic choice of the modality of care. Nurse:patient ratios, target nursing hours of care per patient day, or recommendations from a nursing-patient classification system are the three most popular guidelines that managers use to determine the amount of total staff to supply for a given group of patients. Other considerations focus on the skill mix of the staff—some combination of unlicensed, licensed, or professional personnel—and the distribution of the total staff over several tours of duty to provide care around the clock or whenever the department is open to clients.

The simplest option for suggesting the total amount of staff may be the nurse:patient ratio. The types of patients commonly housed on a given nursing unit are reviewed to discover their usual nursing-care needs and the estimated workload they place on the nursing personnel. A reasonable nurse:patient ratio or staff:patient ratio that will support the care delivery system chosen is determined for each tour of duty and that will be the basis for daily assignment patterns on the unit.

Another method of planning for the total amount of staff establishes a standard of the average amount of nursing care a patient will receive in a 24-hour period. This is expressed in a numerical value of nursing care Hours Per Patient Day (HPPD). The expression of a daily HPPD figure is calculated using the following formula:

$$HPPD = \frac{\text{Total Number of Shifts Worked/Day} \times \text{Hours of Care/Shift}}{\text{Average Number of Patients/Day (Census)}}$$

For example, if everyone worked an 8-hour tour of duty, and the staff supplied to a given unit in a 24-hour period broke down to 6 staff on day shift, 4 staff on evening shift, and 3 staff on night shift, then the total of 13 staff would have worked a total of 104 hours. If, during that same 24-hour period, the staff cared for 24 patients, then the 104 hours of care supplied to a total of 24 patients would have resulted in an average amount of care per patient of 4.33 HPPD. Fitting the numbers into the formula results in the following solution:

$$HPPD = \frac{13 \text{ Shifts Worked/Day} \times 8 \text{ Hours of Care/Shift Worked}}{24 \text{ Patients/Day}}$$

$$HPPD = \frac{13 \times 8 \text{ Hours of Care/Day}}{24 \text{ Patients/Day}}$$

$$HPPD = \frac{104 \text{ Hours of Care}}{24 \text{ Patients}}$$

$$HPPD = 4.33 \text{ Average Hours of Care per Patient}$$

Although this formula is considered to be a classic in the industry, there are some definite problems encountered when managers attempt to compare their HPPD statistics with those of other units or hospitals. There may be subtle differences in identification of the formula's elements.

First, just who is counted in the number of total staff? Some institutions include the head nurse, unit secretaries, and everyone assigned to the unit; other departments may count only those staff members who are involved in the direct, hands-on care of the patients.

Second, can we expect any staff member to be fully productive during the entire tour of duty for which the nurse or aide is being paid? Most hospitals acknowledge that the employee needs a coffee break in addition to a meal break, and many institutions' personnel policies identify two 15-minute breaks per tour of duty as the normal expectation. That would reduce the expected work time from 8 full hours to 7.5 hours. Beyond the scheduled break times, industrial and management engineers often acknowledge an additional "personal fatigue and delay" factor that should be considered in conjunction with mentally, emotionally, and/or physically taxing work.

The third component of the standard formula—"average census"—can also be questioned. Does the institution use a midnight, afternoon, or morning census figure? What about those patients who may be transferred in or out of the unit during the normal course of the day? With the fluctuations in occupancy rates experienced in many settings and the number of transfers logged in some nursing units, it is difficult to understand how the simple census or patient day figure can be used as a measure of nursing workload. Finally, the number of beds occupied does not recognize any variations in care needs of those patients.

Some of the most extensive research done in an attempt to compare nursing-hour figures across hospitals was performed by the National Association of Children's Hospitals and Related Institutions (NACHRI). The NACHRI Nurse-Staffing Data Program collected detailed information for a hospital profile and an individual patient care unit profile, in order to view data consistently and make more appropriate comparisons between units. Even with this most sophisticated approach, the variations in nursing hours per patient-day standards between like units caring for like patients was astounding:

> The total hospital median or worked nursing hours per patient day was 11.8 hours. Individual hospital values ranged from 8.2 to 14 hours. The median of worked hours per patient day for the medical-surgical units was 9.3 with the intensive care units recording a median value of 22.6 hours. The ranges in worked hours per patient day for the medical-surgical units and intensive care units were 5.9 to 14.7 hours and 16.2 to 30 hours, respectively (Gorman and Borovies, 1985).

Patient classification systems, the third possible method for assisting administrators in assigning the total number of staff, were born in an attempt to project the workload for nursing from some assessment of the acuity level (or level of illness) of the patients in question. In the course of their clinical experience, nurses comprehend very quickly that the number of patients housed on a given unit may not be as significant as the types of patients counted in that department's census. As clinicians, nurses appreciate that medical and nursing diagnoses are only the *basic* factors that may provide some inkling of the amount of nursing care needed by an individual patient. The patient's age, anxiety level, dependency needs, intellectual capacities, and cultural background will have impact on the individualized plan of care. Underlying diseases, past health history, previous hospital experiences, amount of family support, language barriers, psychological trauma, emotional stability, and/or relationships with other health care team members will also influence the priority level of the nurse's involvement with that client.

Giovannetti (1979) supplied the pertinent definitions related to this complex topic:

In nursing, the term *patient classification* means the categorization of patients according to some assessment of their nursing care requirements over a specified period of time. The most common purpose has been for determination and assignment of nursing care personnel. . . . To encompass both the definition and the purpose, the term *patient classification system* is commonly used. It refers to the identification and classification of patients into care groups or categories, and to the quantification of these categories as a measure of the nursing effort required.

There are a multitude of patient classification schemes in use today, employing varying levels of sophistication, background research, reliability and validity studies, and philosophical approaches. Moreover, the actual use of classification systems varies from a token use during accreditation visits to daily use for the purposes of variable staffing decisions and, in a few settings, variable patient billing.

In an institution where the patient classification system(s) is taken seriously and its data applied to management decision making, the accuracy and reliability of the periodic classification results may be of paramount importance. The data may serve as a guideline for annual staffing budgets, shift-to-shift assignment of staff across nursing units, and intradepartmental assignments of individual staff nurses to their specific caseloads of patients. In these settings, one would not expect to see staff nurses on the same unit and the same tour of duty necessarily assigned to equal numbers of patients; their caseloads of differing numbers of patients might vary according to the acuity information and other management parameters, such as the expertise of the individual staff member or other duties assigned.

Giovannetti (1979) reminds the industry that "patient classification systems are based on a unidimensional [sic] and partial assessment of patient requirements for care." It would be impossible to document every iota of care required by every individual patient; an attempt to do so would result in tools far too cumbersome for the staff to use in periodic assessment. Further, most patient classification schemes focus on the quantification of care supplied through the existing practice of nursing on a given unit, not necessarily the *ideal* practice. To account for this potentially major difference, separate quality monitoring systems or performance evaluation mechanisms would have to be in place in order to look at the quality of the outcomes of care.

The final important issue likely to affect plans for appropriate staff, and the budgetary impact of such plans, is the specific collection of personnel policies and scheduling practices unique to each setting. The distribution of staff around the 24-hour time frame may be influenced by the amount of shift differential, if at all, that is promised and paid to employees. Weekend and holiday scheduling patterns, some of which may involve bonus pay, must be taken into account. Policies related to sick, vacation, and holiday time, and which employees are eligible for how much, may influence the number of part-time workers the organization will attempt to hire. The availability (or lack of availability) of supplemental staff, who might fill in temporarily during periods of high census and acuity, might influence the administration to employ fewer (or more) full-time staff assigned to a given unit.

Staffing and scheduling decisions represent a major effort in the budgeting process of the organization. Executive level financial negotiations often center around the number of part-time, full-time, permanent, temporary, per diem, or float staff that will be approved for the next fiscal year for each department. The staff nurse needs to understand as much as possible the specific institutional process of these decisions and contribute to the accurate collection of pertinent data that may influence key decision- and policy-makers.

HIDDEN HUMAN RESOURCES COSTS

Finally, there are other related personnel costs incurred by the institution that are not as obvious as the salaries and benefits received by the employees. Hoffman (1985) identified the top four as:

1. Advertising/recruiting costs
2. Hiring costs
3. Orientation/training costs
4. Turnover costs

Advertising and recruiting costs might include everything from the salaries of recruiters and the cost of classified advertisements in professional journals to attendance at school career days and special externship programs that hire senior nursing students. Hiring involves interviewing time, the processing of applications, many types of correspondence, and the payment of moving expenses for some workers. Hoffman's list of several major costs related to orientation and training includes the salaries of the educational staff, costs of supplies, the overhead on the building space used in education, and the preceptor time of the experienced staff who are often used to orient new employees. When an employee leaves the organization, personnel policies may dictate that the individual be compensated for some amount of accrued benefit time that had not been taken. If the vacated position is not filled in a timely manner, the institution may be forced to pay hundreds of dollars in replacement staff costs for temporary workers or overtime paid to regular staff who work extra duty.

The New Nurse's Role in Health Care Finance

UNDERSTANDING THE NEW ORIENTATION OF HEALTH CARE

For a variety of complex economic reasons, the hospital industry is entering a maturing stage characterized by "substantial overcapacity; greatly restricted access to new capital; [and] an increasingly competitive atmosphere, in which price is rapidly becoming the dominant factor for purchasers" (Go, 1986). Nurses will need to understand the meaning and accept the usage of the terms "profit" and "productivity" as part of their everyday language. The clinical professionals must keep an open mind to the business side and the new trends of health care. It is important to be an educated consumer as well as an educated provider of health services.

When the industry's new directions are recognized, it is easier to accept the expanded role now thrust upon the staff nurse. Ganong and Ganong (1980) have viewed the changing times in the following manner:

> Professional nurses, by virtue of being licensed to practice, have always been expected to assume responsibility for supervising the work of others in lower job categories. From this point of view nurses always have had the responsibility of managerial leadership and its attendant accountability. But in today's work world, professional nurses have both expanded opportunities and more clearly defined responsibilities to apply management principles and practices....
>
> This dual role of nurse and manager applies at every job level in nursing. Whether as staff nurse, head nurse, or administrator, the professional nurse necessarily is both nurse and manager with the emphasis shifting according to need.

One prominent nurse executive, who realizes that nurses and physicians may control up to 80% of the resources used in patient care, has rallied her nursing staff to the concepts of case management and more collaborative practice patterns with physicians (Twyon, 1985). The staff nurse, as a case manager in this system, "is accountable for meeting outcomes within 1.) an appropriate length of stay, 2.) the effective use of resources and 3.) established standards." (Zander, 1985)

UNDERSTANDING THE MARKETING ASPECTS OF THE NURSE'S JOB

It may be necessary to remind some nurses that the patient's perceptions of the quality of care is critically important to the marketing of the institution's services—even if those perceptions are not at all consistent with an agonizingly developed nursing definition of quality. True, the latter may have a greater effect on patient outcomes but, in this competitive environment, the former may have a greater effect on *hospital outcomes* (or survival).

Patients expect competence from health-care professionals and through "guest relations" programs and other promotions, hospitals are becoming more attentive to the impressions that employees may leave with the patient. Professional Research Consultants, Inc., of Omaha, in conjunction with *Hospitals* magazine, compared the results of 1984 and 1985 surveys on patient satisfaction with inpatient hospital stays. In 1985, 81% of those who responded were very satisfied with their nursing care, as compared to 73.4% in 1984. The number of patients who were very satisfied with the "attitudes" of non-nursing personnel rose only slightly from 77.7% in 1984 to 79.8% in 1985 (Powills, 1986).

Nurses can be in the best vantage point to help discover exactly what patients want from their health-care providers and to help generate ideas for new and appropriate services that will increase the attractiveness of the institution in the local community. If, as individuals or in groups, physicians still hold the key to large numbers of admissions, the nursing staff may again play a pivotal role in advising administration on the best strategies with which to approach those physicians. The kind of care supplied by the nursing staff itself, or the creative ideas of the clinical care-givers that come to fruition, may develop into the strongest draw for physicians and consumers alike.

UNDERSTANDING CHANGES BROUGHT ABOUT BY ECONOMIC REALITIES

The health-care industry is experiencing a form of "reality shock" all its own—and on a national scale. The political climate may change somewhat under each new presidential administration, but health-care philosophy and economics will undoubtedly continue to evolve as society faces difficult funding and access decisions. In addressing the issue of paying for health care, other countries have opted for socialized medical systems and other variations on that theme. The United States economy, however, is built upon a capitalistic belief structure and the principles of an open market. Some aspects of this free market system are now being used to regulate the health care industry.

An organization's "accountability to society" is measured in part by its profit and by its ability to deliver goods or services of a quality and at a cost that society will embrace. How "embraceable" will the health-care industry become and how much change will those involved have to endure (or enjoy)? The understated response is that the changes are happening fast and that the system is evolving slowly.

Del Bueno (1985) described the impact of "change in the social or environmental contexts" and two examples of the fall-out that may hit nurses close to home:

> The concept of the clinical specialist was introduced when hospital expenditures were not restricted by reimbursement systems and when quality patient care was the guiding principle, at least on paper. Job enrichment was introduced when qualified people were hard to find or replace and employee satisfaction was high on organizational priority lists. Both of these conditions have changed. Nurses are fortunate to find jobs in many areas, and hospitals are forced to cut expense and payroll budgets. The trend now seems to be away from clinical specialists, at least as independent practitioners, and productivity demands have replaced employee satisfaction needs.

Summary

Nursing practice patterns and behaviors do indeed impact the financial picture of the health-care agency. It would be wise for the staff nurse to keep abreast of the changes taking place in the political arena, the marketplace, and the work setting, so that there can be some attempt to comprehend the pressures coming to bear on the entire system and the role of the nurse. Change is inevitable and economic realities will drive the change. With the proper understanding and skills, we in nursing can participate in and contribute much to this evolutionary process.

Bibliography

Benner P: From novice to expert. Am J Nurs 3:402–407, 1982

Berman HJ, Weeks LE: The Financial Management of Hospitals. Ann Arbor, University of Michigan Health Administration Press, 1982

Boyer NN: Nursing sense saves dollars. Nurs Manage 15:15–17, 1984

Churchill NC: Budget choice: Planning vs. control. Harvard Bus Rev 62: July/ August 1984

Cleverly WO: Handbook of Health Care Accounting and Finance. Rockville, MD, Aspen Systems, 1982

Covaleski MA, Dirsmith MW: Budgeting in the nursing services area: Management control, political and witchcraft uses. Health Care Manage Rev 6 (Summer 1981, 17–24)

Covaleski MA, Dirsmith MW: Building tents for nursing services through budgeting negotiation skills. Nurs Adm Qu 8:1–11, 1984

Curtin L, Zurlage C: DRGs: The Reorganization of Health, p 17–24. Chicago, S-N Publications, 1984.

Davis CK: The federal role in changing health care financing. part II: Prospective payment and its impact on nursing. Nurs Econ 1, September/October 1983

Davis CK: The federal role in changing health care financing. Part I: National programs and health financing problems. Nurs Econ 1:10–17, July/August 1983

Del Bueno DJ, Bridges PB: Providing incentives while reducing costs: An employee suggestion plan. Nurs Econ 3:221–215, July/August 1985

Del Bueno DJ: Bandwagons, parades, and panaceas. Nurs Outlook 33:98–104, 136–138, 146, May/June 1985

Edwardson SR. Measuring nursing productivity. Nurs Econ 3:9–14, January/February 1985

Ethridge P: The case for billing by patient acuity. Nurs Manage 16:38–41, August 1985

Eusebio E, Louisignau K, Horger-Scheuber M et al: Product selection in the hospital: Controlling cost. Nurs Manage 16: 44–46, March 1985

Finkler SA: Budgeting Concepts for Nurse Managers, Orlando, Grune and Stratton, 1984

Franz J: Challenge for nursing: Hiking productivity without lowering quality of care. Mod Healthcare 14:60–68, September 1984

Ganong JM, Ganong WL: Nursing Management, 2nd ed. Rockville, MD, Aspen Systems, 1980

Giovannetti P: DRGs and nursing workload measures, p 88–91. Comput Nurs 3:88–91, March/April 1985

Giovannetti P, Mayer GG: Building confidence in patient classification systems. Nurs Manage 15:31–34, August 1984

Giovannetti P: Understanding patient classification systems. J Nurs Adm 9:4–9, February 1979

Go RA: How to court success in a maturing industry. *Hospitals* 60:112, January 5, 1986

Goddard NL: The Workbook on Financial Management, Staffing, and Budgeting for Nursing. Houston, Goddard Management Resources, 1985

Gorman M, Borovies DL: Comparative nursing hours in tertiary pediatric facilities. Nurs Econ 3:146–151, May/June 1985

Herzlinger RE: Fiscal management in health organizations. Health Care Manage Rev 2:37–42, 1977

Hicks LL, Boles KE: Why health economics? Nurs Econ 2:175–180, May/June 1984

Hoffman, F: Cost per RN hired. J Nurs Adm 15:27–29, February 1985

Hoffman F: Financial Management for Nurse Managers. East Norwalk, CT, Appleton-Century-Crofts, 1984

Jackson BS, Resnick J: Comparing classification systems. Nurs Manage 13:13–19, November 1982

Jarrard JK: Engineered standards in hospital nursing. Nurs Manage 14:29–32, April 1983

Jelinek RC: The relationship between productivity and cost containment. In Jaeger BJ (ed): Evaluating Hospital Productivity. Durham, NC, Department of Health Administration, Duke University, 1979

Jensen J: Hospitals "manage" purchasing in efforts to control supply costs. Mod Healthcare 15:72–73, July 19, 1985

Kaye GH:, Utenner J: Productivity: Managing for the long term. Nurs Econ 16:12–13, 15, September 1985

Lauver EB: Where will the money go? Economic forecasting and nursing's future. Nurs Health Care 6:133–135, March 1985

Malloy JM, Skinner DB: Medicare on the critical list. Harvard Bus Rev 62:122–135, November/December 1984

Norkett B: The role of nursing in marketing health care. Nurs Adm Q 10:85–89, 1985

Nursing expertise enhances revenue base. Hospitals 58:59, December 1, 1984

O'Sullivan PS: Detecting communication problems. Nurs Manage 16:27–30, November 1985

Okorafor H: Hospital characteristics attractive to physicians and the consumers: Implications for public general hospitals. Hospital Health Services Adm 28:50–65, March/April 1983

Peterson C: Reducing stock piles improves cost effectiveness. Nurs Manage 16:12, February 1985

Powills S: Consumer gripes about hospital services drop. Hospitals 60:60–61, April 5, 1986

Quinn, CC: Health care regulation and market forces. Nurs Econ 2:204–209, May/June 1984

Riley W, Schaefers V: Nursing operations as a profit center. Nurs Manage 15:43–46, April 1984

Riley W, Schaefers V: Costing nursing services. Nurs Manage 14:40–43, December 1983

Smalley HE, Freeman JR: Hospital Industrial Engineering. New York, Reinhold Publishing, 1966

Sovie MD, Tarcinale MA, Vanputee AW, Stunden AE: Amalgam of nursing acuity, DRGs and costs. Nurs Manage 16:22, March 1983

Sovie MD: Managing nursing resources in a constrained economic environment. Nurs Econ 3:85–94, March/April 1985

Suver JD, Neumann BR: Management Accounting for Health Care Organizations. Oak Brook, IL, Hospital Financial Management, 1985

Swenson B, Wolfe HB, Schroeder R: Effectively employing support services the key for increasing nursing personnel productivity. Mod Healthcare 14:101–104, December 1984

Twyon S: Fiscal environment—1985. Network Q Newsletter, Massachusetts Organization for Nurse Executives, August 1985

Wilkinson R: Murders get the press, but theft is the problem. Hospitals 60:97–98, April 5, 1986

Zander K: Defining nursing . . . roots and wings. Definition published by The Center for Nursing Case Management of the New England Medical Center Hospitals, Fall/Winter, 1985

Zander K: Achieving the Goals of Primary Nursing Care. Presented at Baptist Hospital of Miami, Florida, May 11, 1979

Chapter 9

Risk management and quality assurance

MARILYN B. CHASSIE

In many respects, effective quality assurance and risk management efforts parallel the dimensions of effective financial management introduced in Chapter 8. Both quality assurance and risk management represent additional aspects of the management control function. In the management process, control refers to actions taken to ensure that actual outcomes are consistent with those planned and anticipated (Gibson, Ivancevich, and Donnelly, 1979; Schmude, 1985). The institution's quality assurance and risk management programs are mechanisms by which the organization ensures that standards for care and departmental operation are established, reviewed, and are consistent with currently accepted practice; that standards are consistently achieved or under scrutiny, and that threats or potential threats to organizational survival are prevented, reduced, or contained. The term *quality assurance* refers to a system for monitoring outcomes of professional interventions and departmental activities compared with established standards to evaluate and document appropriateness and effectiveness of practices. Historically, quality assurance efforts reflected a desire of professionals to improve practices through peer review directed at protecting the interests of service recipients (Carroll, 1984). The term *risk management* refers to a system for anticipating and maintaining skills, technology, communication, and resources necessary to avert mishaps and to address incidents and accidents that occur. Goals of a risk management program are generally related to protecting the financial position of the institution (Devet, 1985; Hopkins, 1985, LaCava, 1985).

Underlying programs of quality assurance and risk management is the

principle of professional and organizational responsibility and accountability for the safety, quality, and appropriateness of all services delivered. In protecting the interests of the patient, the interest of the professional care-giver and the assets of the institution are protected as well.
If a risk management program is to be effective, quality of care issues
and peer review processes must be considered. Trending data analyzed
for risk management purposes targets areas for intensive quality assurance evaluation (Oulton, 1984). Quality assurance and risk management
functions are not mutually exclusive, but overlap in such a way that each
is affected by and affects the direction and emphasis of the other (Figure
9-1).

In bringing into focus the professional nurse's responsibility for quality assurance and risk management, a helpful analogy can be drawn
between responsibility to the patient and responsibility to the institution. A primary professional responsibility to the patient is support for
recovery and optimal health through intervention to reduce environmental and physiologic threats to well-being and survival. In acting as
the patient's advocate, the clinician monitors key indices of health status
and scans for potential dangers. Continuous evaluation is carried out to
assure that the regimen of care is sufficient to effect the desired patient
outcome or to initiate modification of the prescribed regimen at the ear-
liest sign that it is ineffective. Nursing diagnoses of specific problems or

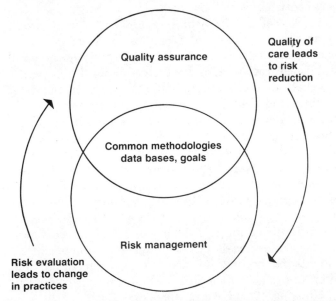

Figure 9-1   Relationship between quality assurance and risk management.

responses frame the strategy for intervention and follow-up. The professional nurse assesses the patient's environment to ensure that all resources needed for patient support are present and functioning properly and to eliminate hazards that might interfere with optimal health. The patient's personal resources are identified; the nurse clinician seeks to support the patient's individual strengths and to intervene to protect the patient's social and physiological resources.

In essence, quality assurance and risk management activities are undertaken to result in similar outcomes for the institution at the unit, departmental, or organizational level. That is, a basic institutional responsibility is to ensure that subunits within the nursing service domain are operating appropriately and are protected from environmental and internal threats to optimal functioning. Quality assurance and risk management programs provide the framework and define the processes by which nursing service scans the external environment for changes in definition of safe practice and identifies potential consequences of noncompliance with legal, professional, and external regulatory standards. Through quality assurance and risk management programs, mechanisms are established for monitoring key indices in the internal environment to identify dangerous situations or practices that may result in harm to the patient, employees, visitors, or property, and hence, suboptimal, ineffective institutional operation. Systematic assessment of policies, procedures, and practices in the light of established professional and institutional standards affirms that conditions within the institution are appropriate to address patient requirements in a manner consistent with accepted patterns of care. Monitoring may give rise to problem definition and subsequent modification of standards or practices based on evaluation follow-up. Quality assurance and risk management programs that provide for continuous monitoring of critical indices, feedback relative to defined standards, and reappraisal of professional and departmental practices enhance effectiveness and efficiency of unit, departmental, and organizational operation. Ultimately, these systems support the public image and financial health of the institution by ensuring that practices and services result in outcomes planned and anticipated by health-care providers and consumers.

The purpose of this chapter is to describe incentives for implementing quality assurance and risk management programs, to describe the professional nurse's responsibility in support of the nursing quality assurance and risk management programs, to identify factors that pose professional and organizational risk, to suggest dimensions appropriately addressed in a nursing quality assurance program, and to propose strategies for reducing risk factors that result in institutional vulnerability.

At the completion of this chapter the professional nurse will be able to

1. Conceptualize quality assurance and risk management functions as components of the nurse's responsibility to the profession and to the institution.

2. Identify professional, regulatory, and governmental entities that guide, support, and review quality assurance and risk management programs.

3. Enumerate factors critical to implementation of effective quality assurance and risk management programs within nursing services.

4. Describe processes by which problems identified through quality assurance and risk management monitoring efforts might reasonably be addressed.

5. Critique existing quality assurance and risk management programs in nursing.

Incentives for Quality Assurance and Risk Management Programs

The impetus for implementation of relevant and effective quality assurance and risk management programs in general, and particularly in nursing, has gathered momentum in recent years due to multiple economic, professional, and sociopolitical forces operating in the health-care services environment. Forces providing incentives for expansion of quality assurance and risk management activities and application of quality assurance and risk management findings to hospital operations are discussed below.

ECONOMIC

Historically, health-care institutions and providers have been in the unique financial position of being able to pass on costs of providing services to recipients of care and third-party payers with very little control placed upon the actual dollar figure charged for services provided. In 1983 a dramatic shift in health-care financing occurred as a result of specific governmental efforts to contain rapidly escalating health-care costs (Carroll, 1984; Devet, 1985; Felton, 1985; Kaplan, 1980; Mushlin, 1985). Since the government is the nation's primary third-party payer for hospital services, the impact of modification in its reimbursement program is pervasive. Revision of public policies for financing acute health care through implementation of the Tax Equity and Fiscal Responsibility Act of 1982 (TEFRA) shifted hospital reimbursement away from traditional payment systems based on the provider's costs for services rendered (Carroll, 1984). Medicare reimbursement for care delivered is now based upon predetermined payment schedules that reflect historical costs for treatment of specific patient conditions. In other words, reimbursement for care is decided prospectively, regardless of the actual current costs incurred by the institution providing that care. This fiscal approach, known as *prospective payment,* provides incentive for the health care institution to control service delivery costs relative to reimbursement schedules in order to maintain or improve its financial position. Cost containment programs are now being emphasized in many institutions (Mushlin, 1985).

Although external pressures to control costs are substantive, arbitrary decisions to reduce services or to modify accepted patterns of care in order to realize a strong financial position carry with them an inherent risk, unless decisions to cut costs are carefully weighed against potential adverse consequences for the patient (Donabedian, 1984). The institution bears a corporate responsibility for those who deliver care under its sponsorship and can be held to account for inadequate and inappropriate practices undertaken on its premises (Carroll, 1984). The costs of one court case can obliterate savings realized by implementation of numerous cost containment measures (Devet, 1985). The question, then, is one of identifying conditions under which services can appropriately be curtailed or modified without attendant reduction in quality of care (Donabedian, 1984; Mushlin, 1985). Data from quality assurance and risk management activities can be used to document patient outcomes under various patterns of care, under care delivered by different individuals and categories of care-givers, in alternative settings. Further, quality assurance and risk management data can be merged with financial data to determine cost effective strategies for structuring health-care services (LaCava, 1985; Mushlin, 1985). Without the quality assurance and risk management components, cost containment decisions regarding services offered may be made on the basis of incomplete and inadequate data.

Escalation in health-care costs also precipitated repercussions in the private sector as businesses and labor groups became concerned about resources required to support health insurance premiums and medical benefits. To seek relief from soaring health-related costs, these payer groups have initiated cost-containment strategies, such as self-insurance, second opinions for specified surgical procedures, preferred provider, and health maintenance organization arrangements. As consumers purchasing entire programs for health care, businesses and labor groups have become increasingly sophisticated in requiring documentation that cost-effective health care is also quality-effective health care (Felton, 1986). Programs and institutions seeking to attract health-care purchasers can capitalize on quality assurance findings that verify consumer satisfaction and a high caliber of patient care when marketing their services to businesses and labor groups.

PROFESSIONAL

A traditional and valued responsibility of nursing, as with other professions, is development of standards against which professional practice is measured and by which the profession holds itself accountable to the public (Steel, 1985; Phaneuf and Lang 1985; Schroeder, 1984 b). Standards of nursing care developed by the American Nurses' Association (ANA) and speciality organizations have historically emphasized criteria that measure quality in components of the nursing process. As technology changed and results of the nursing process were emphasized, revisions of general and specialty nursing standards of care have increasingly included structural and patient outcome standards in addition to nursing process standards. The addition of structural and outcome criteria to process criteria in measurement of nursing care has expanded the defined scope of professional nursing practice.

Continuing development of professional standards, definition of valid and reliable criteria for measuring performance relative to those standards, and application of assessment methodology to nursing quality assurance activities will likely receive greater emphasis from nursing professional organizations in the future (Steel, 1985; Schroeder, 1985 a). This thrust for standards development comes only partially from altruistic concern for optimal patient care. As long as the nursing profession controls the definition of standards of care against which practice of the profession is defined and measured, the profession maintains autonomy in self-determination and self-regulation. Such autonomy is essential to survival of the nursing profession within the health-care services environment. Standards developed to reflect the practice and scope of nursing today reflect the evolving definition and nature of professional nursing (Carroll, 1984; Schroeder, 1984 a).

Incorporation of professional nursing standards of care into nursing service standards for practice reinforces the current definition of professional nursing within the institution. Moreover, incorporation communicates the standards to which nurses in the organization hold themselves accountable and responsible for their practice and the criteria by which nursing care is evaluated. Quality of care may be assessed as excellent, good, or poor when measured against valid standards of performance (Carroll, 1984). Use of professional standards in evaluation of nursing practice serves to verify and reward effective clinical performance of outstanding professional practitioners. Further, development of nursing service standards for practice and associated valid criteria for measuring practice patterns against resultant patient outcomes affirms the accountability of the profession for self-evaluation and self-regulation (Carroll, 1984; Steel, 1984; Phaneuf and Lang, 1985).

Effective implementation of the nursing quality assurance program reflects nursing competence in applying appropriate managerial control to professional clinical responsibilities (Devet, 1985). Results from monitoring activities that verify nursing's contribution to achievement of anticipated patient outcomes and unit, department, and organizational goals inspire confidence and pride among members of the nursing staff. When quality assurance findings serve as the basis for rewarding clinical competence, desirable target behaviors are emphasized among members of the professional nursing staff. Further, criterion-referenced quality assurance methodology is applicable to evaluating and justifying use of professional nurses as primary care-givers in alternative care settings and in expanded roles. Finally, results of quality assurance activities can be applied by nursing management to influence and justify distribution of financial and personnel resources across institutional subunits and within the nursing department itself (Thompson and Thompson, 1984).

SOCIOPOLITICAL

Prior to governmental entry into health-care financing, nurses, other health care professionals, and the health-care industry had gradually and voluntarily instituted measures for assessing the quality of care delivered to patients. Florence Nightingale herself helped lay the foundation for quality assurance efforts by promoting the collection and report of hospital statistical data (Schmude, 1985). As early as 1913, a systematic, objective approach for measurement of patient outcomes was advocated as the basis for hospital evaluation by E. A. Codman, one of the founders of the American College of Surgeons. Hospitals sought recognition as institutions providing high quality care and invited review and approval through evaluation mechanisms established by the American College of Surgeons. Eventually, the college merged with other professional and health industry associations to form the Joint Commission on Accreditation of Hospitals (JCAH), the vehicle by which hospitals still voluntarily undergo review against established standards to obtain accreditation (Shanahan, 1985; Carroll, 1984; Kaplan and Hopkins, 1980; Schroeder, 1984).

When soaring health-care costs and unprecedented demand for health-care services accompanied federal entry into health-care financing, accreditation by JCAH was initially designated as the criterion to verify compliance with federal conditions for reimbursement of hospitals. At this juncture the JCAH substantively modified quality of care standards and became more diligent in survey and review practices. Social and political pressures gradually led to creation of additional programs of utilization and quality assurance review to verify hospital eligibility for publicly funded reimbursement (Carroll, 1984; Grimaldi and Micheletti, 1984). Currently, hospitals must document that quality care is accessible to all segments of the population and delivered on the same basis for all patients, regardless of ability to pay. The combination of quality assurance and financial data provides documentation that the patient's health problems, rather than payer status, determine services provided.

As consumers become more knowledgeable about health promotion and services available for health maintenance and illness intervention, segments of the population demand alternatives to traditional medical intervention and expect third-party payers to reimburse them for the cost of alternative services utilized (Steele, 1985; Leininger, 1981). Quality assurance and risk management programs built into alternative care programs document their equivalence to existing services and verify consumer satisfaction with selected alternatives.

The consumer public has become increasingly sophisticated and knowledgeable regarding patients' rights and considers recourse through the courts when outcomes of professional intervention are not those anticipated (Creighton, 1985; Devet, 1985; Hoyt, 1985; Leininger, 1981). Trial juries are awarding huge monetary settlements resulting from medical mishaps and seemingly insensitive, irresponsible professional practice. Nurses are being held accountable for their unique professional responsibility to the patient (Hoyt, 1985). The cost of professional malpractice insurance is rising, especially for selected nursing and medical specialties. The patient can no longer be considered a passive recipient of health-care services (Levine, 1981; Steele, 1985). As a health care consumer, the patient desires and often demands active involvement in deciding the course of treatment, the extent of intervention, and the schedule and conditions under which aggressive care is discontinued (Leininger, 1981; Creighton, 1985).

In light of the present sociopolitical environment, health care institutions are in a position to receive additional benefits by documenting quality of care related to accreditation and reimbursement eligibility. When quality of care deteriorates, the care provider's reputation suffers. In this consumer-oriented society, a health-care organization cannot afford to develop a reputation for poor or mediocre care. A high quality of nursing care is integral to the institution's reputation (Devet, 1985; Harrell and Frauman, 1985). Summary data from quality assurance and risk management efforts that document the quality of care delivered may be used in marketing efforts to attract prospective patients and purchasers of health care (Carroll, 1984). In addition, positive institutional evaluations resulting from the use of valid, patient-relevant criteria are reflected in public goodwill and "word of mouth" marketing for the institution.

The Professional Nurse's Responsibility

Nursing's role in quality assurance and risk management involves the full range of management activities (see Figure 9-2). Responsibility for planning includes consideration of factors in the environment that place the patient, care-givers and institution "at risk," sources of internal organizational support for the nursing quality assurance and risk management programs, and resources applicable to refinement of quality assurance and risk management efforts. Through goal development for the quality assurance and risk management programs, focus is placed on

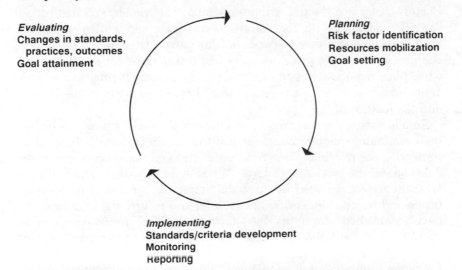

Evaluating
Changes in standards,
  practices, outcomes
Goal attainment

Planning
Risk factor identification
Resources mobilization
Goal setting

Implementing
Standards/criteria development
Monitoring
Reporting

Figure 9-2   Managing the nursing quality assurance and risk management programs.

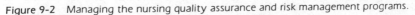

dimensions of nursing practice that carry the greatest risk, activities that occur with relative frequency, and standards that reflect state-of-the-art nursing practice.

Responsibility for implementing the nursing quality assurance and risk management programs includes identifying professional staff members' appropriately assigned leadership and supportive roles in the quality assurance and risk management efforts, establishing mechanisms for measuring, reporting, and integrating outcomes of the nursing quality assurance and risk management activities, and selecting means for applying findings to the modification of nursing services and hospital operations. In controlling program implementation, the application of findings to modification of nursing service and hospital operations is evaluated. Finally, in conjunction with the management control function, the effectiveness of the nursing quality assurance and risk management programs themselves is reviewed. Program effectiveness is assessed relative to the pre-established goals for performance developed within the scope of program planning. And so, even the quality assurance and risk management programs are subjected to evaluation in order to assure program integrity and applicability. In considering the new nurse's role in support of quality assurance and risk management program implementation, attention is directed toward an examination of related nursing management concerns.

PLANNING THE PROGRAMS.

Factors that place the patient, professional practitioner, and institution "at risk" usually result from failure to anticipate and address problems in delivering health care to patients. The perspectives of the consumer, the professional care-giver, and the institution must all be considered when planning quality assurance and risk management programs to prevent, modify, or eliminate practices that threaten patients, professionals, and the institution.

In addressing the interests of its citizens, the state authorizes licensing examination requirements for health care professionals directed at protecting the public at large from untrained and unsafe care-givers. As discussed in the section above, the JCAH and the various levels of government have developed institutional standards for acquiring accreditation and reimbursement for care rendered. Professional organizations have established standards by which health-care professionals hold themselves accountable for their practice. Within the scope of implementing a plan to anticipate and address problems of practice that place the patient, nursing professional, and organization at risk, knowledge of state statutes, regulatory agency standards, and professional standards for safe and appropriate practice is essential.

RISK FACTORS

Noncompliance with Standards

When a patient requires professional health-care services, that individual seeks care which he is unable or unwilling to self-administer. In essence, the patient trusts the competence of another to monitor and evaluate health status, recommend modification in health practices, and intervene or refer when health status warrants intervention (Levine, 1981; Schmude, 1985). Public law defines aspects of care that citizens of the state entrust to professional nurses and to every other category of licensed health-care worker. By practicing within statute-defined parameters, the professional is accountable to the public trust. Patient-care activities that extend beyond those encompassed by the regulatory statutes governing professional nursing place the patient, the care-giver, and the health care institution at risk. The patient is at risk because no assurance exists that proper training, evaluation, and credentialization of the practitioner has occurred relative to the dimensions of practice in question. The care-giver is at risk because practice exceeds that described in the regulations and therefore is not within the scope of authorized practice. Finally, the institution is at risk because it is accountable for care rendered inappropriately on its premises and under its auspices (Carroll, 1984). The professional nurse is responsible for assuring that ministrations fall within the scope of the *Nurse Practice Act* of the state within which care is rendered.

Copies of the state's "Nurse Practice Act" and "Rules and Regulations Governing the Practice of Professional Nursing" may be obtained from the State Board of Nurse Examiners (SBNE) or its counterpart, the body authorized to license professional nurses in the state. The SBNE is responsible for proposing and implementing modifications in rules and regulations related to the practice of professional nursing, hearing cases on licensure issues and revocation of licensure, and overseeing the entire licensing process. Periodically, the SBNE proposes changes in the rules and regulations governing nursing, typically published in the state *Register,* accompanied by a period for comment prior to implementation. In order to remain abreast of proposed changes impacting nursing practice and to comment on proposed changes prior to implementation, the institution's nurse executive typically screens the *Register* or reviews commentaries on proposed changes received from professional and institutional associations monitoring the regulatory environment. Anyone interested in proposed changes to regulations governing the practice of professional nursing may screen the *Register* and comment upon the proposed changes in writing or at public hearings. Following the comment period, approved modifications in the rules are published. Periodically, updated copies of the "Rules and Regulations Governing the Practice of Professional Nursing" may be obtained from the SBNE.

As part of the quality assurance responsibility, nursing management plans and implements systems to verify that the practice of nursing in the institution is consistent with the definition of professional nursing practice appearing in the state statutes and regulations. Nursing policies and procedures are designed to verify that incumbents in positions requiring licensed nursing personnel are in fact licensed by the state to practice their profession. Further, job requirements for all nursing positions must be consistent with the scope of nursing practice defined in the statutes. When nursing activities border on or encompass functions and responsibilities described in practice acts of other health-care professions, the professional nurse carrying out these functions has a responsibility to determine how rules and regulations governing nursing address participation in these activities. When nursing activities border on or overlap the practice of medicine, specific protocols for training and supervision should be delineated to protect the patient, the nurse, the physician, and the institution. Select categories of nursing personnel may be described in the institution's Medical Staff Bylaws as adjunct members of the medical staff. On rare occasions, an opinion from the state's attorney general may be necessary to clarify statutes governing the practice of nursing and medicine prior to extension of nursing practice into controversial dimensions of patient care.

JCAH and professional standards have been drafted to result ultimately in positive patient outcomes (Joint Commission, 1986). Noncompliance with these standards has potential to result in patient injury and poses a threat to the practicing professional and the institution. Copies of the JCAH "Standards for Nursing Services" and "Standards for Quality Assurance" may be obtained directly from the Joint Commission. Professional standards of care may be obtained from the ANA and from respective professional specialty associations. These resources will be discussed in greater depth later in this chapter.

Exclusion of Patient and Family

Failure to include the patient and family in decision making regarding plans for health maintenance, professional intervention, and care planning places the care-giver and institution in a vulnerable position (Creighton, 1985). Unless the patient is clear about the personal commitment demanded for wellness and recovery from illness, the care-giver cannot determine whether that patient is willing or likely to carry out activities required by the regimen for care. Without education adequate for making an informed decision regarding alternative options for treatment, the patient can feel manipulated and coerced, even if the intervention selected is optimal in the opinion of involved health-care professionals. A preliminary discussion of hazards associated with particular interventions reflects the commitment of the professional care-giver to provide the patient and family with an understanding of possible consequences of alternative decisions. The professional nurse may educate the patient regarding procedures, assist in obtaining informed consent, verify that the patient has accurately interpreted information pertaining to treatment plans, risks and potential outcomes, and facilitate communication between the patient and other health-care providers involved in decision making processes. Failure adequately to inform and include the patient and family in decision making creates an atmosphere of distrust and suspicion in a relationship principally grounded in trust (Creighton, 1985; Schmude, 1985). Efforts directed toward inclusion, communication, and education in the formative stages of the patient-professional relationship serve to reinforce patient confidence in the professional practitioner and to avert development of an adversarial position of the patient toward the health care provider.

Ignoring Problems

Within every institution, management information exists to monitor business aspects of the institution's operation. JCAH standards regarding safety of the physical plant, medical staff quality assurance, infection control, and utilization review require documentation pertinent to risk prevention and problem identification within nursing services. Nursing management accesses documentation that provides feedback on effective patient care and information regarding untoward or unexpected occurrences within subunits for which nursing management is operationally responsible. Failure to review, chart, and communicate management data that reflects inappropriate or ineffective operation places the patient, professional practitioners, and the institution at risk. For example, staffing plans for patient units are structural standards derived from a system that reflects patient requirements for nursing interventions. If that system is valid, consistent understaffing will likely be reflected in errors of omission: missed treatments, delayed medications, reduced response to patient requests for assistance, incomplete patient education, and so forth. If the number and timing of interventions defined in the standard is appropriately and reliably associated with patient outcomes, a reduction in patient satisfaction and delayed recovery will be observed over time as a consequence of understaffing or inappropriate staffing (Donabedian, 1984). Although many assumptions underlie the argument, one can see how the potential for adverse consequences may be documented through monitoring, charting, and correlating key indices of organizational effectiveness. The relationship between management information and patient outcomes must be evaluated, communicated, and acted upon when untoward consequences are documented (Greeley and Stearns, 1984; Fine, 1986; Decker, 1985). Evaluation of management information for applications related to quality control and risk prevention can be initiated while planning for implementation of nursing quality assurance and risk management programs.

Absence of Systems

Unless systems exist to support problem resolution within the institution, problem identification alone does nothing to reduce potential injury to patients and subsequent adverse consequences for the professional practitioner and the organization (Fine, 1986). A system must be in place to address problems as problems, without attendant "finger pointing," "blame placing," and "buck passing." Focusing attention on corrective action to resolve problems helps maintain a positive employee attitude toward risk management activities. Opportunities for rapid report and follow-up of serious errors focus attention on problems before errors are repeated. Suggestions for new and safer processes for providing care may be evaluated prospectively. Open communication to the highest levels of administration facilitates problem resolution for difficulties unresolved at lower organizational levels (Rifkin et al, 1984). Mechanisms for establishing muiltidisciplinary task forces to address interdepartmental problems must be clarified and communicated. Without systems to support problem resolution through corrective action, reduction in risk to patients, professionals, and the institution cannot be accomplished. These systems must include processes for re-education of hospital personnel regarding modification of standards, policies, and procedures resulting from problem evaluation and resolution activities (Greeley and Stearns, 1984; Decker, 1985).

Internal organizational support and resources may be used to ensure that nursing efforts are consistent with institutional quality assurance and risk management plans. Data collected through existing institutional and medical staff programs may be applicable to nursing quality assurance and risk management analysis with minor modification in the way findings are reported (Oulton, 1984; Donabedian, 1984). Individuals identified within the institution as the risk manager, the DRG coordinator, the utilization review coordinator, the quality assurance coordinator, or the medical affairs coordinator may be very helpful in identifying existing data sources. They can evaluate and share reports generated as a part of their organizational responsibilities and help to determine how specific data are applicable to appraisal of nursing service activities. Further, the mechanism by which these individuals communicate findings and recommendations through the organizational hierarchy to the governing body will likely parallel the mechanism for communicating nursing quality assurance and risk management conclusions and suggestions to upper levels of management. Knowing the communication systems for problem resolution can reduce frustration with institutional change processes.

RESOURCES PROVIDING SUPPORT

In addition to individuals assigned overall responsibility for quality assurance and risk management within the institution, a number of external resources provide support for establishing and revising nursing quality assurance and risk management programs. Some written materials and resources may be in the possession of the nurse executive, other members of the administrative staff, and nurse managers. Quality assurance and risk management resource materials are likely to be distributed selectively to interested employees. Published resource materials are available and may be acquired through the institution's library or the regional medical library. Once the topics of quality assurance and risk management become salient to the new nurse, applicable material is likely to be identified in professional journals and publications. Some potential resources for nursing quality assurance and risk management program implementation are addressed below.

Joint Commission on Accreditation of Hospitals

The JCAH annually publishes the *Accreditation Manual for Hospitals,* which delineates the standards for JCAH accreditation (Joint Commission, 1986). An entire section of this manual is devoted to "Standards for Nursing Services." Other sections pertinent to nursing include those related to anesthesia and surgical services, medical staff, quality assurance, special care units, and utilization review, among others. In addition to the manual, the JCAH publishes other materials to update health-care professionals on pertinent quality assurance and risk management topics. These include a newsletter that periodically summarizes Joint Commission action, books such as "A Guide to JCAH Nursing Standards" (Kranz and Ware, 1983), and a journal designed to disseminate information about quality assurances approaches, activities, theory, research, and related aspects of patient care (Kaplan and Hopkins, 1980). In addition, the JCAH regularly conducts seminars on quality assurance, nursing standards, and other topics and provides consultation services to institutions regarding program development to attain and maintain compliance with the JCAH standards (Kaplan and Hopkins, 1980).

Professional Organizations

Professional nursing organizations develop and publish standards for the practice of professional nursing and nursing specialties (ANA, 1973, 1975). Quality of care issues are addressed in clinical nursing and professional journals directed at nursing managers, practitioners, and educators. Journals that address issues of appropriate clinical practice relative to specific patient problems and nursing diagnoses provide data pertinent to evaluation of nursing quality assurance and risk management efforts.

Private Consulting Firms

In addition to consultation services available through the JCAH, hospital associations, and professional associations, numerous private consulting firms offer support for hospital quality assurance and risk management efforts. Periodically seminars are presented by consultants to acquaint potential users with their services and to promote written materials produced for professionals responsible for implementing quality assurance and risk management programs. Some consulting firms publish advisory newsletters to update quality assurance coordinators and risk managers regarding innovative approaches to implementing quality assurance and risk management functions. Printed materials include examples of monitoring tools and specific recommendations for implementing the quality assurance and risk management functions in general, with applications for nursing (Integrating Hospital Quality, 1983; Schmude, 1985; Devet, 1985; Thompson and Thompson, 1984). Use of such resources capitalizes on the creativity and expertise of individuals who specialize in designing quality assurance and risk management tools for assessing compliance with specified standards. Those responsible for program implementation within nursing services can select and modify model tools to evaluate and improve nursing care and management practices under specific institutional conditions.

GOALS FOR QUALITY ASSURANCE PROGRAM

Since planning is future oriented, part of the planning process is related to determining and predicting outcomes of program implementation for some point in the future (Schroeder, 1984 b). In doing so, planning involves delineating specific program goals and devising systems necessary for goal attainment (Rowland and Rowland, 1985). Participation of individuals directly responsible for implementing each facet of the nursing quality assurance and risk management programs is essential to this aspect of the program design. Understanding of, confidence in, and commitment to programs result from active involvement in goal setting during program planning (Decker, 1985).

Those in key leadership positions have a responsibility to see that goals for the nursing quality assurance and risk management programs are consistent with institutional and departmental goals, are comprehensive in that they encompass structural, process, and outcome standards, and reflect a philosophy of continuous evaluation for early problem identification and resolution (Decker, 1985). Through goals established for nursing quality assurance and risk management programs, nursing administration communicates commitment to effective and efficient departmental operation.

The language of management, which frames the development of goals for the nursing quality assurance and risk management programs, is concrete, specific, and quantitative (Nornhold, 1986). Goals stated in a concise and measurable manner facilitate evaluation of goal attainment. Goals salient to each specific unit enhance program relevance. Goals that are attainable and realistic permit employees to experience success and pride. Goals that exceed present performance levels stimulate growth and challenge high achievers to excel. In summary, goals for the nursing quality assurance and risk management programs should be concise, measurable, salient, attainable, and challenging (Decker, 1985).

INVOLVEMENT OF THE NEW NURSE

Involvement of the new nurse in planning nursing quality assurance and risk management programs is focused predominately at the unit and personal level. First, the new nurse is expected to assist in specifying the general goals for the nursing quality assurance and risk management programs at the unit level. Each nursing unit varies with the respect to patient population, rates of compliance with standards, credentials and skills of nursing personnel employed, and so forth. Unit goals should emphasize the issues most relevant to that unit within the broader scope of the nursing services quality assurance and risk management plans (Schroeder, 1984 b).

The new nurse participates in unit meetings to predict, identify, and prioritize problems for further evaluation within the nursing unit, between units within nursing services, and between the nursing department and other institutional entities. The new nurse suggests alternative strategies for standards attainment when results of monitoring activities reveal unacceptable unit performance, and assists in planning changes in unit practices to address deficiencies. Finally, in conjunction with the immediate supervisor, the new nurse establishes individual performance goals to enhance care within the nursing unit patient population and to reduce risks associated with employment in the health-care setting.

IMPLEMENTING THE PROGRAM

Implementation of the nursing quality assurance and risk management programs begins with identification, selection, or development of standards against which nursing care is evaluated. Associated with strategies for risk reduction, these standards are categorized as structural, process, or outcome oriented (Phaneuf and Lang, 1985; Kaplan and Greenfield, 1984; Schroeder, 1984 b). Standards for nursing practice are based on identified values and frame development of specific, relevant criteria for objectively measuring standards attainment. Data sources required to provide documentation relative to criteria are identified, and monitoring is initiated. Analysis of data collected verifies that current practice supports standards attainment or targets specific areas for intensive evaluation. These dimensions of quality assurance and risk management program implementation are discussed below.

GENERATING STANDARDS OF PRACTICE

A standard is an agreed-upon base line condition or level of excellence that comprises a model to be followed and practiced. Within the context of nursing services, standards define the scope and dimensions of professional nursing practice within the institution. Standards are relatively general and may be categorized as structural, process, or outcome oriented (Phaneuf and Lang, 1985; Schroeder, 1984 b; Mayers *et al*, 1977).

Structural standards deal with the systems by which delivery of nursing services is framed and organized. The nurse staffing system establishes the standard for nursing personnel requirements relative to patient care needs for nursing resources. Portions of nursing job descriptions define the education, experience, credentials, and abilities required for placement of applicants in nursing positions. Utilization policies determine patient subpopulations placed and cared for on select nursing units. Equipment, supplies, and medications standards define essential resources required to support patient care relative to the anticipated patient mix. Safety and infection control policies describe environmental considerations and controls essential to patient and personnel safety. All may be considered structural standards integral to providing safe and effective nursing care, but distinct from the actual content and processes of nursing practice, *per se.*

Process standards describe the manner in which nursing care is to be delivered and nursing activities to be carried out. Nursing process standards are comprised of the actions, behaviors, and content of nursing practice in general, often specified to select patient subgroups. For example, Standard 1 of the American Nurses' Association "Standards of Nursing Practice" states, "The collection of data about the health status of the client/patient is systematic and continuous. The data are accessible, communicated, and recorded." The eight general standards of nursing practice defined by ANA are stated in similar, succinct fashion (ANA, 1973, 1975).

Process standards, if not explicitly delineated as such by nursing service, are reflected in many sources and formats generated to direct, describe, and document the content and activities of nursing care. Process standards are communicated through modalities such as standard care plans, nursing protocols, nursing procedures, performance appraisal portions of nursing job descriptions, and specific standards of care for target homogeneous patient groups. Prior to the initiation of any monitoring activities, process standards must be extrapolated from these frameworks and stated succinctly.

Process standards serve a useful purpose when attainment of outcome standards is particularly difficult to measure and verify. Circumstances appropriate for evaluation through use of process standards include those in which adverse outcomes occur infrequently, outcomes are ascribed to numerous factors beyond nursing control, patients have complex problems with multiple outcomes, long term care is likely, terminal care is anticipated, and the population is small (Kaplan and Greenfield, 1984).

Outcome standards, the most patient-specific, refer to results of nursing interventions as reflected in patient status (Greeley & Stearns, 1984). Outcome standards are drafted in terms of what the patient will do, know, express, or experience, and reflect nursing goals for physiological, emotional and mental well-being. In a sense, outcome standards may be conceptualized as long term goals for patient knowledge and physical, social, and emotional functioning (Kaplan and Greenfield, 1984).

Criteria Development

Criteria are the specific assessment factors, critical elements, indicators, or essential components required to operationalize and measure attainment of a given standard. Criteria that reflect the intent of the standard may include working definitions of terms used in the standard, statements about behavior, circumstances, or clinical status that explicitly describe what is generally implied or addressed in the standard (Mayers et al, 1977; Devet, 1985; Phaneuf and Lang, 1985; Shanahan, 1983;

Schroeder, 1984 b). Criteria relative to Standard 1 of the ANA "Standards of Nursing Practice" are presented below.

CRITERIA RELATED TO STANDARD 1, ANA STANDARDS OF PRACTICE

Standard 1: The collection of data about the health status of the client/patient is systematic and continuous. The data are accessible, and communicated, and recorded.

STANDARDS OF NURSING PRACTICE

General Criteria

Assessment Factors

1. Health status data include:
   Growth and development
   Biophysical status
   Emotional status
   Cultural, religious, socio-economic background
   Performance of activities of daily living
   Patterns of coping
   Interaction patterns
   Client's/patient's perception of and satisfaction with his health status
   Client/patient health goals
   Environment (physical, social, emotional, ecological)
   Available and accessible human and material resources

2. Data are collected from:
   Client/patient, family,

STANDARDS OF ORTHOPEDIC NURSING PRACTICE

Orthopedic Practice Criteria

1. Health data include, but are not limited to:
   Current medical diagnosis and therapy
   The individual's perceptions and expectations that relate to his health-illness state and health care services
   Information about previous use of and access to health services
   Environmental, occupational, financial, educational, recreational, and spiritual information as it relates to the individual's habits and social and work roles
   The individual's mental and emotional response
   Interview history:
   Onset of symptoms and/or recognition of alteration

continued

STANDARDS OF NURSING PRACTICE	STANDARDS OF ORTHOPEDIC NURSING PRACTICE
General Criteria	Orthopedic Practice Criteria

significant others.
Health care personnel
Individuals within the
    immediate environ-
    ment and/or the
    community.

3. Data are obtained by:
    Interview
    Examination
    Observation
    Reading records, reports,
        etc.

4. There is a format for the
    collection of data
    which:
    Provides for a systematic
        collection of data
    Facilitates the complete-
        ness of data collection.

5. Continuous collection of
    data is evident by:
    Frequent updating
    Recording of changes in
        health status.

6. The data are:
    Accessible on the client/
        patient records
    Retrievable from record-
        keeping systems
    Confidential when
        appropriate

Mechanism and time of
injury, type of first-aid,
and transport to health
care facility
Progression of
    symptoms
Limitation of function
Description of pain:
    Location
    Radiation
    Quality
    Time of occurrence
    Causative factors
    Methods of relief:
        position, medica-
        tions, use of external
        supports
Other pathophysiologi-
cal conditions:
    Infection
    Congenital
        abnormalities
    Diabetes
    Heart disease
    Peripheral vascular
        disease
    Upper respiratory
        infection
    Chronic obstructive
        pulmonary disease
    Urinary tract disorder
    Gastric/duodenal ulcer
    Gallbladder disease
Pharmacological
history:
    Any previous use of
    steroids

continued

STANDARDS OF ORTHOPEDIC
NURSING PRACTICE

Orthopedic Practice Criteria

Current medications
Allergies
Pertinent family history
Social habits:
  Tobacco
  Alcohol intake
Physical examination:
Orthopedic:
  Joint range of motion
  Position and appear-
    ance of extremities
    and trunk
  Relative measure-
    ments of musculo-
    skeletal structures
  Growth and
    development
  Gait
  Sensation
  Circulation
  Muscle strength
General physical
assessment:
  State of hydration
  Skin moisture and
    temperature
  Body temperature
  Status of pressure
    points
  Skin petechiae
  Weight in relation to
    height
  Fatigue/activity
    tolerance
  Mental acuity
  Sleep/rest pattern
    interruption
  Nutritional status:
    appetite, nausea/
    vomiting

continued

STANDARDS OF NURSING PRACTICE	STANDARDS OF ORTHOPEDIC NURSING PRACTICE
General Criteria	Orthopedic Practice Criteria
	Bowel sounds, diarrhea/constipation
	Chest pain, shortness of breath
	Tachycardia, heart rate, respiratory rate
	Homan's sign (calf tenderness)
	Urinary output
	Localized edema
	Blood balance
	Limitations of sight and hearing
	Diagnostic findings:
	X-ray
	Special radiographic diagnostic studies
	Complete blood count
	Serum chemistries
	Latex fixation
	L. E. prep
	Sedimentation rate
	Serum salicylate level
	ECG
	Blood coagulation studies
	Uric acid
	Alkaline phosphatase
	Fluid aspiration
	2. Health data collected by appropriate methods
	3. Health data collection is complete

• From Standards of Nursing Practice (1973) and Standards of Orthopedic Nursing Practice (1975). Kansas City, MO, American Nurses' Association

The first column describes criteria related to patients in general and the second describes criteria to define compliance with the same standard for a subset of orthopedic patients (ANA, 1973; 1975). Similar modifications in general criteria might be anticipated for other subpopulations depending upon factors most relevant to specific patient conditions and health problems.

Derived from established standards, relevant criteria focus on significant nursing actions, identify meaningful observations, reflect competent nursing judgment, are accurate, realistic, and accessible. All criteria selected for measuring standard attainment are considered critical and, as such, evidence of the presence of all must be documented through the monitoring process unless specific exceptions are delineated (Greeley and Stearns, 1984). In other words, if the key elements are not present, noncompliance with a given standard is reflected in review documentation.

When criteria are established, a target figure, a value, usually stated in the form of a percentage, is selected as an indicator that the standard is attained. If the goal for compliance with standard is 100%, a decision must be made as to whether a 95% compliance figure is acceptable or whether efforts must be directed toward improving the compliance figure (Greeley and Stearns, 1984).

Data Collection

Data retrieval is classified as concurrent or retrospective, depending on the relationship between the time at which care is delivered and the time at which data collection for evaluation takes place (Kaplan and Hopkins, 1980; Kaplan and Greenfield, 1984; Greeley and Stearns, 1984; Maibusch, 1984). Concurrent review is conducted while the patient is still under treatment and retrospective review is conducted after discharge. Although subject to interruption by pressing unit demands, concurrent review has an advantage over retrospective review in that immediate feedback is provided and an opportunity exists to initiate corrective action in each specific case included in the evaluation process. Furthermore, a variety of data sources can be used to acquire a comprehensive picture of the issue in question (Kaplan and Hopkins, 1980; Maibusch, 1984).

Since retrospective review involves examination of data permanently stored in medical records or other documents, the process is not particularly sensitive to interruption. However, scheduling data collection and analysis under retrospective review is critical. Data too old are no longer meaningful due to changes in staff, standards, or systems. Furthermore, only rare opportunity exists to alter care found deficient through the retrospective review process. In a retrospective system, nonpermanent supplemental documentation is no longer available to justify discrepancies between findings and standard, and the methodology is limited to review of documentation without the presence of the subject for observation (Greeley and Stearns, 1984; Kaplan and Hopkins, 1980; Kaplan and Greenfield, 1984).

Typical data retrieval methods include document review, interview, observation, and questionnaire (Carroll, 1984; Decker, 1985). In concurrent review, open charts may be examined, patients interviewed, patient care observed, and staff observed or interviewed. In retrospective review, closed charts may be audited, discharged patients interviewed or surveyed, and staff interviewed for recall data. Several concurrent and retrospective audit systems for evaluation have been developed over the last 20 years and are currently marketed for use (Kaplan and Hopkins, 1980; Kaplan and Greenfield, 1984; Maibusch, 1984). The nursing department may choose to use or modify existing systems in developing mechanisms for evaluating nursing care of patients within the institution.

In addition to the conventional sources of data for quality assurance monitoring, incidence reports can also serve as sources of data documenting deficiencies in practice. However, untoward occurrences recorded through incident reports typically reflect exceptions to the rule and do not result from systematically monitoring compliance with standards. The value of incidence reports is derived from extensive documentation describing circumstances in a way that enables evaluators to address the question of how an incident occurred. Trending of reported untoward occurrences through the incident report mechanism points to areas for further investigation.

Monitoring compliance with standards of practice must occur in a planned, systematic manner with regularly scheduled data collection (Decker, 1985; Carroll, 1984; Schmude, 1985). According to Carroll (1984), three issues should be considered when determining the types of review to perform. These issues include (1) the time frame in which review is to be conducted, (2) the subject matter under review, and (3) the data sources available. Choices should center on collecting key indicators with predictive value at intervals that anticipate normal phases of the planning cycle (Decker, 1985). Furthermore, data collection can occur in conjunction with other activities for which data sources are scanned. For example, data collection relative to criteria outlined on pages 172–175 can occur at the time of patient transfer to another unit, during a multidisciplinary conference, at a change of shift, at discharge, or at some point following discharge when the medical record is audited for reimbursement coding or financial purposes. Each criterion is sufficiently specific so that a simple yes/no response will reflect deviation from targeted compliance.

Data Analysis

If criteria can be considered reasonable expectations for practice decided in advance and used to measure performance, the degree of compliance attained will reflect and operationally define the quality of care provided (Thompson and Thompson, 1984). Analysis of criterion-related data can be kept simple in considering the development of strategies to address deficiencies identified (Carroll, 1984). Data broken down by criterion, unit, day, and shift will essentially address the questions, "What?", "Where?", "Who?", "When?". The question of "How?" is a manner of interpretation, can be addressed through specifically designed evaluation research, and will need to be asked in planning strategies to correct deficiencies found.

Interpretation of data involves deciding whether a person or systems problem exists in the delivery of care to patients. Does the staff lack knowledge, motivation, skills, or caring? Are the mechanisms in place to support the staff in acquiring resources necessary to carry out the care demanded by the patient needs?

The corrective step is the most important step of the implementation process and includes feedback to staff about results, continuing education, individual counseling, purchase of new equipment, revisions of policies, procedures, and standards, and changes in job content for categories of nursing personnel (Greeley and Stearns, 1985).

THE NEW NURSE AND PROGRAM IMPLEMENTATION

Significant professional care is provided by staff nurses directly involved with the patient. Staff nurses assess patients, plan care, develop priorities, organize time, and evaluate efforts on the daily basis (Decker, 1985). It is only reasonable that members of the nursing staff be involved in identifying and selecting criteria for measurement of patient care through monitoring activities. Staff nurses should be most sensitive to the aspects of clinical care that need appraisal, sensitive to deterioration in proficiency relative to technical skills, and to the kinds of patient outcomes that reflect appropriate nursing intervention. Under the nursing manager's supervision in team meetings, staff nurses can negotiate to develop criteria related to specific standards, discuss methodologies for intervening relative to specific problems in order to achieve desirable patient outcomes, target questionable or apparently unnecessary practices for evaluation and possible elimination, and discuss unit strengths and weaknesses candidly.

Through development of criteria for assessment of compliance with standards for nursing practice, staff nurses become proficient in using the concrete, specific, and quantitative language of business (Nornhold, 1986). Through evaluation of staffing patterns and practices, new nurses may realize that increased productivity doesn't preclude quality, but may even enhance quality when work loads are neither too heavy nor too light relative to patient care demands (Harrell and Frauman, 1985). Through monitoring personal and peer practices, the new professional is intimately involved in reinforcing desirable and appropriate nursing care.

The consequences of continued deviation from excepted standards of care include suboptimal care of patients, potential for financial losses if claims are denied due to inappropriate admission, treatment, and documentation, jeopardizing accreditation status and licensure approval, and danger of exposure to malpractice or personal injury claims (Carroll, 1984). Through participation in implementation of the nursing quality assurance and risk management programs, the new nurse is in a position significantly to influence the likelihood of such occurrences.

EVALUATION OF PROGRAMS

Evaluation asks the question, "What change has taken place and was it meaningful?" Criterion-referenced monitoring processes and associated modifications in practices should document that deficiencies in care are remedied and that overall quality of care consistently improves. Documentation of improvements is found in reported results of audits, surveys, and monitoring activities. Results are reflected in minutes of meetings reviewing quality of care throughout the institution.

In evaluating nursing quality assurance and risk management programs themselves, consideration needs to be given to program structure, process, and content. To be effective, programs must include the appropriate components. Did mechanisms exist for monitoring and evaluating care rendered? Were findings from data collection incorporated into revised systems for care delivery? Did the mechanisms exist for follow-up on important problems and for problem resolution? Were findings documented and reported?

The *nursing* quality assurance program and risk management program must be integrated into the overall *institutional* quality assurance and risk management programs. Furthermore, all levels of nursing staff must be involved in planning, implementing, and evaluating structural, process, and outcome oriented components of nursing care delivery. Content monitored through quality assurance and risk management programs must be relevant and applicable to decision making at all levels of nursing care.

Summary

The nursing quality assurance program is aimed at supporting patient care practices by verifying that nursing interventions are appropriate and applicable to the patients' health status or are reevaluated and modified. Nursing risk management programs are aimed at protecting the interest of the institution through maintenance of a safe and supportive milieu for patients, families, and care-givers. Inspiring confidence in the institution through provision of consistent quality care reduces the probability of litigation (Thompson and Thompson, 1984). Quality assurance and risk management programs are integrated to the extent that both focus evaluation on the same structures, processes, outcomes, and content to achieve program goals.

Effective quality assurance and risk management programs define structural, process, and outcome standards for patient care to reflect prevailing social, ethical, and professional values and current technological capabilities (Phaneuf and Lang, 1985; Schroeder, 1984). Through program implementation, review and evaluation of patient care against established standards results in development of new and improved practices and interventions on behalf of patients and their families. The health-care environment becomes a safer place to provide and receive care.

Many incentives exist for development of effective, integrated nursing quality assurance and risk management programs. Rapid change in health care technology demands regular and critical review of standards and practices to assure the very best outcomes for patients within financial constraints imposed by finite resources. Data retrieved through quality assurance and risk management monitoring can assist nurse managers in addressing issues related to regulatory demands, expanding legal liabilities, aggressive competition between institutions and professional providers, and cost containment. To be viable, professional nursing decisions and practices must withstand rigorous review, testing, and reevaluation. Through development of nursing quality assurance and risk management programs, the nursing profession assumes its responsibility for self-evaluation and self-regulation. Such professional accountability can only lead to improvement in patient care and validation of nursing contributions within the institution.

The new nurse needs both clinical and business skills to practice effectively in the modern health-services environment (Nornhold, 1986). A part of the business of professional nursing is contributing to evaluation; to control of services rendered to the patients in care. Decisions about standards, criteria, interventions, and modifications in practice and performance expectations are influenced significantly by staff nurse perspectives. By embracing the goals of quality assurance and risk management, the new nurse begins to participate in the evaluation and modification of nursing operations critical to survival of nurses as managers and administrators in the health-services environment.

Bibliography

American Nurses' Association: Standards of Nursing Practice. Kansas City, American Nurses' Association, 1973

American Nurses' Association: Standards of Orthopedic Nursing Practice. Kansas City, American Nurses' Association, 1975

Carroll JG: Restructuring Hospital Quality Assurance: The New Guide for Health Care Providers. Homewood IL, Dow Jones-Irwin, 1984

Creighton H: "Relatives sue for putting patient on life support." Nurs Manage 16:56, 60, 1985

Decker CM: Quality assurance: Accent on monitoring. Nurs Manage 16:20–24, 1985

Devet C: The Monitoring Sourcebook: Vol 2: Nursing Practice. Chicago, Care Communications, 1985

Donabedian A: Quality, cost, and cost containment. Nurs Outlook 32:142–145, 1984

Felton G: Harnassing today's trends to guide nursing's future. Nurs Health Care 7:211–213, 1985

Fine RB: Conceptual perspectives on the organization design tasks and the quality assurance function. Nurs Health Care 2:101–104, 1986

Gibson JL, Ivancevich JM, Donnelly JH: Organizations: Behavior, structure, processes, Dallas, Business Publications, 1979

Greeley H, Stearns G: Primer on retrospective outcome audit. Qual Rev Bull 10:438–441, 1984

Grimaldi PL, Micheletti JA: Implementation of the peer review organization program. Qual Rev Bull 10:340–346, 1984

Harrell JS, Frauman AC: Prospective payment calls for boosting productivity. Nurs Health Care 6:535–537, 1985

Hopkins G: Integrating staff resources results in higher productivity. QRC Advisor 2:5–6, 8, 1985

Hoyt EM: The great nurse emancipation case. Tex Med 81:48–51, 1985

Integrating Hospital Quality Assurance. Chicago, Interqual, 1893

Joint Commission on Accreditation of Hospitals: Accreditation Manual for

Hospitals. Chicago, Joint Commission on Accreditation of Hospitals, 1986

Kaplan KO, Hopkins JM: The QA Guide: A Resource for Hospital Quality Assurance. Chicago, Joint Commission on Accreditation of Hospitals, 1980

Kaplan SH, Greenfield S: Criteria mapping: Using logic in evaluation of processes of care. Qual Rev Bull 10:462–466, 1984

Kranz D, Ware A: A Guide to JCAH Nursing Standards. Chicago, Joint Commission on Accreditation of Hospitals, 1983

LaCava FW: The role of legal counsel in hospital risk management. Qual Rev Bull 11:20–24, 1985

Leininger M: Sociocultural forces impacting upon health care and the nursing profession. In Change: A Conference on the Future of Nursing Care. Washington, D.C., US Government Printing Office, 1981

Levine AS: The influence of social and cultural evolution on the relation between professional and patient. In Change: A Conference on the Future of Nursing Care, Washington, D.C., US Government Printing Office, 1981

Liebler JB, Levine RE, Dervitz HL: Management Principles for Health Professions, Rockville, MD, Aspen Systems, 1983

Maibusch RM: Evolution of quality assurance for nursing in hospitals. In Schroeder PS, Maibusch RM (Eds.): Nursing Quality Assurance: A Unit-Based Approach. Rockville, Md, Aspen Systems, 1984

Mayers MB, Norby RB, Watson AB: Quality Assurance for Patient Care. New York, Appleton-Century-Crofts, 1977

Mosby RB, Freund LE, Wagner B: A nurse staffing system based upon assignment difficulties. J Nurs Adm 7:2–24, 1977

Mushlin AI: The analysis of clinical practices: Shedding light on cost containment opportunities in medicine. Qual Rev Bull 11:378–384, 1985

Nornhold P: Power: It's changing hands and moving your way. Nurs 86 16:40–42, 1986

Oulton R: Use of incident report data in a systemwide quality assurance/risk management program. Qual Rev Bull 10:583–587, 1984

Phaneuf MC, Lang MM: Standards of nursing practice. pp 1–18. In Issues in Professional Nursing Practice Monograph Series. Kansas City, MO, American Nurses' Association, 1985

Rifkin M, Lynne C, Williams R, Hilsenbeck C: Managing quality assurance activities in a large teaching hospital. Qual Rev Bull 10:418–422, 1984

Rowland HS, Rowland BL: Nursing Administration Handbook, 2nd ed. Rockville, MD, Aspen Systems, 1985

Schmude J: Nursing Services. In Continuous Monitoring and Data-Based Quality Assessment, Vol. 3. Salem, WI, Greeley Associates, 1985

Schroeder PS: Trends in quality assurance: A vision for the future. In Schroeder PS, Maibusch RM (eds): Nursing Quality Assurance: A Unit-Based Approach. Rockville, MD, Aspen Systems, 1984(a)

Schroeder, PS: The quality assurance process. In Schroeder PS, Maibusch RM (eds): Nursing Quality Assurance: A Unit-Based Approach. Rockville, MD, Aspen Systems, 1984(b).

Shanahan M: The quality assurance standard of the JCAH: A routine approach to patient care evaluation. In Luke RD, Krueger JC, Modrow RE (eds): Organization and Change in Health Care Quality Assurance. Rockville, MD, Aspen Systems, 1983

Steele JE: Challenges to Nursing Practice, pp 1–13. In Issues in Professional Nursing Practice Monograph Series. Kansas City, MO, American Nurses' Association, 1985

Thompson RE, Thompson JB: Nuts and Bolts of Hospitalwide Accountability. Elmhurst, IL, Thompson, Mohr, 1984

SECTION II

FOCUS ON EMPLOYMENT

Chapter 10

Becoming a successful employee

DONNA RICHARDS SHERIDAN

Your responsibilities as a nursing employee begin on your first day of reporting to work for your first paid nursing position. No doubt this moment is filled with excitement, enthusiasm, a willingness to do well, and perhaps a touch of apprehension. Your are ready to be a good nurse providing quality patient care. It's not new; you did it as a student, you tell yourself.

What *is* new is the commitment you are making also to be a good employee. You have been hired by an organization that exists for a purpose. You have become part of a unit that contributes to the overall organizational purpose. And you will be expected to contribute both to the organization and to the unit while providing excellent care for your patients.

On your way to becoming a good nurse, you learned to be a good student (or you would never have made it to this point). As a student your nursing goal was to learn. Your focus had to be on yourself—obtaining the necessary knowledge and skills to become a professional nurse. Now your focus needs to shift so that you can use that knowledge and skill within the framework of an organization. Although your primary focus will shift, much of what you learned about succeeding as a student will help you succeed as a nurse.

This chapter will enable you to

1. Explain the relationship between a good student and a good employee.
2. List ten characteristics of good employees.
3. Describe the written sources of job expectations in a health-care setting.
4. Explain how to assess the cultural, informal expectations in a health-care setting.
5. Describe the interrelationship of motivation, goal setting, and performance appraisal.
6. Explain how to take responsibility for your own professional development.

What is the relationship between your role as a good student and your role as a good nursing employee? Edna Neumann, dean of professor at City College School of Nursing in New York, asked her students this question. The replies she received showed great overlap between "what makes a good student?" and "what makes a good nurse and employee?". Because of this overlap, much of what you have currently been doing well will be useful in your role. Neumann's students from City College responded that good students and good nurses

Work from a good knowledge base

Have excellent clinical skills

Are willing to accept responsibility

Can communicate with and support (help out) peers (in one case members of the health-care team, patients, and family members; in the other case classmates)

Complete assignments (in one case patient assignments, in the other case class assignments)

Enjoy their work

Participate in team efforts

Are involved and committed

Have a genuine interest in and for patients/peers

Understand their role and fulfill the requirements

Set goals

Are assertive and nonjudgmental

Work hard

Are caring

Explain to and teach others

Are loyal

Stand up for beliefs and principles

Follow rules yet are independent thinkers

Project a positive nursing image

Collaborate

Take pride in their work

Demonstrate a high level of self-esteem

Are self-disciplined

Are punctual

Reach out to others

Have determination

Are honest

Are pleasant

Produce quality work (nursing care or classwork)

Show warmth and concern

Are ambitious and curious

Are accountable

Have a sense of satisfaction and achievement in work done

Are motivated

Strive for upward mobility in their careers

Are eager to share with and learn from others

Are receptive to new ideas

Evaluate themselves frequently to continue to grow

Show empathy and compassion toward others

Are flexible

Show enthusiasm

Can "fit" into a variety of situations

Can delegate/share responsibility

Are neat, polite, and courteous

Are efficient and organized

Take pride in their work, their job, and their organization

Are able to follow and to lead

Learn about and contribute to their profession

Seek out challenges

Respect fellow students/workers regardless of grade or job level

Are patient

Have a probing mind and ask questions

Have the courage to challenge injustices

Care equally for people regardless of religion, race, or sex

Contribute to the school/hospital

Are dedicated

Have a sense of humor and are cheerful (Neumann, 1985)

Looking over the above list, it becomes apparent that learning to be a good employee is lifelong learning. What makes a good student also makes a good nurse and a good employee. They are the amorphous characteristics that make a good person. You have been working on this all your life and hopefully will continue to grow in this way throughout adulthood and your nursing career. These characteristics will help you now to be a good employee.

Pol (1986) highlights the key points: "I think a good employee is one who has goals (long-term and short-term) both personal and professional. This employee must also be loyal, flexible, and kind. This person should be able to accept the client (patient) at client level of education and background. The employee should be a person interested in people and their dignity.[11]

Expectations of the Employer

Besides the amorphous "good" characteristics defined above, what does your employer expect? An employer, any employer, has a responsibility to get a quality product "out the door" in a way that keeps the employees happy, or satisfied enough to make them want to continue "churning out the product." In health care, the product is service. In nursing, the product is bringing people to the highest possible level of health and self-care, within the constraints of the economy, the law, and other imposed limitations. No organization can exist unless it operates within these limitations. So the job of your hospital employer, no matter what level, is to produce quality patient care. This is accomplished indirectly by using employees. So actually, the employer is responsible for producing satisfied employees—nurses—who produce quality patient care.

Your direct employer (boss) probably is a nurse administrator. This person defines what quality patient care "looks like" for your unit. The organization adds what quality patient care looks like for your institution. The expectations your employer has of you come from a variety of levels and are found in a variety of places.

A job description will offer you the fastest clues as to your employer's expectations. Your job description will tell you your job classification (title), a brief description of the job, the specific qualifications for the job, to whom you report, and your functions and responsibilities in the job. It clarifies what your role is in contributing to the overall purpose of the organization. Weber (1978), "the father of modern bureaucracy," recognized the need for rules to guide bureaucracies and the need to break down an organizational purpose into tasks. Weber then proposed hiring only persons qualified to serve the organizational purpose for jobs described by these delineated tasks. Thus, your job description contains tasks essential to the organization's goals.

Your organization's job descriptions may list expectations very specifically, such as "obtains and documents a nursing history upon admission of each assigned patient through a planned interview." In this case, your learning needs are very clear—what form or format is used for the nursing history and for the documentation? Your organization may not have job descriptions that delineate your tasks quite clearly, and may state your job expectations very broadly, such as "uses the steps of nursing process to deliver quality patient care." If this is the case, other procedural documents may be available to clarify your job, "standards of care" that define "quality patient care" for your unit or organization.

Although very often much of your job expectation is explained to you in orientation, it is a good idea to know if and where expectations are written to serve as a resource to you as needed.

Reviewing policies and procedures may be helpful in understanding your job if you have broadly written job descriptions. Review policies and procedures related to the specific functions of your job. For example, if you want to know if it is your job to administer a certain type of chemotherapy drug, "who" can administer the drug is stated in a policy. Further, you can find "how" to administer the drug in a procedure. Policy and procedure manuals are located on each nursing unit.

Job descriptions in your organization may be in the form of a clinical ladder. Clinical ladders recognize the fallacy of the old concept "a nurse is a nurse" or "all nurses have the same skills." A clinical ladder differentiates and defines the clinical expectations of each nursing level. Of three or four levels, each one increases in responsibility and authority. Usually a Staff Nurse One is a new graduate. This person is still learning how to be a nurse in a particular organization. A Staff Nurse Two is a fully functioning staff nurse who performs the expected daily operational tasks of a nurse that are necessary to the organization's purpose. Staff nurses on levels three and four make additional contributions to the organization, often in the form of educational or beginning management functions. For example, a Staff Nurse Three or Four may conduct an inservice on developing a care plan for one of the unit's difficult patients or an update on care of a patient with a problem not usually, but currently, on that unit. A Staff Nurse Three or Four may have unit management responsibilities. She may be charge nurse for a particular shift or she may contribute to the organization through interdisciplinary committee or task force work, advising a clinical issue such as development of a policy addressing continuous morphine sulfate drip.

In addition to your job description and/or clinical ladder, you can find out about your employer's expectations by reviewing the organization's purpose and mission statement. These statements offer a broader perspective of your employer's expectations. They give you an overall sense of the organization's purpose and goals, and how your job fits into these goals. Stoner (1982) differentiates an organization's purpose from the organization's mission. According to Stoner (1982) "The *purpose* of an organization is its primary role as defined by the society in which it operates . . . a broad aim that applies not only to a given organization but to *all* organizations of its type in that society." It would seem obvious, then, that the purpose of a hospital is to provide health care. Your organization probably has this purpose stated in some way. Your role as a nurse in this organization is congruent with this health-care purpose.

The mission, according to Stoner, is "the unique aim that sets the organization apart from others of its type . . . it can be described in terms of the product and market—or the service and client served." For example, your organization may be a hospital that specializes in ambulatory care. With this mission, you need to consider again if you "fit" with the organization. Certainly nurses are needed in ambulatory care—the role is congruent. But if you are a pediatric nurse you may need to find out more about the patients this organization serves in order to determine if you belong there, that is, to see if your knowledge and skills match the organization's tasks.

You may be in a public corporation hospital, a community hospital, a university medical center, or a government hospital. Each of these organizations exists for the purpose of providing health care. Each has a mission to meet a wide range of health-care clients' needs, yet each may have a very different mission to meet in addition to providing health care. A public corporation hospital (whose stock is publicly traded) also has as its mission the making of profits in order to attract and keep its stockholders and thus to continue as a public corporation. A community hospital must define care based on local health-care needs considering community population descriptors such as *age*. For example, are more obstetric services or more gerontology services needed? A university medical center needs to conduct research and offer learning experiences for nursing and medical students. A government hospital may exist specifically to serve veterans or to perform research.

Your job as a nurse will change, based on these missions. The various organizations even have a different "feeling." University centers buzz with the academic activities of students, interns, residents, instructors, and researchers. Community hospitals often are less complex, smaller organizations where everyone may know each other. Public corporations may have more rigid materials management systems and lower staffing ratios. Recently, however, many of these differences have disappeared. Major economic constraints in health care have forced nonprofit hospitals to streamline their organizations and become more efficient. Due to technology, many community hospitals may have some areas of complexity surpassing similar areas in medical centers. And as negotiating and contracting for services becomes more common by third-party payers, even populations of patients are shifting. Because of these major changes in health care, your mission statement may not accurately reflect the current objectives of your organization unless it has been recently rewritten.

Another way of looking at your organization's mission is to ask, as Drucker (1974) does, "what is our business?" Satisfying the customer is the mission of every business, says Drucker. To know what the customer (patient) sees, thinks, believes, and wants, at any given time, and to meet those needs is the basis of customer satisfaction. As an employee with daily patient contact, your role is very important in carrying out the mission of the hospital. You can meet patient needs directly through nursing care and indirectly by communicating and coordinating patient needs with other members of the organization, such as dietitians, housekeepers, physicians, administrators, and so forth. You may do some of the communication directly and some indirectly through your supervisor.

Besides a purpose and a mission, organizations have objectives. An objective is a target ... more specific than a mission statement, in fact, the translation of the mission into specific, more concrete terms with measurable results. Objectives may be written on an organizational level, then made more specific on a unit level. For example, an objective by your organization might be "to provide quality patient care." Your orthopedic unit might define this in relation to total hip replacements.

Perhaps your hospital uses a planning system to address its future direction. This document also offers you clues about your job. The document also offers you clues about your job. The document may be in the form of a strategic plan, a Management by Objectives (MBO) system, or annual goals. These documents offer key current information relating to the larger picture of the expectations your employer has of you. By understanding this larger picture, you often have a better framework for performing in congruence with the organization in your day-to-day job.

Strategy is the "broad program for achieving an organization's objectives and thus implementing its mission" (Stoner, 1982). Strategy creates a unified direction for the persons in an organization. Strategy defines "how" the mission will be accomplished. According to Stoner, "every organization has a strategy—although not necessarily a good one—even if that strategy has not been explicitly formulated." If your organization has a written strategy or defined objective, you should read it and take some time to consider the implications of the organization-wide strategy on your own role. For example, if one objective for this year is related to cost containment, you may know of a less expensive way to provide care for a particular patient that will not reduce quality. You can take this information to your employer who may be able to help implement it. Or perhaps just recognizing the need to complete all your charge slips for your patients' supplies, or limiting how much you take into an isolation room that later may need to be discarded will help your organization reach its objectives.

In addition to the purpose, mission, objectives, and strategy statements that you explore, another way, in fact one of the best ways, of discovering what expectations your employer has of you, is to ask your employer. Ask the person to whom you report, "What are your expectations of a nurse on this unit? . . . What are your expectations of me?" Sheridan, Bronstein, and Walker (1984) suggest to head nurses that they should clearly communicate both their own philosophy of care and their specific expectations to their nursing staff. They list examples of some expectations a head nurse may have that should be made quite clear to her staff:

"I expect you to develop collegial relationships with physicians.

I expect you to model excellence in patient care on this unit.

I expect (or do not expect) extra supplies to be at a patient's bedside.

I expect overtime to be an exception.

I expect all patients to understand the medications they are taking.

I expect all nurses to take a lunch break off the unit."

If you are not receiving these clear messages, ask. These expectations are often less easily discovered than the more formal written "rules" found in job descriptions, policies, and procedures.

Asking about expectations others may have of you need not be limited to your employer. You should also ask colleagues, "What is expected from a staff nurse on this unit . . . *really?*" Or simply ask, "How will I succeed as a staff nurse on this unit?" The answers to these questions will lead you into a more difficult, but not less, important assessment to make regarding employer expectations. A key to surviving and thriving in a particular organization lies in understanding the cultural aspects of that organization.

Culture is defined by Short and Ferratt (1984) as "an elusive concept generally explained in terms of company-wide values and beliefs and the behaviors of employees resulting from them." Bower, former managing director of McKinsey and Company and author of the *Will to Manage,* describes corporate culture simply as "the way we do things around here" (Deal and Kennedy, 1982). Robson (1984) defines culture as a value system made up of customs that shape the company's self-image and mold its employees. It is a distinct personality that each institution develops and fosters over time (Savings and Loan News, 1983).

Understanding this informal part of the organization is essential to your success. Although you can't "look it up" in a policy or procedure manual, information about your new work setting's culture is available by asking questions, listening well, and observing behaviors. What do nurses wear? How detailed is shift report? What is included in a patient-care plan? How do employees help each other? Who can "get things done" with the laboratory or with housekeeping? How do you "win" the support of nursing assistants? Who goes where for lunch . . . and for how long?

If you don't bother to assess the culture of your organization and your unit, you will find out what it is by falling into "culture pits." A "culture pit" is the hole you fall into while blindly exploring the cultural terrain. It is the violation of a cultural norm. For example, perhaps the norm on a unit is to walk out of report and take vital signs. You think it would be more efficient to gather your treatment supplies and check IV solutions before you take your patients' vital signs at the beginning of your shift. A unit clerk who records vital signs likes to chart them within the first 15 minutes of the shift. Since yours are not completed by that time, she doesn't record them . . . nor does she communicate this to you. You don't find out that the signs are not recorded until later in the shift when there is a problem with a patient and information is not "where it is supposed to be."

Whether norms are good or bad, they *are,* they exist. Don't violate norms without being aware of the consequences. Sometimes if you disagree with a norm, you don't have to address it directly but can begin changing it in a less threatening way. For example, you notice no one uses the intercom to answer lights except night shift. They do it because they have less staff. You think this is the worst time to answer a light by intercom, intruding loudly into the darkness and frightening the patient or bothering a sleeping roommate. In lieu of telling others they "shouldn't do that," you might make yourself available to answer more lights in person and thus role model a more desirable behavior. Or you might open a friendly discussion with colleagues by saying, "I wonder how patients feel when we. . . ."

After exploring what is expected of you by your employer and by the organization, you should have a good idea of what your job is. You have considered expectations others have of you from organizational and unit levels. You have considered both formal, written expectations, such as your job description and purpose statement, and the informal, unwritten, expectations found in the culture and norms, or discovered through observations and questions. This clearer definition of your job will help you contribute to "getting a quality product out the door." Next, consider what you expect of your employer.

Expectations of the Employee

Remember your employer's job goes beyond "getting the quality product out the door." Your employer does this indirectly, through you, and therefore needs satisfied, willing and able, committed and enthusiastic employees, that is, motivated employees, to produce quality patient care. How does your employer try to motivate you? What can you expect from your employer?

Fitzgerald (1984) claims "the key in determining workers' needs and developing motivational programs or processes is the workers' own perceptions of their needs." What motivates *you* may not be a motivator for someone else. For example, you may enjoy the responsibility and accountability of a relatively autonomous primary care system to meet patient needs. Another nurse may prefer being part of a team and finds working in this more interdependent way with colleagues more rewarding. You may find caring for a greater number of patients more challenging than two clinically demanding, unstable patients or vice versa. You may want to represent your unit on a clinical task force seeing it as a change from routine and opportunity to help problem solve something important to you . . . or you may see the same assignment as "pulling you away from the bedside" and the reason why you are a nurse. Think about what motivates you. There will be opportunities, especially during orientation and performance appraisals, to let your employer know what motivates you. It is your responsibility to spend some time thinking about and communicating your motivators to your employer. Even the best employer cannot motivate someone else. The best the employer can do is help to supply the motivators to those employees who make them known.

After reviewing expectations of your employer and the organization as a whole, it is easier to think of motivators that not only meet your needs but also the needs of your organization. For example, if you would enjoy some management responsibilities, and your regular charge nurse is going on vacation, offer to fill in. Volunteer to help solve a problem related to dispensing of medication if you'd like to do more interdepartmental activities or if you'd like to see the problem solved. Watch for opportunities to meet your needs in a way that also meets your unit's or organization's needs—then offer to help.

Your employer, who is trying to understand what motivates you, may use Maslow's framework of needs to explore staff motivations. Maslow (1943) suggests that an unmet need is a motivator. He presents a hierarchy-of-need levels, claiming that lower-level needs must be met before higher-level needs can be met. Using this framework, your employer tries to understand your needs and meet them, beginning at the lower end of Maslow's hierarchy. For example, as a new employee, you may have relocated to take this job so you need to find suitable housing or even find the cafeteria for lunch. These are physiological needs, Level One, not uncommon to a new employee. Even an established employee has Level One needs, such as needs for lunch and coffee breaks. After Level One needs are met, according to Maslow, Level Two needs for safety and security become motivators. New employees want to find out how often and how much they are paid and figure out how to live within this constraint. Long-term employees may be interested in retirement benefits or how downsizing might affect their jobs. Level Three, social needs, are very important to new employees trying to understand and "fit" the culture of their new environment. Other social needs may be met by night shift potlucks or solving a unit problem over coffee with colleagues. Level Four needs are related to self-esteem and motivate employees to share expertise with each other through unit inservices or preceptorship of new graduates. Level Five, self-actualization needs, are creatively addressed by such programs as unit journal writing clubs, by unit-based nursing, and by designing new systems to increase unit quality or productivity.

No one stays on one level of the hierarchy but most people spend some time there. For example, you may move from Level Five to Level One an hour after lunch time when you still haven't received lunch relief as an operating room nurse. Often nurses enter a new organization with some Level One needs. However, most nurses spend most of their time between Level Three and Level Five. There are circumstances that can change this. If a hospital begins closing beds due to decreased revenue generation and layoffs result, the entire nursing staff may drop to safety-security needs and motivators should be aimed at this level.

Herzberg (1966) used the term "hygiene factors" to describe the two lower-level needs of physiology and safety/security. Herzberg claims employees are dissatisfied if lower level needs are not met. For example, health-care benefits are not adequate. However, meeting lower-level needs does not motivate or satisfy an employee. It merely removes dissatisfactions. Where health-care benefits are inadequate, adding benefits will remove this dissatisfaction. However, adding more and more health-care benefits after removing the dissatisfaction will not increase job satisfaction. Job satisfaction can only be increased by meeting upper-level needs. Removing dissatisfiers is essential to job satisfaction but will not, in itself, motivate employees. Satisfiers, according to Herzberg, will motivate employees after the dissatisfiers have been removed. Some job satisfiers you may want to seek out include greater autonomy, responsibility, and accountability. Remember that these satisfiers/motivators are different from one nurse to the next.

There are some consistencies mandated that address lower-level motivators. On a basic level, employees expect to be treated fairly. Over the years, fairness abuses by industry have led to unions and legal actions that now ensure basic employee expectations as legal rights. Personnel departments and union representatives (where there is a nursing union) can inform you of your rights should you have a grievance against your employer. In these situations it is important for you to seek assistance because both employee and employer must follow the policies and procedures exactly. Beyond basic fairness, another consistent factor in motivation that addresses higher level needs is stated by Fitzgerald (1984): "Workers will be motivated if they have jobs that make them feel good about themselves. Individuals need to feel they have a future in the organization and their work load must be perceived as reasonable."

Besides spending time thinking about what motivates you, think about the future in your organization. Look for "fits" between what the organization needs, what your employer expects, and what motivates you.

Performance Appraisal

Any deficits between the job expectations of your employer and your current abilities constitute your growth needs. You and your employer need to assess your strengths to do the job and how you "fit" with the unit and the organization. When you do not yet have the ability to do the job or to do it within your new setting, you and your employer need to plan together how you will gain this needed knowledge and/or skill. Identifying and planning how to meet the needs you have in this new job should be done with your employer. This establishes a baseline for your performance and for your future performance appraisals. Considering the organizational unit and patient needs along with your motivations should be part of a goal setting process with your boss. Setting goal priorities and realistic time frames are important to your success in growing and moving ahead. Your goals should include subgoals and feedback sessions with your employer so you can be sure you both have the same understanding of where you are going and how soon you will get there. Both of you should be clear about your goals and how you will accomplish them. Goals need to be stated in measurable, behaviorable terms and have realistic time frames with subgoals rewarded and celebrated along the way.

Performance appraisal sessions are your opportunity to share with your employer your perceptions about your progress. Together you can look at how you have grown and look for new goals or areas in which you need to grow. A performance appraisal session offers the opportunity to receive individualized feedback, a pat on the back, some shared concerns, and some chances to grow. Performance appraisals should not be a shock to either party. There should not even be surprises. If you have a problem, or see a problem developing, go to your employer and discuss it in a timely manner. Ask your employer to do the same with you.

Summary

One of the most important aspects of being a good employee is taking responsibility for yourself. Use your initiative to understand and "fit" into your organization—to grow, to learn, and to look for your own goals. Be proud of your profession and your organization and seek out ways to contribute—that's what makes a good employee.

Bibliography

Deal TE, Kennedy AA: Corporate Cultures. Menlo Park, CA, Addison-Wesley, 1982

Drucker PF: *Management Tasks, Responsibilities, Practices.* New York, Harper & Row, 1974

Fitzgerald P: Workers perceptions: The key to motivation. In Health Care Super, October, 1984

Herzberg F: Work and the Nature of Man. New York, World Publishing, 1966

Maslow AH: Motivation and Personality. New York, Harper & Row, 1959

Newmann E: Unpublished work. Survey of What Makes a Good Student and What Makes a Good Employee. New York, City College School of Nursing, 1986

Pol M: What makes a good employee. Stanford Nurse, Spring/Summer, 1986

Sheridan, DR: Bronstein JE, Walker DD: The New Nurse Manager: A Guide to Management Development. Gaithersburg, MD, Aspen Publications, 1984

Short E, Farratt TW: Working unit culture: Strategic starting point in building organizational change Manage Rev. August, 1984

Stoner JA: *Management,* 2nd ed. Englewood Cliffs, NJ, Prentice-Hall, 1982

Successful Mergers Require A Mesh of Corporate Cultures: *Savings and Loan News,* Vol 104, No 3, p 94 March, 1983

Weber M: Bureaucracy. In Shafritz JM, Whitbeck PH (eds) Classics of Organizational Theory. Oak Park, Ill, Moore Publishing, 1978.

Chapter 11

Strategies for professional success

KATHERINE W. VESTAL

Persons who enter nursing have made a choice. Entering the nursing profession is a decision to initiate a career in a field that offers numerous opportunities. The nursing field is growing, diversifying, and changing in such a way that nurses have almost limitless career options. The key to career success is deciding in which direction to go and then strategizing ways in which to reach your goals.

This chapter will enable you to

1. Describe the difference between a job and a career.
2. Construct a career map to serve as a development guide.
3. Prepare the tools, both written and as verbal presentations, necessary for career success.
4. Define the methods for career evaluation.

While career planning may sound easy, the diversity in nursing has, in fact, made it more difficult. Many nurses begin their professional life simply looking at a job. They soon find that there are many jobs and the decision is only which one to accept. Despite an over-supply of nurses in small geographic pockets, the general job situation for nurses remains good. There are jobs, although the hours or locale may not be ideal. Nevertheless, a nurse *can* get a *job*.

Then there are those nurses who want a *career*. A career is a means of finding professional growth, satisfaction, and self-fulfillment. More clearly stated, it is a progression of jobs that lead to rewards and recognition. Having a career implies a type of commitment that entails constant effort and progress toward achieving success. In order to know if you are successful, you must clearly understand what success means to you. Success is subjective; it is a set of achievements that you define for yourself. Persons often define success in terms of what others want, such as, "my mother wants me to teach nursing," or "my husband says the only way to make it is to be a manager." In the final analysis, the person who must define success is you. What are the achievements to which you aspire, and what measures will you use to know if you have arrived?

Another interesting facet of success is that it is dynamic. The criteria for success will probably change many times in your career. As you achieve one milestone you will reexamine your personal expectations and move forward. Or you may reach the point you strive for and discover that you no longer find it an indicator of success. So you rethink your goals.

Career planning and strategizing is an ongoing process that is a part of your overall professional activities. It should be looked upon as fun and an opportunity to be creative, to let others advise you, and to determine directions that you want to take. One thing is clear: no decision is in reality a decision; rather than actively participate in your own career planning, you let others do it for you. And you may not like the results.

Career development is not easy. A sense of cautious optimism is probably reasonable. It is a conscious and deliberate process that attempts to match the trends of the profession to the personal and life stages of the nurse, and to mesh these often divergent patterns into a planning model. Out of this analysis may come a contract with yourself about the pace you wish to pursue, the people you will impact, and the price you are willing to pay for your success. Many nurses find that the price, either in time, energy, or trade-offs is higher than they are willing to pay, and revise their career goals accordingly.

In a 1985 survey conducted by *RN* Magazine, nurses were asked why they entered the nursing profession. Job security and opportunities for professional advancement were both ranked high. The other reasons nurses work are to follow a strong drive toward a goal and to work at what they perceive is personally rewarding. From that standpoint, work can be the ultimate seduction in life. Work can become a passion, but that is not necessarily bad. If you find it to be rewarding, and are able to do it successfully, how can it be bad? A tendency to overwork is a risk that nurses take when embarking on a career. For some, becoming work directed is comfortable; for others, uncomfortable. Each person will adjust as she finds a way to balance her personal life and her professional life, or until they are one and the same.

Another important factor when considering a career in nursing is the rapidly growing health-care system. Models of delivery organizations and forms of nursing care are evolving at such a rapid rate that they will give rise to unprecedented opportunities. The economics of the time have placed increasing emphasis not only on cost containment, but also on innovation and the creation of new delivery models. As they have always been, nurses will be the framework for these systems. Nurses will venture more into nurse-controlled, nurse-owned, nurse-compensated, and special-function roles.[1]

Career strategizing requires a commitment to a future in nursing. The dilemmas of career women are inherent in a nursing career, but present many manageable challenges. Career moves are rewarding, fun, and always a part of a bigger picture. At the start of your career in nursing, begin to plan your strategies for success. All nurses are the same in that they want to do well, to progress, and to feel that they are making a difference. These aspects of career accomplishment are important and can be best accomplished with clear goal setting and career strategizing for success. A job may "just happen," but a successful career is made. The new graduate must determine how this can be done.

Career Development

When growing up, virtually no one has any idea what "career" means Inaccurate perceptions of what specific careers entail often keep persons from fully exploring options and, in the long run, they may be cheating themselves of rewarding experiences. Once a person does choose a career, she may find that even the good choices have many rough edges. Nurses may spend 6 to 8 years "getting into a role." Once they feel truly competent, they often become apprehensive. Suddenly they find themselves asking, "Is this all there is?" They feel they should be running the second lap, yet they don't know where to go.

Career anxieties are common. These anxieties play havoc with the amount of control a person wants over her life. Having high career expectations places pressure to move ahead very quickly. In addition, it is common knowledge that your future, in part, depends on helping your employer to succeed, so young workers tend to sacrifice a good deal to help ensure that the organization will succeed as well.

The work force in America today reveals interesting demographics. One half of the U.S. work force is now under 35 years of age, up from just over one third at the end of the 1950's. The work force is increasingly better educated. It is composed of flexible, mobile, and highly skilled workers who are intensely aware of the changes taking place in the labor markets.[2] Traditional wage structures have broken down and been replaced by new structures. Partly in response, young workers have become more interested than ever in acquiring new skills and are willing to change jobs, including location, to seize opportunities. In addition, they also tend to speak highly of their current employers. They may have their gripes but their post-depression work ethic has produced new attitudes toward employers. A new generation of young workers who have grown up with kaleidoscope changes are in the middle of these changes, learning whatever new skills they have to learn, moving a hundred or a thousand miles in order to find a job, keeping the wheels of the economy turning.

These trends are important when considering career development because the nursing profession as a whole, the health-care trends, and the national state of the economy are inextricably intertwined. The new nurse entering the work force must not only be competent, but must also be competitive with others who are vying for the same career advancement. Developing careers becomes a matter of strategy and good decisions, not a matter of luck. The nursing license is not a ticket to nirvana but rather to a way of life that can be as difficult as it is rewarding, and that comes with demands as well as privileges.

A CYCLICAL PROCESS

Career development is a cyclical process. It is a method not only of developing career options but also is a process of continual reassessment and redevelopment. The frequency of the reassessment and redevelopment will depend on your level of ambition, the pace at which your career is moving, and the changes that occur around you that may prompt you to reconsider your needs. So while you may occasionally assess your career position daily, it is more likely that you will formally assess it yearly.

The process of career strategizing is best compared to the nursing process. There are four basic components: assessment, definition of goals, implementation, and evaluation. These components will provide structure for the process that is necessary to avoid a cursory or shallow analysis of career issues. Being methodical in your analysis will yield higher quality results in the long run.

As a new nurse, career planning will provide you with a sound direction for the initial steps in your profession. In time, you may feel that your career is stalled and you may need to make considerable efforts in order to advance it.

Throughout the career development process, it is useful to keep in mind that there are three basic competencies necessary for success. The first is *analytical competence*. This is the ability to identify, analyze, and solve problems without complete information. The second is *interpersonal competence,* which is the ability to influence, supervise, and control behaviors, while the third is *emotional competence* or the capacity to be stimulated by emotional and interpersonal crises rather than be debilitated by them. These attributes will become the framework for career success, and the strategies will become the catalysts.

Career Mapping

Career mapping is a method of creating a master plan. Similar to the strategic plan that is developed by a business, a career plan can serve as a map for your career advancement. Persons rarely take adequate time to plan and, consequently they react haphazardly to opportunities that arise. Just because an opportunity becomes available does not mean that it will fit into your personal plan for your career.

A career master plan should serve as a methodical future mapping system. It can prescribe whether or not you will need more education, what types of experience are necessary to meet your goals, and it can identify targets for income that you want to reach. These plans pinpoint opportunities in your own field, project potential opportunities in other fields, and define career movement patterns. They can also provide direction concerning the type of networking you will need, professional association involvement, and continuing education requirements. In addition, the plan introduces the element of time, in that certain career stages should be achieved, within set time limits. The element of time is important because it can easily elude you until you suddenly realize that too many years have passed with no real advancement. Then you become frustrated at an outcome you could very well have controlled.

CAREER FOCUS: NARROW OR BROAD

A frequent dilemma of the new nurse is how to choose a clinical area in which to work. The educational experience has provided many diverse clinical experiences, most of which you liked. So how can you possibly pick just one area in which to work?

First of all, recognize that your first job is just that—a *first* job. You will hold many others in your career, each of which will enrich your total nursing knowledge. So look at the initial job as the first opportunity in a series of many.

Second, new nurses often face the dilemma of the pressure to specialize in a narrowly focused area. This, too, can be dealt with by assuming that the decision to develop a narrow or broad focus will evolve through your dynamic career planning. The ultimate need for a broad background may already be evident, but a current practice that is narrow may well suit the situation. For example, if your goal is to be a director of maternal child services and you know this will require a broad base of experience in all maternal and pediatric services, it is understandable why your first job will be in labor and delivery. You must start somewhere. Later, the planning for broad experience will be critical to career development.

PRODUCING A MAP

The process of producing a map involves four steps: 1) accessing your skills and interests; 2) determining your goals; 3) creating a map, and 4) developing strategies to support the map. These processes are simple and in the end produce a written plan that you can reflect on, and that you can share with others for their advice.

Assessing Your Skills and Interests

As a new nurse, it is particularly important that you realistically determine your present set of skills. Initially, you may assess that they are few, but upon closer examination you should find that you have a long list. This list may look like a basic inventory of strengths and interests.

Table 11-1.   List of Skills and Interests

SKILLS	INTERESTS
Interest in people, especially children	Pediatrics
Easy to establish rapport	Families in crisis
Good knowledge of nursing process	All MCH areas
Great skill at writing nursing care plans	Management of people
Good communication skills	Learning new things
ICU nursing skills good	
Even-headed in crisis	
Good organizational skills	
Able to manage time well	

It is important to write down these items and make the lists as detailed as possible (as done in Table 11-1). You will utilize this information not only for the map but also for interviews.

Determining Your Goals

Next, you must give thought to what you want to accomplish. This may be done in the form of a one-year, five-year, or ten-year plan. Some new nurses are absolutely certain of their ultimate career goals when they enter the profession, while others are quite confused. Knowing that this plan is dynamic and can be changed any time you want, permits you to establish goals and develop a plan without feeling committed forever.

Creating a Map

The map should begin with where you are now and end with your goal. The steps outlined in between will be those steps you will need to take, in terms of experience and education, in order to meet your goals.

A typical career map is seen in Table 11-2. Notice that the new nurse starts in a staff nurse position, and ultimately aspires to be a director of maternal child nursing in 10 years. This seems to be a reasonable goal that could be met if all of the preparatory elements were accomplished. Obviously, this nurse will need varied clinical experiences, additional education, and hard work to meet the goal. The map shows that she worked and went to school for her master's degree at the same time in

Table 11-2.   A Ten Year Career Map

EXPERIENCE YEARS	2 YRS.	2 YRS.	1 YR.	2 YRS.	3 YRS.	YEAR 10
New Graduate B.S.N.→	Labor and Delivery→	Postpartum Staff Nurse→	Pediatric Staff Nurse→	Pediatric Head Nurse→	Pediatric ICU Head Nurse→	Director MCH
Education	MCH Continuing Education		Masters in MCH		Management Continuing Education	

order to reach her 10-year goal. If she had elected to stop working in order to go to school, her experience factor would be different, or the time factor would need to be lengthened to compensate.

If the map were designed to prepare a teacher, or clinical specialist, or home health care nurse, the process would be the same. Determining the goals and then putting a map on paper is essential in converting dreams to realities.

Developing Strategies to Meet the Goals

Once the goals and map are in a form that can be shared, it is useful to talk to other persons about it. Ask nurses who have accomplished goals similar to yours how they did it and what advice they could give you. Explore educational programs, both formal degree and continuing education, to determine your options. Will you have to move to another area in order to get either the experience or the education?

Then develop an active list of activities to be accomplished, such as special skills to be learned, leadership roles to fill, ways to achieve visibility in the organization, and ways in which you can market yourself in a positive manner. These plans can be incorporated into an overall strategy for developing your career.

Sounds like a lot of work? It may be, but compare it to the amount of work you will do that may not contribute to your career goals if you don't have a plan. This time will be well spent and may save you years of random progress.

LATERAL OR DOWNWARD MOVEMENT

Lateral and downward movement is becoming a more openly employed and less stigmatized method of managing people in today's changing organizations. In fact, under certain circumstances, lateral and downward movement can be good for you as well as for the organization.

With the movement of the baby boom generation into the ranks of middle management and mid-level roles in organizations, a phenomenon of slow upward movement has developed. The youth of the work force and the economic recession are also factors that have provided fewer available jobs for young people, resulting in tight upward mobility. Recognizing these factors is important in career planning, because if a specific experience requirement exists and constant upward involvement is not possible, both lateral and downward moves may be the answer.

In your parents' career, lateral or downward movement indicated that career growth was virtually over and advancement unlikely. In *your* career period, this stigma should not prevail because the job market and organizational designs are drastically different. Instead of dwelling on whether a move is up, down, or sideways, focus on whether or not the *experience* is essential to your career plan. If that experience is *essential* for your future plans, then there is no question that you should pursue it. A temporary lateral move to put you in a better position for future growth is a small price to pay now for a much larger reward later. For example, in the case of the nurse striving for the MCH role, if she had not had labor and delivery experience, which is essential for the role, she may have had to return to a role as L&D staff nurse after her tenure as a pediatric head nurse. A one year "downward move" as L&D staff nurse would prepare this nurse for the role of director. One year is not a high price to pay. By keeping the long-range goal in mind, the stops along the way make sense. Thinking long term shows that you are willing to delay gratification and take risks. You will take a job that is not easy because you understand that you need the experience.

IS MANAGEMENT THE ONLY WAY UP?

Another dilemma often faced by nurses is their perception that the only road to advancement is through managerial jobs. Obviously this is not true, but this misconception can easily be assumed when looking at many hospitals and clinical settings. It would be nice to believe that all health-care institutions have also developed routes upward through clinical work, education, and research but it still remains a phenomena of a few enlightened organizations.

This is why it is important to map your career. If you can clearly show your goals as that of education or research or clinical work, then you can plan your moves accordingly. Becoming a manager only because you want a promotion will generally result in disaster. Like all work, you must enjoy it to do well.

In order to progress in other areas you may have to select for work an organization that has those tracks for advancement. Or you may need to find alternative career options such as consulting, or specialty companies, or self-employment. Don't buy into the idea that management is the only way up until you do some research to validate or invalidate your assumptions.

Tools for Career Building

Career building is a composite of theory, practice, and evaluation. Designing a career entails an enormous amount of time and energy, and even more to implement one. There are several critical tools that are essential in career progress. These include developing a professional presence, presenting yourself in writing, and promoting yourself in person. These factors are often critical in whether or not you progress.

DEVELOPING A PROFESSIONAL PRESENCE

It is probably not possible to define the term "presence." It is a subjective feeling that one either has or does not have. If a nurse has "presence," she can enter a room, and everyone will know she is there before any words are spoken. A nurse with presence always projects a professional image through her attire, her language, and her conduct. Nurses with this nebulous quality of presence can work at the staff level or the executive level; they may be in positions of little or great power. Presence is not a function of role, but rather a function of demeanor.

A useful way to look at presence is to identify those persons who, you think, possess this quality. Then analyze the behaviors they exhibit that promote this aura, and decide which of those behaviors might be useful for you. Individualize them to fit *your* personality. The aura of presence can be learned, and in fact, *must* be learned for career success.

Research has shown that attractive people are generally viewed positively and this attitude follows over into the job market. That does not mean that you have to look like a model, but grooming, from hairstyle to clothing, will be paid as much attention as your resumé. You should dress for the role you want to play on the job. Research has shown that recently graduated students who dressed more formally for job interviews were noticeably more assertive. They believed that they made a favorable impression on the interviewers.

Career confidence requires that you no longer act like a student when you are looking for a job. Career confidence means you are ready to step forward without stepping on the wrong toes. Positive attitudes rather than super aggressive methods work best. Think through the encounters you are about to have, plan as many details as possible, and be mentally prepared to deal with the mini-crisis that may occur. Above all, be as calm, cool, and collected as possible. It helps promote your image as a true professional, at ease with your new role.

PRESENTING YOURSELF IN WRITING

A great portion of your professional life will involve writing. The writing may be clinical, as with nurses' notes or nursing care plans; managerial, as with memos or requests, or educational as you develop teaching plans and tools, or research-oriented materials. In addition you will be required to perfect the act of personal writing in the form of letters and thank you notes. An often overlooked business tactic, the thank you note should be carefully examined from the standpoint of both etiquette and business.

The habit of writing a note to persons you meet at a conference, colleagues who help you with a problem, or to let someone know you are aware of a recent accomplishment is a powerful tool in business. Thank you notes are appropriately written after interviews to reiterate your interest in the job, and to thank the interviewer for her attention. This is an important way to keep your name up front.

Another important written presentation is the resumé. An essential tool when applying for a job, the resumé is useful for many other professional activities as well, so spending time to develop a concise resumé is essential.

The Resumé

The resumé is a summary of your qualifications and accomplishments and contains a concise account of your work history, interests, and goals. The *curriculum vitae* (CV) is a form of resumé used mostly in academic circles to summarize educational, professional, and scholarly accomplishments. While the two terms, resumé and CV, are generally used interchangeably, this text will use the term "resumé."

A resumé will be presented to prospective employers or others who want a concise history of *you*. It summarizes years of pertinent experience in a few pages. While many persons advocate a one page resumé, as your accomplishments accumulate it may be impossible to condense the information into one page and still do yourself justice. Be as concise as possible, but at the same time mention all important aspects of your career.

The format of a resumé may vary but it must look professional and be accurately typed on a top quality paper; these are essentials. There are many books that show different formats for resumés. Select the format that appeals to you; after all, it is your personal career tool. More important, make sure that all the information is completely honest, correct, and complete. Misrepresentation of information is easy to spot, and can lead to immediate dismissal.

Information Files. It is important to begin immediately to keep accurate files of your accomplishments so that you can easily retrieve information when it is needed. While you may update your resumé only once a year, it is necessary to keep the information needed for updating in a safe and convenient place. A simple means of doing this is to use a manila folder labeled "Personal File 1987." Place all pertinent pieces of information into this file, such as brochures of programs you attended during that year, copies of projects you developed, important letters, and so forth. On the file cover list the committees of which you are a member, professional organization involvement, and speeches you may have made. At the end of 1987, file the folder in a safe place, and start a new one for 1988.

In this way, you will always be able to reconstruct important activities of each year. You may rewrite your resumé many times to refocus it, and accurate information is essential. There is always a tendency to forget details and without solid data it will be impossible to reconstruct your career activities over time.

Resumé Information. The resumé is your personal marketing tool, so you must make important decisions about what you want to include in it. There are no rules that dictate content. For example, if you want to include your age and feel that it will be helpful to you, do so. If you feel it would be detrimental, do not.

The basic components of a resumé are your name, address, phone, education, experience, continuing education, honors, professional work and personal interests. These components can be arranged in any order, but keep in mind that the reader will go from top to bottom and left to right on the page. So strategically arrange the information that is most important to you. An example of a resumé for a new nurse is seen on the opposite page.

Note that Mary Smith, R.N. is applying for her first job in nursing, so her resumé is designed to reflect that goal. After more experience, Mary will redo the resumé, adding new material. In future years, her resumé goal will read "to become director of maternal child nursing in a large teaching hospital."

At the present time, Mary's job experience in retailing and as a student nurse are included because they reflect her ambition and accomplishments as a valuable employee. Again, as years of nursing experience grow she may elect to start her chronicle of work experience with her first professional nursing job and to add committee work and other professional activities.

In summary, resumés are important tools for career success. Be sure they are free of typographical errors or misspelled words, and that they

A Resumé

MARY A. SMITH, R.N.
1206 Edison
Houston, Texas 77000

PERSONAL DATA:

Birthdate: 6/27/63
Place of Birth: North Carolina
Marital Status: Single
Health: Excellent

PROFESSIONAL GOAL:

To practice as a staff nurse in Labor and Delivery.

EDUCATION:

Place	Degree	Year
University of Texas	B.A. English	1983
University of Kansas	B.S.N.	1987

OCCUPATIONAL EXPERIENCE:

Sales Associate, Neiman Marcus, Dallas	1980–1983
Student Nurse, Kansas General Hospital	1984–1987
(Worked as staff on weekends)	

PROFESSIONAL MEMBERSHIPS:

American Nurses Association	1987–present
Sigma Theta Tau	1987–present

CONTINUING EDUCATION:

Nurses Role in High Risk Delivery	University of Kansas	1985
NAACOG Convention	Atlanta, Ga.	1986
Grand Rounds in OB	University of Kansas	Monthly

INTERESTS:

Writing articles for publication
   Painting
   Marathon running

References Upon Request

are absolutely accurate in content. Top quality originals and copies are essential, and are easy to make, using the word processors available today.

Cover Letters.   A cover letter to a prospective employer should accompany your resumé. This cover letter serves to introduce you, express your interest in the organization, and explain briefly what you can offer it. Like the resumé, it should be flawlessly typed, professionally constructed, and addressed to the *proper person.* (See the sample opposite.)

Asking for information to be sent to you ensures a reply and will be an indication to you that your letter has received some attention. You want to follow up with a phone call.

PRESENTATION IN PERSON

Presenting yourself *in person* to an employer typically happens in the form of a job interview. This is a structured discussion, usually taking place in the work setting, in which you assess the organization and it assesses you. What each of you is probing are strengths, weaknesses, and the potential "fit" within the organization. Depending on the job, any interview could have different formats, such as the individual interview, serial interviews, group interviews, stress interviews, and reinterviews. It is important that you be prepared for the interview and know in advance the form it may take, so that you can be prepared.

Individual Interview

This is a one-on-one interview, usually between a nurse recruiter or nurse manager and you. During a specified amount of time, each of you will have the opportunity to ask and answer questions. Because you may be nervous, it is helpful to write out your questions in advance and take notes during the interview. It is easy to say "I'm a little nervous and I want to be sure I remember the things we discuss. Would you mind if I make notes as we go along?" Then take only the notes necessary to trigger your memory—do not take notes as if you were attending a lecture. Eye contact and interaction with the interviewer is imperative.

This interview should include a brief tour of the area in which you may work, and an overall discussion of work benefits. It may not include salary negotiations, especially if there are other interviews to follow.

Enter the interview with confidence and with professional presence. At the end, if you feel that certain aspects of the interview did not go well, review and rehearse these points before your next interview. There should be few surprises in the interview because the questions are almost standard:

A Cover Letter

1206 Edison
Houston, Texas 77000
January 1, 1987

Dr. Sandra Smith, R.N.
Vice-President for Nursing
General Hospital
Salem, California 44000

Dear Dr. Smith:

   I am interested in joining a progressive nursing organization that has a need for my skills and can provide opportunities for my professional growth. I understand that the Maternal Child Services at General Hospital offer opportunities that meet my interests.

   I have a B.S.N. from the University of Kansas. The attached resumé further outlines my qualifications. As you will note, I am seeking an entry level position as a labor and delivery nurse, but would be willing to discuss other MCH openings you may have. I would eventually like to progress to a nursing management role in the MCH field.

   If you would like to discuss my experience in detail, I would be glad to come for a personal interview. I would appreciate receiving information about your hospital, and in particular its nursing organization.

   I look forward to hearing from you.

Sincerely,

Mary A. Smith R.N., B.S.N.

Enclosure

- Why do you want to work *here?*
- What are your strengths and weaknesses?
- What are your nursing goals?
- What will you bring us as a professional nurse?

In turn your questions should focus on the organization and what it can offer you, its promotional policies, career philosophies, orientation practices, and commitment to professional growth.

The important thing is to relax and let the interviewer structure the meeting. However, be sure you have met your own informational needs before you leave. In addition, determine when you can next expect to hear from the organization and when it can expect to hear from you.

Serial Interviews

These interviews are designed to reduce the risk of hiring the wrong person. In this situation all of the major individuals you will work with interview you. This may include persons from personnel, recruitment, nursing, and administration. While serial interviews are uncommon for staff nurse positions, they are frequently utilized as you move up in the organization. The interviewers generally ask questions that have a specific job relationship within their area of responsibility. They want to be sure you have the knowledge but, more important, that you "fit in."

Serial interviews can sometimes get out of hand with as many as 15 to 25 persons interviewing the candidate before a job offer is made. Advice for serial interviews is to be sure you are consistent throughout the many sessions and that you treat each interviewer as if he were the key person in the decision-making process.

Group Interviews

These interviews are frequently used in the health care profession and involve meeting with 5 to 20 persons at one time. Each person may have been assigned an area of questioning, or the interview may simply be an open session. A group interview can be a useful test for a job that requires sophisticated communication skills or people skills. Your strategies should include frequent eye contact with each person and projection of a professional but relaxed manner.

Stress Interviews

A few years ago stress interviews were popular. The theory was that, by subjecting candidates to a stressful situation, their ability to react properly under stress was tested. For example, while the candidate was filling out an application, persons would interrupt or create distractions, then watch to see the applicant's reaction. The problem with stress interviews was that top candidates were often turned off and could not imagine why an organization would subject prospective employees to such treatment. If you are subjected to a stress interview, project self assurance, and remain poised. Recognize it as a test, not a personal affront.

Reinterviews

It is common today for organizations to request a reinterview after some initial screening has taken place. Once all applicants have been seen, the top three or four are called back for interviews that are more precisely focused. Treat all the interviews as essential. They are a valid means of selecting qualified employees. The time lapse between the initial interview and the actual hiring may be much longer than you anticipate. Check back often with the organization to determine if you are still under consideration. Never assume you are not until you receive confirmation that you are no longer a candidate.

Presenting yourself professionally in writing and in person are essential tools for success. Prepare your written materials carefully before mailing them. Practice your interview skills, arrive on time, and participate enthusiastically. The organization will make every effort to select the applicant with the most interest and potential. You want to be that person!

THE NEXT STEP: PROMOTION

Every nurse who strategizes for career advancement looks forward to the day when she is promoted. A promotion involves the same process of submitting your resumé, interviewing, and competing for a job. Only this job provides upward mobility rather than entry level possibilities. The stakes may be higher in that you might be an internal candidate vying for promotion over your peers or competing directly with a colleague for the job.

It is important to recognize that the organization will want to select the best candidate for the job and that while being an internal candidate may offer an initial advantage it will not ensure promotion. You must be competitive and meet the new job requirements, just as all other candidates must. So the same factors of education, experience, maturity, and other requisite skills will come into play. In addition, there will be the inevitable and ever present office politics.

If you are seeking promotion, you must take an active part in your own career planning. You must also have a clear view of your immediate supervisor's views. Assuming added responsibility, establishing and pursuing goals, and acquiring the education needed at the next job level will contribute toward your chances of advancement. If chosen for the job, you will experience excitement, challenge and, ultimately, opportunities to advance even further.

You can increase possibilities of promotion by being visible and promoting yourself in strategic ways. The more persons who know who you are, what you do, what you know, and what you can offer, the more opportunities will come to you. These new opportunities are crucial to your success, so become comfortable talking about yourself; regard self-promotion as a benefit to others.

An important aspect of self-promotion is to market yourself, rather than merely bragging. Prepare by writing down every possible detail about yourself; and become adept at retrieving such information when it is needed. Describe in detail *who* you are, what you do, what you know, and what you want. Probe deeply to find the heart of the information, your values, attitudes, enthusiasm, and confidence.

Evaluating Job Offers

If you are offered a new job, you will need a way to determine whether or not it is an advantage to you to accept the position. Ginsberg recommends the seven C's for systematically assessing realistic job opportunities.[3]

1. *Content of the position:* Will this train and position me for advancement?
2. *Challenge of the position:* Is the challenge too much, too little, just right?
3. *Climate of the position itself and within the organization:* The work environment is critical to success.
4. *Chemistry:* What is your feeling about how well you will get along with your immediate supervisor?
5. *Concern for results and people:* What importance does the organization place on those who work for it?
6. *Compensation:* Is the total monetary package with benefits satisfactory for you?
7. *Community:* Is the job in a community where you would want to live?

In the final analysis, when making a critical decision about a new job, be sure you possess as many facts as possible. Just because the job is offered to you does not mean you should accept it. Weigh the factors carefully before making a decision.

If You Are Passed Over

Being passed over for promotion can be a big disappointment. You felt you were the perfect choice, and now feel rejected and slated for obscurity in the organization. How can you recover and go on to be highly productive, a candidate for future promotions?

It is helpful to have open communication with your supervisor during the entire selection process. He is in a position to diffuse some of your distress and reassess your current role in the organization. Assuming he wants you to continue to work in that capacity, it is useful to seek the counseling or assistance needed to deal with your feelings.

Then work with your supervisor to evaluate options for increased involvement in your own work setting. Assume more responsibility or new opportunities so that you feel you are still progressing. Talk with the persons who did *not* hire you in a candid, nonthreatening manner, in order to determine the areas in which you were not competitive. Using this information, shore up your deficiencies. Then you will be ready the next time! The employee who is passed over is by no means passed by, and opportunities in the future will arise.

CHANGING JOBS

All nurses will change jobs at some point in their career, and probably at many points. Changing jobs may not necessarily mean changing organizations, because it is possible, over time, to have many roles in the same organization. However, some job changes may involve going to a new setting, a different part of the country, or entering a new facet of the health care field. These changes can be positive experiences if handled well, or negative if handled poorly.

In the past persons who changed jobs too frequently (that is, more than 3 times in 5 years) were regarded as job-hoppers. This stigma often made employers reluctant to hire the individual for fear they would invest significant resources in training and orientation, and never reap long-term productivity. However, in the past few years the economy and business world have dictated a new set of circumstances. It is common now to see mergers, acquisitions, closures, and consolidations, all of which lead to a reduction in staff. Persons lose jobs more frequently, and the search in the job market is more fluid.

Thus, the nurse who changes jobs must have a clear statement about why the changes occurred. Was the job change due to an organizational restructuring that eliminated your position, or to career development needs, or to a relocation? As long as the explanation is factual and plausible there is little problem. However, if you have changed jobs 3 times because you didn't like your supervisor, the prospective employer will look more critically at you.

Job Dissatisfaction

Job dissatisfaction may one day become a reality for you. It may be that you lose interest in your job, or that the demands are too high for the rewards. Or it may be that you envision yourself in a different role or setting. Whatever the reason for your dissatisfaction, the result will be that you begin to search for another job. Statistically, persons change jobs at least 3 times in their worklife.

Be sure you distinguish *job* dissatisfaction from *career* dissatisfaction. In the former, you change jobs and put your current knowledge and skill to work in a different milieu. In the latter, the nature of the work itself, the tasks to be performed, the purpose to be served, have become so distasteful that you begin to think about a different career. Often nurses mistakenly believe they are dissatisfied with nursing as a career, when in the final analysis a problem exists simply with their current job. Obviously, the answer for each dilemma is vastly different.

In the case of job dissatisfaction, you must take time to analyze the cause of the dissatisfaction. Otherwise, it is highly probable that you may change jobs and find the same set of circumstances in another setting. What are the causes of your problems? Goal blockage? Uncertain expectations? Contradictory demands? Poor relationships with coworkers? Organizational restrictions? Policies of the institution? Recognition gaps? A sense of being overworked or undervalued? The answers to these questions will help you determine whether the problem is simply job dissatisfaction or a more serious discontent—career dissatisfaction.

Risk Management in Career Planning

The concept of risk management that you are familiar with in health-care delivery can also be applied to the management of your career. There are five steps involved in this process:[4]

1. *Risk Identification:* What is important in your life and how can you posture yourself for success, rather than increased risk? By identifying where you want to be at certain stages of your career, you can then identify those issues that might prevent you from reaching each plateau.
2. *Risk Evaluation:* After you identify the risks, you can estimate the probability of an adverse outcome due to the risk.
3. *Opportunity Identification:* Besides identifying potential risk situations, you can identify and evaluate potential opportunities.
4. *Implementation:* Once action steps are identified, you can be in control of your career progress. Timing is an important factor and one that should be given due consideration.
5. *Monitoring:* Since situations can change, and a decision made on today's facts may not hold up tomorrow, you must try to keep on

top of events as far as career risks and opportunities are concerned. Once you set up a monitoring process, it is important to use it.

Acting Roles

One job opportunity that needs special explanation is the "acting role." This is a situation in which you assume a temporary role or responsibility without an official title or commitment. There are advantages and disadvantages to accepting an "acting" role, and as long as you understand both components clearly you can make a good decision.

First of all, keep in mind that an acting role is not the real thing. It is considered "acting" because the supervisor is not in a position or not ready to commit the job to you in total. Being asked to take a job is seductive and you can easily be caught up in the glamour and drama of perceived advancement, when in reality the advancement is not permanent.

The issue of permanency is at the heart of the problem when considering an acting role. While you may gain valuable experience, and may actually be an official candidate, there is always the risk that you will not get the job. Not being selected for the job on a permanent basis means you must return to your former job, if it is still there, and become a peer once again to persons who were for a time subordinates.

This is difficult. In addition, the person who has acquired the job on a permanent basis may resent you because you still retain some of the characteristics of supervisor but have moved back to a subordinate position. That places you at great risk with the new person who is himself struggling to assume power.

So when assuming an "acting" role, be sure you know what is to be gained—experience, a chance to prove yourself, another level of visibility—and what is to be lost—you may have to leave the setting when the acting role is over, or you may find you liked the role so much you do not wish to return to your former status. If you assume an acting role, determine how long you are to fill the role—6 months or 1 year—so that the supervisor will have a time frame and impetus to hire a permanent person.

If you do assume an acting role, you cannot view every decision as if it were temporary. Expand your resource base, nurture new contacts, and visibly do the job well. Be sure you negotiate the title you will use and any compensation changes you desire. Once you accept the "acting" role your ability to negotiate options diminishes dramatically.

When You Quit

Quitting a job is a highly sensitive and political act. Never think that the quitting process is any less important than the hiring process. The way you behave at the end of a job will be what persons will remember about you. Plainly put, no matter what the reason for your leaving may be, the process should be professional, discrete, and well thought-out.

Often a person who quits a job is in the midst of great emotional turmoil. It is immaterial whether this is a result of disappointment, rage, or righteous indignation. No matter how "right" you are about leaving, the only memory among coworkers will be the style with which you depart. Keep in mind the old adage that "the organization will survive." This should emphasize to you that although you feel that "they can't survive without you," in fact, they will!

So whether your departure is positive or negative, it is important that you conduct the process in such a manner that you are viewed as a professional, well-mannered person.

Review the personnel policies carefully and understand the procedures to follow for severance of employment. Such details as the required number of days' notice and the required actions that must be taken are important and may determine your future eligibility for rehire. Keep in mind that organizations change, and that while you may not think you would ever rejoin that organization, you never know. So do not burn bridges, and carefully meet the termination requirements.

You will need to submit in writing a note to your supervisor indicating that you will be leaving, the exact date, and a brief explanation stated in a positive manner. A positive statement about your time on the job or your reluctance to leave is appropriate. Do not make the mistake of using the letter of resignation as a place to vent your litany of complaints. After all, this letter goes in *your* personal file and could be used adversely in the future.

If you want to air your concerns, do so in an exit interview. Make an appointment with the appropriate persons to discuss your reasons for leaving and share your feelings. In this way, you have your say, you inform them of issues, but you do not place the problems in your permanent file.

EVALUATION OF CAREER PROGRESS

Evaluation is a critical part of career success but is usually the area in which you tend to spend the least amount of time. Evaluation is important because it reminds you of how well you are doing, where you need improvement, and keeps you cognizant of needs for additional development.

Evaluation takes place at many points, and should be consciously recognized as such. For example, each time you update your resumé, look it over carefully for gaps and needs. Arrange to round out your experiences, so as to round out your resumé. At the time of your annual employee evaluation you have an opportunity to consider your strengths and needs, and discuss them candidly with you supervisor. As you review your career map annually, the areas for development should be quite clear.

Additionally, you may want to review your accomplishments and aspirations with mentors, colleagues, and superiors. Talk with your teachers and other professionals about opportunities. Never assume you can build a career by yourself because it is ultimately the result of your contributions to a bigger entity; assistance from others will support your career growth.

Your career evaluation should take place at least annually in a formalized and comprehensive manner. If you do not do so, the years are likely to slip by and you will find yourself looking back and wondering how time got away from you. Career success requires strategizing and restrategizing. It is the evaluation process that allows you to keep on track in both role and time.

SUMMARY

Most careers, no matter how carefully planned and executed, include a number of surprises, both pleasant and unpleasant. Most persons tend to attribute the happy events, promotions, and rewards to their own capabilities; they place the blame for unpleasant happenings such as job problems, demotions, or dead-end positions as circumstances beyond their control or the fault of others. Nurses must begin to see that most career developments reflect not only their own performance, but also their relationships with other persons and the circumstances of the particular time.

Career advice usually focuses on keeping your options open and being prepared to take advantage of promising opportunities. For a successful career, however, a strong commitment must be made to the task at hand; sooner or later a heavy investment of intellectual and emotional energy will be needed.

The sooner a new nurse gains a positive perspective of her career the better. Early planning can result in better outcomes. While nurses know that all careers have ups and downs, the intent of career strategizing is to maximize the ups and minimize the downs. With the overwhelming amount of change and turmoil in health care today, it is important that new nurses begin to develop a clear vision of where they are headed. Otherwise, the chances of becoming a victim of the confusion are great.

Career strategizing is a formal, informal, and methodical process. It takes time, energy, and commitment to the concept. But considering the alternative of being adrift in an uncertain environment, the time is well spent. New nurses who understand this concept can do a good deal in charting their careers. The chances of success are phenomenal. After all, isn't that the goal of every nurse? Success is no accident; it is planned every step of the way.

REFERENCES

1. Coleman J, Dayani E, Simms E: Nursing careers in the emerging systems. Nurs Manage, p 19, January 1984
2. Brody M: Meet today's young American worker. Fortune, p 90, November 1985
3. Ginsburg S: Evaluating job offers: Seeking the seven C's. Super Manage, p 25, May 1983
4. McEwan B: The risk management approach to career planning. Super Manage, p 12, January 1984

BIBLIOGRAPHY

Arrington C: Lies from the locker room. Savvy, p 35, July 1982

Blotnick S: The Corporate Steeplechase: Predictable Crises in A Business Career, Facts on File, 1984

Browdy JD: Career planning for the newly appointed health care supervisor Health Care Super. 3(4): p 31–41, July 1985

Burton C, Burton D: Job expectations of senior nursing students, JONA, p 11, March 1982

Day C: The who, how, when, and why of the promotion decision: A middle management perspective in hospitals. Hosp Health Serv Adm p 31, July 1983

Drodney DL: For professional advancement: Your resumé. Nurs Manage 15(8), p 13, April 1984

Hall D, Isabella L: Downward movement and career development. Organizational Dynamics, p 5, 1985

Horton T: Self management: Key to knowing where to go and how to get there. Manage Rev, p 2, July 1984

Kaye B: Six paths for development. Nurs Manage 13(5), p 18, May 1982

Larwood L, Gattiker U: Study shows first job is key to career success. AMA Forum 73(7), p 29, July 1984

Lee N: Targeting The Top. New York: Doubleday, 1980

Levenstein A: Career dissatisfaction. Nurs Manage, p 61, November 1985

Lewis H: Specialism: The best career path? RN, p 40, June 1984

Margerism C, Kakabadse A: How American chief executives succeed. AMA Survey Report, 1984

Mendelson R: Female career development. Occup Health News 33(4): 194–196, April 1985

Nurse Executive Managing Strategies: Career Advancement for RN's in Hospitals, Part I, No. 6. American Hospital Association Publication, Division of Nursing, 1984

Robinson-Smith G: Alternative Careers in Nursing. Nurs Econom 2(1):23–24, January/February 1984

Scott P: Executive career planning. Nurs Econom 2:58, January/February 1984

Smith M: Career development in nursing: An individual and professional responsibility. Nurs Outlook, p 128, February 1982

Spitzer R: The nurse in the corporate world. Super Nurs, p 21, April 1981

Strickler J: Resumé preliminaries. The Executive Female, p 29, March/April 1984

Strickler J: Resumé preliminaries. The Executive Female, p 29, March/April 1984

Sullivan EJ, et al: Management screening in an assessment center. Nursing Success Today 2(1): 31–34, 1985

Taking the fast tract to nowhere. Manage Rev, p 55, January 1982

Vestal K. In Stevens K (ed): Power and Influence: A Sourcebook for Nurses. New York, John Wiley & Sons, 1983

Chapter 12

Networking strategies for the new nurse

GAYE W. POTEET

A hundred times everyday I remind myself that my inner and outer life depends on the labors of other men, living and dead, and that I must exert myself in order to give in the measure as I have received and am still receiving[1]

Albert Einstein

The Challenges and Pitfalls of Networking

A network is defined as a system of interfacing lines, tracks, or channels: a network of arteries, or any interconnected system.[2] Networking was defined in 1980 by Welch as "the process of developing and using your contacts for information, advice, and moral support as you pursue your career."[3] This adaptation of the good old boy or buddy system has occurred among women as a direct result of the women's movement and the increased awareness among women of the importance of significant contacts in career advancement.

227

This chapter will enable you to

1. Summarize the importance of professional networking
2. Identify the three types of networking
3. State action steps for successful networking

Women, including nurses, have recognized in the 1980's that network-ing successfully is essential to career success. It has been estimated by many business leaders that fully one half of all positions are filled by word-of-mouth personal contact. The failure to cultivate a network of well-connected individuals is paramount to being excluded from this 50% of all employment opportunities. In the author's opinion an even higher percentage of key nursing positions is filled through personal con-tacts, especially in the area of nursing service administration.

Contrary to popular opinion, the income gap between men and women is widening. In 1983, women working full-time earned fifty-nine cents for every dollar earned by a man, with the gap expected to widen even more through the decade of the eighties.[4]

However, women are increasingly committed to movement into the mainstream of professional life in America. By abandoning the so called Cinderella complex, women are increasingly more realistic about the likelihood of remaining in the labor force throughout life. Young girls choosing a career or profession are moving into areas such as medicine, law, and business in unprecedented numbers. Other young women in the traditional female professions such as nursing are demonstrating far more commitment to their profession and to the advancement of its members.

Traditionally denied the opportunity to develop teamworking skills via organized sports, women very often have to learn networking skills later in life than do men who, from childhood, participated in team sports. Title VIX of the Higher Education Amendments opened the door for women to participate in organized sports. From elementary school through post secondary education, opportunities for women to partici-pate in team sports, such as basketball and soccer, have increased dra-matically since the passage of the law in 1976.[5] It can be hypothesized that these young women will learn the skills of networking through organized team sports; in the meantime, however, the approximately 79,000 nurses entering the profession each year need assistance in mastering the strategies of successful networking.[6]

The basic purpose of networking is to improve one's personal and professional effectiveness. Networking itself refers to a system of interconnected and cooperating individuals.[7] When applied to nursing, networking (or the utilization of contacts for information and advice) is an essential part of the process of developing and expanding a tested base of knowledge, which then constitutes and governs professional nursing practice.[8] Networking has the potential to become a vital link in the quest toward advancement of nursing practice. Basic to successful networking is the knowledge and understanding of the various categories of networks, the advantages and disadvantages of alliances, and the process of information brokering.

Networking in nursing falls into three categories: personal, political, and research. Within each of these networks three types of networking relationships are possible. Nurses can network among nurses in their own institution, they can network outside the home institution (but still within the nursing profession), and third, they can network with persons in other disciplines and professions outside the home institution. The major focus of this chapter is to describe the challenges of developing a personal network. Additionally, it discusses the status of political and research networks in the nursing profession, and offers practical strategies for increasing one's personal power.

PERSONAL NETWORKING CHALLENGE

The process of networking successfully is only one strategy for personal and professional success. While you are urged to develop sincere, trusting, support relationships with your nurse colleagues and with persons in other disciplines, you are also cautioned to avoid an over reliance on this activity. The current flurry of interest in networking in nursing and other women's groups serves to remind us that, yes, we are indeed our brothers' and our sisters' keepers. However, a concentrated effort to develop a personal support network may or may not be successful. It is difficult to relate to someone who has not experienced successful networking how the traditional network really works. Network relationships are like friendships. Just as a friendship requires attention and care, so do networking relationships. A personal network is not an object that can be seen, yet it is a very real, although unidentifiable, structure. Network relationships are not preordained, they develop according to one's natural needs and interests. The entire process is almost always informal, complete with all the nuances of any other human interpersonal relationship. The challenge is to gain an awareness of networking opportunities by being sensitive to and knowledgeable about those individuals who have the power, influence, and direction to assist you as you seek to improve your personal and professional effectiveness.

The current interest in networking among nurses is both a source of pride and a cause for concern to this author. The heightened interest in nurses helping nurses succeed and achieve career goals is a source of pride. The naivety with which it seems to be undertaken is a cause for concern.

Bonnie Garson captured the essence of this concern when she wrote

> You can't assume that the successful woman in an organization is going to be on your side. You can't assume that the liberal male manager is going to be on your side. Assumptions like that get you into a lot of trouble. Pick allies who have a record of being in favor of a woman. . . . So, if you can find a good person, male or female, that can set an example for you, you are very lucky.[9]

Nursing administrators, colleagues, and faculty can assist young nurses in utilizing the informal support process that exists in the nursing profession as well as in individual organizations; however, caution is urged. Just as you cannot assume that every successful nurse wishes to assist the novice, one cannot assume that merely joining a networking group or organization will lead to a clear understanding of how networks really function.

Networks, like relationships, develop out of mutual goals, needs, and desires. And just as relationships have the potential for positive and negative results, so do the contacts formed through the process of networking. Anyone participating in such an endeavor is cautioned to be aware at all times that other participants are constantly evaluating the risks and benefits of opening up their world of contacts or their personal network to the newcomer. How interested others are in networking with the newcomer will always depend on their perceptions of what the newcomer has to offer. The benefits and costs of entering into a new networking relationship are certainly being measured by all involved parties.

The novice may ask a colleague or faculty member for guidance in this process. The nurse colleague or the individual faculty person considers the benefit/cost ratio in the decision of whether or not to extend one's self to the newcomer. Individuals differ in their willingness to help others and in their actual ability to assist others in launching a successful career.

Merely attending a class on power or networking conveys on the person attending the class neither power nor a powerful networking relationship. The subtlety of mutual needs expressed through informal support networks is captured in part in the following description:

Being aware of the informal world is being aware of the changing [interpersonal] . . . relationships, the person-to-person sensitivities, the informal political values and taboos and the informal understandings between functions and among people within the function as well as knowing what thou shalt and shalt not do. Arrangements within the unstructured world are seldom written down; there are no descriptions of the informal interpersonal credit bank—in fact, the entire power dimension is never fully described. You must gain your awareness by tuning in to the arrangement to sense who has the clout, power, influence, direction.[10]

By keeping the mutual needs in mind and by always serving to give more than she gets, the staff nurse's chances for success will be greater.

For most staff nurses a distinction exists between a personal support group made up of friends from outside work, family, or neighbors, and a professional support network. Around the country women's networks are forming generally for the purpose of providing professional information and support to women. As the new nurse matures and advances in her career, joining such a group may be beneficial.

NETWORKING GUIDELINES FOR THE NEW NURSE

In addition to developing an understanding of networking relationships, certain organizational strategies also have the potential to enhance the likelihood of personal networking successfully. Successful networking requires planning and follow-up (see Table 12-1). Identify individuals that have the potential to assist you and who can give you the information you need for success. Keep records regarding people who may be

Table 12-1   Steps in Successful Networking for the New Nurse

OBJECTIVE	ACTION PLAN
Join American Nurses' Association.	Attending local and state meetings will provide opportunities to meet nurses in leadership positions.
Join specialty organizations such as NAPNAP, NACOG, AACN.	Involvement can lead to relationships with other nurses in your specialty area.
Volunteer for committee memberships in your workplace.	An outstanding performance brings you to the attention of nurse leaders in your organization.
Demonstrate commitment and competence in the staff nurse role.	A work record characterized by competence and integrity is an essential base for future career advancement.
Attend national ANA conventions or specialty conventions.	This provides an opportunity to keep your knowledge current and allows you to know who's who in nursing and in your area.

able to help you obtain the information you are likely to need. Write down names, addresses, and phone numbers. Attend presentations given by individuals whom you have identified as potential resource persons. Introduce yourself to the individual, follow-up with a call or letter and always be appreciative of any help given to you. The recommendations or components of successful networking listed below can assist you in evaluating the present status of your personal network. Your network includes all of the individuals, students, employees, and employers who have influenced your personal and professional life. In part your success will depend on how competently you utilize your personal network.

One means of systematically keeping track of the individuals you meet is to exchange business cards. The cost of having business cards printed is minimal. Although the actual cost may vary from place to place, 1000 cards usually can be purchased for $25 to $30. When you meet persons at conferences or other meetings, you can ask them for a business card and give them one of your cards.

Business cards should always be printed on paper of good quality similar to that of a fine wedding invitation. White cards are acceptable as are off-white and cream. At no time should business cards be printed on cheap paper or colored paper; such choices indicate poor taste on the part of the cardholder. The information to be printed on business cards varies with personal preference; however, the following is one example for the staff nurse:

Karen Jones
Registered Nurse—Critical Care
Mercy Hospital
110 Summerset
Someplace, USA
919-441-9262

COMPONENTS OF SUCCESSFUL NETWORKING

Recordkeeping:
Keep organized files and business cards of people who can assist you in the future.
Follow-up:
Write letters after workshops and conferences expressing your appreciation for a suggestion or a contact.
Extend yourself to others:
Assist your colleagues when they need help.

Keep the cards you receive in an organized fashion. Most business supply stores have folders designed to assist in the organization, storage, and easy retrieval of business cards. It is important to invest early in a handy folder for business cards and other names and addresses that could be important to future success. Any office supply store has an assortment of folders to attractively and conveniently store business cards. Be sure to ask for a business card from key persons you meet at conventions or other meetings. When attending conventions and conferences, try to be present at *all* sessions including cocktail hours, luncheon and dinner meetings. Successful networking requires organization, commitment, and time. A list of networking dos and don'ts compiled in part by Puetz follows:

Do learn how to ask questions.

Do try to give as much as you get.

Do follow up on contacts.

Do keep in touch with your contacts.

Do report back to your contacts.

Do be businesslike as you network.

Don't be afraid to ask for what you need.

Don't pass up any opportunities.

Don't tell everything to everybody.

Don't share personal information.

Don't ask personal questions.[11]

The long-term goal in building a personal network is to increase one's base of contacts and one's personal power. According to Josefowitz, there are two aspects of power. The first view of power refers to the traditional, finite idea of power, that is, there is just so much power and no more. The second view of power, referring to effectiveness, is more elastic and relates more to the nurse's potential personal power. In this sense power can spread out or change its shape depending on the needs of the individual or organization.[12] The derivation of the word *power* is *pouvoir*, a French word meaning *to enable*.[13] In order for the new nurse to enpower others, the new nurse must first acquire some power of his or her own.

The health-care industry increasingly is going to need and value nurses who know what they want and where they are going with their careers, nurses who can develop goals, action plans, and timetables for implementing the goals. Few nursing education programs have concentrated on helping students set professional and personal goals. Institutions such as hospitals need nurses who can balance the competing demands of work and personal responsibilities.

Establishing professional and personal goals is one way of determining where you want to go with your career. According to one author the process of developing clearly stated goals involves all of the following:

> . . . understanding the difference between goals and activities, learning to state goals in specific terms, brainstorming a comprehensive set of goals, refining and ranking them, categorizing them according to career, personal development or family orientation, and recognizing the relative importance of these categories for you.[14]

The next consideration is how to attain the goals. An action plan that is clear, simple, and realistic is an action plan that is likely to work. An action plan that is ambiguous, complex, and beyond the scope of the resources available is an action plan on a collision course with failure. This is not to suggest that the plan cannot be an ambitious one nor is it to suggest that it be one absolutely guaranteed to succeed. There undoubtedly should be some challenge involved, but the challenge must be a reasonable one.[15] An example of an action plan for the staff nurse is shown in Table 11-1.

Dividing the action plan into specific activities with a realistic timetable increases the likelihood of accomplishing one's goals. Avoid becoming a fanatic over the planned timetable. Persistence and flexibility are ingredients that most often lead to success.

Mentoring and Sponsoring Relationships

Young nurses often establish mentoring and sponsoring relationships with their nursing faculty, head nurses, supervisors, and clinical nurse specialists. The young staff nurse looks to these relationships for support and advice. Generally the relationships terminate when the nurse changes jobs. The relationships are probably not true mentor relationships, but fall more into that of the young nurse seeking a role model.[16]

According to Lucie Kelly, a noted nurse writer and leader, mentoring has not really occurred to any great extent in nursing. She writes that a mentor system is critically needed in the nursing profession.[17]

Political Nursing Networks

As of November, 1980, nurses number approximately 1,603,069 women, with an additional 45,060 men, making the nursing profession the largest predominantly female profession in the United States.[18] Political and health analysts have commented on the potential power of the profession, based on the fact that one out of every 44 voters is a nurse.

Effective political involvement and influence require additional development of all types of political networks. Political networks offer two opportunities for advancing the nursing profession. The value of "connections" or access to the right person is a well-known political strategy; however, political networking also requires the deliberate use of politics or the use of influence and interpersonal relationship to achieve some planned goal or purpose. According to one author these political networks are of three types. The first one resembles an "old boy network," in which older, more experienced nurses assist younger, less experienced nurses in the political process. The second type of political network is a system designed to put expert nurses in contact with legislators. Committee staff and legislators themselves have long relied on this type of contact for advice and information as they seek to make technical decisions. The third type of political network is a grassroots organization designed to allow for the rapid deployment of letters, calls, and telegrams when nursing issues arise. The political clout of nurses and the nursing profession depend in large part on the profession devoting more resources to this process. Unless we do so, nurses will continue to be omitted from health policy decision making process.

Political networking has generally resulted when a group of nurses become very polarized in support of or in opposition to an issue or cause. To date networking in nursing seems to have had the greatest potential when it was used as a vehicle creating a united effort on behalf of a cause or when a vital issue in the profession of nursing was at stake. A call to arms such as the one described in Hauser's description of the Cape Girardeau incident is an excellent example of a nurses' political network.[19] In this example nurses joined together to protest a court decision involving nurses who were accused of practicing medicine without a license. The issue—the use of protocols and standing orders—affects nurses in multiple settings from home health-care and the administration of an enema to the critical care nurse administering lidocaine for a life-threatening arrhythmia.

Still another example of successful nurse networking occurred when the membership of the Virginia Nurses' Association sought to block the introduction of Chelsea beer into the marketplace. An initial television advertisement portrayed teen-agers seated around a table drinking Chelsea beer and eating peanut butter sandwiches. Although the beer had an alcoholic content approaching that of beer, the marketing strategies had targeted traditional soft drink markets. Through the efforts of the involved members of the Virginia Nurses' Association, plans to market Chelsea beer as a soft drink were dropped and, in fact, Chelsea beer was dropped from the Anheuser-Busch Company's product list and resulted in an estimated loss of $5 million in company revenues.

Research Networks

Another example of a successful nursing network is in the area of research. The networking process can provide nurses the opportunity to exchange ideas about research, initiate new projects, and collaborate on ongoing research activities. Opportunities for nursing research exist on a local, state, regional, and national level. Collaboration can advance the quality of nursing research and assist in the dissemination of findings. Multiple approaches and solutions are more likely to be forthcoming when the research process has included the opportunity for extensive collaboration within the profession.

Networking also has the potential to help alleviate the sense of isolation that often accompanies the conduct of independent research projects. Careful sensitive networking does have the potential to improve not only your personal effectiveness but also your professional effectiveness.

Summary

In summary, the most successful networking in the nursing profession has to date centered around nurses uniting for a common purpose involving a political cause or some fundamental issue affecting the profession. Networks of nurses organized around the goal of fostering nursing research interests and activities have also been successful in achieving limited goals. It is in the area of forming individual nurse networks for the purpose of improving personal and professional effective-

STEPS IN THE ANALYSIS OF ONE'S PERSONAL NETWORK

1. Identify individual(s) who have had most influence on your career.

2. Identify successful mentor-protege relationship(s) during your career.

3. Whom would you use as references in applying for a new position?

4. Where do you go for career guidance and counseling?

5. Who are the individuals in your life who share your successes and your failures?

6. Reverse the perspective in questions 1-4 and answer the questions again.
   Whose career have you influenced?
   Whom have you mentored successfully?
   Who uses you as a reference for a new position?
   Who turns to you for career guidance and counseling?
   Who shares her successes and failures with you?

The list of persons generated from answering these questions forms the core of your own personal network.

ness that the greatest attention needs to be focused. This attention must be both supportive and encouraging to young nurses, but also must be realistic and incorporate the subtleties of all aspects of human relationships, including the human support relationship that is the essence of the networking concept. Some steps to help you analyze your own personal network are outlined on the opposite page. Finally, a challenge to all nurses: Strive to be the kind of nurse who does not have to put out another person's light in order that your own may shine more brightly.

References

1. Einstein A: In Wallis CL (ed): The Treasure Chest, p 123. San Francisco, Harper & Row, 1983
2. Mish FC (ed.): Webster's Ninth New Collegiate Dictionary. Springfield, Merriam-Webster, 1983
3. Welch MS: Networking. New York, Harcourt Brace Jovanovich, 1980
4. Statistical Abstract of the United States, 105th ed, p 419. Washington, DC
5. Higher Education Amendments of 1966 U.S. Code 1970, Title 20, S. 711 et seq. Nov. 3, 1966, P.L. 89–752–80 Stat, 1240. Higher Education Amendments of 1968. U.S. Code 1976, Title 20, S 403 et seq. Oct. 16, 1968, P.L. 90–575, 82 Stut. 1014. From Shepard's Acts and Cases by Popular Name: Federal and State 2nd ed. Vol 1. Colorado Springs, Shepard's Inc, 1979
6. American Nurses' Association: Facts about nursing 84–85. Kansas City, MO, American Nurses' Association, 1985
7. Kleiman C: Women's Networks. New York, Ballentine Books, 1980
8. Nicoll LH: Networking: A vital link to the advancement of nursing practice. The Maine Nurse. 69(1):8, 1983
9. Garson B: Views from Women Achievers. A Series of Dialogues from the Management Process, p 116. New York, American Telephone and Telegraph Corporation, 1977
10. Silber MB, Sherman VC: Managerial Performance and Promotability, p 5–6. New York, American Management Association, 1974
11. Puetz BE: Networking for Nurses. Rockville, MD, Aspen Systems, 1983
12. Josefowitz N: Paths to Power. Reading, MA, Addison–Wesley, 1980
13. New Cassell's French Dictionary. New York, Funk & Wagnalls, 1967
14. Carr–Ruffino N: The Promotable Woman, rev ed. Belmont, CA, Wadsworth Publishing, 1985
15. Pollok CS: Adapting management by objectives to nursing. Nurs Clin North Am 18(3):481–490, 1983
16. Puetz BE: Networking for Nurses. Rockville, MD, Aspen Systems, 1983
17. Kelly LY: Dimensions of Professional Nursing, 3rd ed. New York, MacMillan, 1975
18. American Nurses' Association: Facts about Nursing 82–83. Kansas City, MO, American Nurses' Association, 1983
19. Hauser P: Networking: Tactic for the supreme court case. Missouri Nurs 52(3):12, 1983

SECTION III

FOCUS ON CONTEMPORARY NURSING ISSUES

Chapter 13

Licensure, legislation, and health policy

MARGARET MURPHY VOSBURGH

Nurses in practice today are finding that it is not enough to be knowledgeable about their own work setting. As professionals in health care, nurses are affected to a great degree by health policy formulated at national, state, and local levels. In addition, nurses are actively committed to influencing policy formulation so that the outcome is reflective of nursing's professional interests. Nurse practice acts are a part of the total policy picture and must be reviewed on a state-by-state basis. It is imperative that the new nurse understand issues basic to health policy formulation so that she can determine where and how her influence may be directed.

This chapter will enable you to

1. Understand the nature of health policy
2. Identify the governmental process of policy making
3. Describe how nurses can influence policy formulations
4. Identify components of the nurse practice acts

Framework for Policy Decisions

Health policy is an extension of public opinion and social consciousness. The underlying values and beliefs of a society provide the foundation for its health policy.

As America emerged into a nation, its citizens subscribed strongly to a philosophy of liberalism, which emphasizes personal freedom for the individual. The individual rights and freedoms of the citizen were to be the cornerstone for any and all governmental mandates. Liberalists contended that governmental policies existed to enhance the rights and freedoms of citizens. Because of these views the infant American government was designed with checks and balances to prevent it from imposing arbitrary constraints upon its people. Government's sole purpose was to protect the right of the American citizen to make individual choices.

In 1776, Adam Smith published *The Wealth of Nations* and introduced Americans to the philosophy of capitalism. Capitalism contends that the greatest good can be attained if individuals are allowed to pursue their own economic and social benefits. Capitalism represented a departure from the prevailing beliefs of the time. No longer were self-denial and poverty viewed as a measure of Christian piety; individual gain and profit became compelling forces in the new social structure. The new American nation, fresh from its war for independence, found the tenets of Smith's work both compatible and achievable. The philosophy of liberalism and the economic tools of capitalism continue to dominate our lives and influence how we formulate public policy.

Authority for Policy Formulation

Although the constitution of the United States never defines the term "public policy," it is a fundamental tenet of a constitutional democracy that elected representatives of the people should be the ones to shape public policy. Theoretically, Congress, the executive branch, and the judicial branch of government have primary responsibility for separate phases of the public policy process. Constitutionally, Congress is given responsibility for policy formulation through the mandate of making laws. The president, as head of the executive branch, is charged with faithfully executing the laws designed by Congress, and the judicial branch is required to interpret the laws as disputes are litigated in the courts. In practice, each branch of government performs most of the policy functions of formulation, implementation, and interpretation (Kronenfeld and Whicker, 1984). Today the separation of function is less rigid and it frequently seems that the executive branch drafts legislation a supportive congressional leader will introduce to Congress. Courts often formulate policy through common law decisions and court orders.

ROLE OF CONGRESS

While Congress is charged with policy formulation, it is the various committees and subcommittees organized within Congress that put into operation the process of policy formulation. New legislation is assigned to, or originates in, a relevant subcommittee. Subcommittee topics are generally reflective of the concerns and problems of society. With their respective chairmen, subcommittees investigate and formulate laws designed to protect the rights of persons involved in specific issues. Two major congressional subcommittees studying contemporary issues are the subcommittee on aging and the subcommittee on alcohol and drug abuse. Committee and subcommittee chairmen are generally senior members of the dominant party and it is the committee chairmen who choose the agenda items to be studied. The active use of committees allows members of Congress to specialize in topics particularly relevant to their constituencies (Dodd and Scholt, 1979).

ROLE OF ADMINISTRATIVE AGENCIES

Congress frequently delegates policy formulation to administrative agencies. Congress may issue a broad statute, then expect an administrative agency to develop more specific regulations to govern the program. Congress passed Medicaid legislation but it was the responsibility of an administrative agency to draft rules and regulations that made the program functional. It is the interpretation of the statute by an administrative agency which determines the scope and impact of policy (Kronenfeld and Whicker, 1984). The President and Congress have set the direction to control health-care costs but it is the Health-Care Financing Administration that must design strategies and rules to reach this objective.

ROLE OF SPECIAL-INTEREST GROUPS

The power of special-interest groups to influence health policy is formidable. Special-interest groups have no formal governmental position but exert power by influencing the vote of elected policymakers.

Special-interest groups gain support for their position by providing information to policymakers on policy options currently under consideration. The information shared with house and senate conferees is often biased and considerate only of the position taken by the special-interest group. The opinions of the special-interest groups may be further communicated to the public through media coverage and advertising campaigns.

Special-interest groups frequently use campaign funds as a means of influencing legislation. Political action committees raise money for candidates sympathetic to their cause. Whether the special-interest group is the American Nurses Association, a pharmaceutical company, or the American Heart Association, traditional lobbying tactics are used to arouse public opinion in the hopes that federal action will be taken and legislation drafted to support the group's particular position.

Policy Process

If Congress wishes to respond to an issue, a legislative proposal, or bill, is introduced by a member of Congress, hearings are conducted to study options, and a formal record is established. All legislation must be approved by both houses of Congress and then pass through the Budget Committee in the appropriate House before it formally becomes a law. Figure 13-1 illustrates the congressional budgetary process.

Legislation provides a national plan to deal with a specific issue. Once a priority has been established and a law enacted, the Appropriations Committees make funding recommendations to the full bodies of the House of Representatives and the Senate. It is entirely possible that legislation may be approved in principle and rejected in the Appropriations Committees. If a bill is passed by a majority of members in the House and Senate, it is sent to the president for signature. The president has ten days in which to make his decision. If he signs the bill, it becomes law. If he vetoes the bill, it goes back to Congress for consideration of an override vote. The president's veto may be overturned with a two-thirds majority vote by both House and Congress.

Influence of Nursing on Policy Formulation

Policy development is a complex process involving many players. The process is dominated by special-interest groups, the agency in the executive branch that administers the policy area, the congressional committees and subcommittees responsible for the specific area, and the media. The process is complex and wrought with multiple checks and balances. The system was designed to inhibit dominance by any one special-interest group. It was also designed to be a government of the people, for the people. Despite the complexity of the system, citizens are still able to influence the political process. Legislative or administrative decisionmakers frequently seek advice from knowledgeable persons with expertise in areas presently under consideration. Expert testimony, multidisciplinary committees, and task forces are utilized to keep governmental officials abreast of changes within the health-care field (Bradham, 1985). Nurses should position themselves to testify at these hearings and offer advice on health-care issues. Lobbying activities provide feedback to elected officials on the direction their constituencies wish them to pursue. Nurses can and should have regular dialogue with legislators, congressional leaders, and their legislative aides. These individuals are surprisingly accessible and eager to hear from the constituents. Actively supporting political candidates is another very powerful way to influence health policy. Figure 13-2 illustrates how nurses can influence the legislative process. Nurses should remember that elected officials are generally very sensitive to the wishes of a voting body of 1.7 million members.

Federal Influence on Health Policies

HISTORICAL PERSPECTIVE

The role of the government in health-policy formulation has been an evolving one. From 1776 to 1929, the American government played only a minor role in health policy formulation. In 1929, the American economy collapsed and the Federal Government exerted a new influence on American health care. The Great Depression of 1929 left the American people dazed and unable to cope with an enormous need for economic relief (Ripley, 1974). Local tax revenues could not meet the sustained demand for economic relief of the unemployed and when their needs remained unmet they turned to the federal government for help. The federal government intervened and began to establish standardized relief programs for all the states. The government, under Franklin D. Roosevelt's New Deal, recognized that health care constituted a major component of the recovery effort and sought to create programs that would enhance the health and welfare of the general population. The role of the federal government in health became firmly entrenched with the historic report of the Committee on Economic Security that led to the Social Security Act of 1935 (Somers and Somers, 1977). This act rep-

House Committee on the Budget
The Congressional Budget Process

Information Gathering, Analysis, and Preparation of First Budget Resolution

October	November	December	January	February	March
	10	31	Approx. last week in Jan.		15
	President submits Current Services Budget.	Economic Committee reports analysis of Current Services Budget to the Budget Committees.	President submits budget (15 days after Congress convenes).		All committees and joint committees submit estimates and views to Budget Committee.

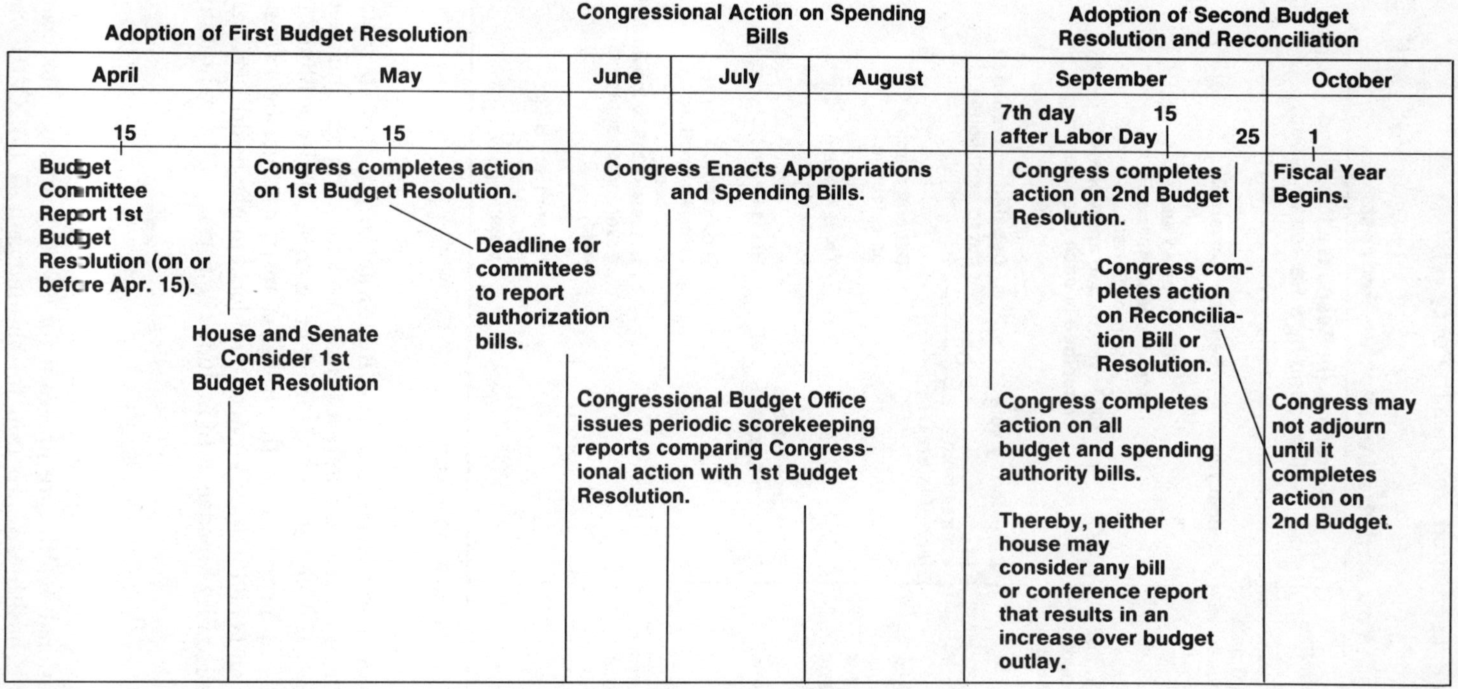

Adoption of First Budget Resolution		Congressional Action on Spending Bills			Adoption of Second Budget Resolution and Reconciliation	
April	**May**	**June**	**July**	**August**	**September**	**October**
15	15				7th day after Labor Day 15 25	1
Budget Committee Report 1st Budget Resolution (on or before Apr. 15).	Congress completes action on 1st Budget Resolution.	Congress Enacts Appropriations and Spending Bills.			Congress completes action on 2nd Budget Resolution.	Fiscal Year Begins.
	Deadline for committees to report authorization bills.				Congress completes action on Reconciliation Bill or Resolution.	
	House and Senate Consider 1st Budget Resolution	Congressional Budget Office issues periodic scorekeeping reports comparing Congressional action with 1st Budget Resolution.			Congress completes action on all budget and spending authority bills.	Congress may not adjourn until it completes action on 2nd Budget.
					Thereby, neither house may consider any bill or conference report that results in an increase over budget outlay.	

Figure 13-1 The Congressional budgetary process.

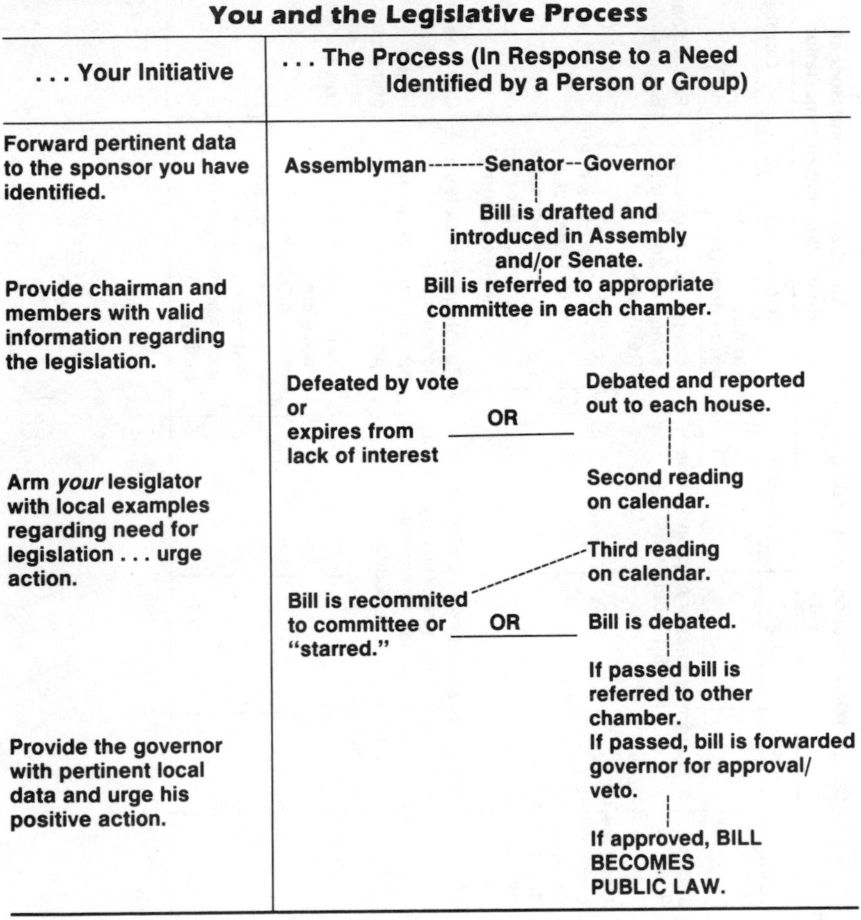

You and the Legislative Process

. . . Your Initiative	. . . The Process (In Response to a Need Identified by a Person or Group)
Forward pertinent data to the sponsor you have identified.	Assemblyman-------Senator--Governor
	Bill is drafted and introduced in Assembly and/or Senate.
Provide chairman and members with valid information regarding the legislation.	Bill is referred to appropriate committee in each chamber.
	Defeated by vote or expires from lack of interest OR Debated and reported out to each house.
Arm *your* lesiglator with local examples regarding need for legislation . . . urge action.	Second reading on calendar.
	Third reading on calendar.
	Bill is recommited to committee or "starred." OR Bill is debated.
	If passed bill is referred to other chamber.
Provide the governor with pertinent local data and urge his positive action.	If passed, bill is forwarded governor for approval/ veto.
	If approved, BILL BECOMES PUBLIC LAW.

Figure 13-2   How nurses can influence the legislative process.

resented the first involvement of the American government in social insurance. The act was to emulate a private pension fund and included programs for the needy, elderly, dependent children, and the blind. It established fiscal incentives for the states to institute their own funds for maternal and child welfare services, and local public health services. In 1950 the eligibility broadened to include the permanently and totally disabled.

Medicare

In 1965, the Social Security Amendment established Medicare (Title XVIII), a national health-care program for the elderly, and Medicaid (Title XIV), a health-care program for the indigent. Title XVIII was added to the original Social Security Bill. Part A of Title XVIII (Medicare) provided for room and board costs of hospitalization and certain posthospital services. It covered up to 90 days' hospitalization during an episode of illness, and psychiatric and inpatient services for up to 190 days in a lifetime. Nursing home care was covered for up to 100 days during an episode of illness.

Part B of Medicare was a voluntary insurance program. Enrollees paid premiums and these contributions were matched from general Social Security funds. Physician's services, laboratory work, equipment, supplies, and additional home health services were covered by Part B of Medicare. Both Part A and Part B were subject to copayments and deductibles.

Medicaid

Title XIX (Medicaid) is a federal–state matching program. Originally, participation was voluntary and coverage across the states varied in scope and in eligibility. Some states extended coverage to families who had borderline poverty level incomes but who earned too much to qualify for federally subsidized welfare. Some states extended benefits to include dental care, extensive mental health coverage, and even ambulance transportation.

With the 1965 enactment of the Medicare and Medicaid programs the federal government assumed major responsibility for the provision of health care to the elderly and the majority of the poor. While the Social Security Administration regulated the Medicaid and Medicare programs, intermediaries such as Blue Cross/Blue Shield handled claims and payments. Congress elected to utilize existing intermediaries to pay hospitals in order to gain cooperation from hospitals and avoid delays in instituting the program. Hospitals and nursing homes received payment, not from the Social Security Administration, but from fiscal intermediaries within their regions.

Congress based reimbursement procedures on reasonable costs and charges. Medicaid reimbursed hospitals for whatever the hospitals quoted as their costs. In an effort to ensure access to health care, Congress adopted a reimbursement methodology that provided no incentives to control costs. Subsequent health-care policy sought to curb federal spending and enhance quality.

Between 1966 and 1971, amendments to Medicare and Medicaid extended the type or amount of services offered in the programs. In 1972 the Professional Standards Review Organizations (PSRO) were created to "avoid overutilization of health-care services and to control costs" (Ditel and Aldridge, 1977). Under the PSRO, physicians formally reviewed the activities of other physicians within institutions. The

PSRO were charged with addressing cost, quality control, and medical necessity of services. In 1981, the use of PSRO by Medicaid was made optional and eventually funding for PSRO was entirely eliminated.

The Reagan Years

The "new federalism" of the Reagan administration sought to diminish the role of the federal government in American life. His health policies were aimed at stimulating competition among health-care organizations by cutting Medicare and Medicaid benefits, phasing out Professional Standards Review Organizations, ending subsidization of medical and nursing education, and of Health Maintenance Organizations (Salmon, 1983).

In 1981, as part of the Omnibus Budget Reconciliation Act, federal funds for Medicare were cut. In 1982, the Tax Equity and Fiscal Responsibility Act (TEFRA) allowed greater flexibility for states to structure their Medicaid programs. TEFRA also provided incentives for hospitals to develop their own health-care programs. Each year between 1981 and 1983 matching federal funds were systematically reduced. As early as 1967, Medicare was directed by Congress to experiment with different reimbursement methodologies (Davis, 1983). In April of 1983, Congress approved Prospective Payment as the reimbursement methodology for Medicare. This legislation represented a major restructuring of the way in which the federal government pays for hospital care of Medicare recipients. Rather than paying retrospective cost-based charges, it pays prospectively according to specific diagnostic-related categories (DRG). Hospitals have an incentive to keep their costs below the DRG rate because they can keep any savings that result. The speed with which Congress passed Prospective Payment legislation and the President signed the bill attests to the American public's desire to curb health-care cost. Under the Reagan plan Medicare beneficiaries assumed a larger share of recipient-paid premiums. The momentum appeared to spread to further shifting of costs to Medicare recipients.

Federal Funding for Hospitals and Research

HISTORICAL PERSPECTIVE

When the federal government became involved as the major provider of health care in America it recognized the need to influence the supply side of the equation. The government began to appropriate funds to ensure an appropriate supply of hospital buildings, and health research.

Hospital construction came to a virtual standstill during the Great Depression. The Hospital Survey and Construction Act of 1946 marked the beginning of many post-World War II federally-funded programs. The Hospital Survey and Construction Act of 1946, or the Hill-Burton Act as it is more commonly called, provided states with the necessary funds to survey their existing hospitals and health centers and plan for additional facilities. Funds for construction were allocated to the states based on the state's total population and per capita income. The grants covered up to one third of the total costs (Kronenfeld and Whicker, 1984). The Hill-Burton Act was amended many times and later provided grants for research related to the development, utilization, and coordination of health services. It also provided monies for the survey and construction of hospital outpatient departments, rehabilitation centers, and nursing homes. The original bill continued to develop and gradually grew to include loan guarantees for construction and modernization of hospitals, communication networks, and emergency rooms. The Hill-Burton Act and its amendments were incorporated into the 1974 Public Health Services Act and subsequently the National Health Planning and Resource Development Act. This act required the Secretary of Health, Education, and Welfare (currently Health and Human Services) to issue national health-planning policy guidelines. Figure 13-3 outlines the agencies within the Department of Health and Human Services. Regional Health System Agencies (HSA) were established to implement the national guidelines. Each regional HSA was to have a population of between 500,000 and 3 million persons. The state's governor had the latitude to establish the HSA as part of the local government, as a public regional planning body, or a special nonprofit corporation. A striking feature of this approach was the stipulation that whatever structure the states chose, the majority of the governing body had to be composed of consumer representatives. The HSA's had the authority to review and approve the use of federal funds within their areas for health services or research.

CURRENT IMPACT

The Reagan administration weakened the HSA system by reducing its funding by 54%. In fiscal 1981 the program was funded at $126.5 million. By fiscal 1983 the funding was reduced to $58.3 million (Kronenfeld and Whicker, 1984). Reagan requested the total elimination of federal aid for health-planning programs in the 1984 budget. The objectives of the Reagan administration were to reduce federal regulation, increase responsibilities of the states and private sector, and promote competition and market-oriented reforms to increase efficiency (Peres, 1985). Reagan's directive was heard by the country's largest for-profit hospital chain. The 10 largest proprietary hospital corporations expanded an average of 42.5% in 1981 alone (Johnson and Punch, 1982). More than 50% of non-

Department of Health and Human Services

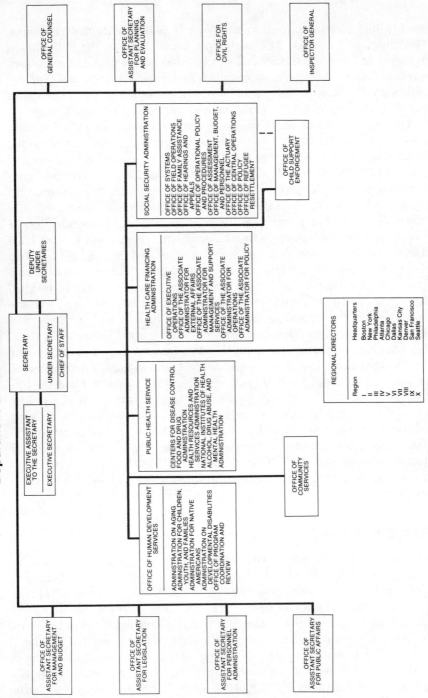

Figure 13-3 Agencies within the Department of Health and Human Services. (From US Government Manual, 1984)

government psychiatric beds are currently owned by proprietary chains (Federation of American Hospitals, 1982). It is estimated that by the end of this decade 25% to 30% of hospitals will be owned by for-profit hospital corporations (Salmon 1983). The rising demand for nursing home care has attracted the interest of proprietary hospital systems and many are diversifying to include for-profit nursing home corporations (Salmon, 1983).

Public hospitals, and particularly those hospitals in the inner cities, have been forced to reduce services and many have been forced to close because of the reduction in federal funds. The American Hospital Association reported that 186 hospitals closed between 1974 and 1980. Between 1980 and 1981, 33 hospitals and more than 3,000 beds closed (Federation of American Hospitals, 1983). Estimates suggest that 1000 additional hospitals may close their doors by 1990 (Wadholz, 1982). An important feature of the Hill-Burton Act was that hospitals receiving funds were expected to devote charity care in an amount equal to 5% of the operating revenue (Bloch and Pupp, 1985). As federal funds for modernization are reduced and urban centers fall into decay, there is growing fear that persons with serious medical problems will not seek care because of their inability to pay or their inability to find health care in their urban neighborhoods. There is some evidence that community hospitals are rearranging their mix of services to maximize profit and minimize losses (Solomon, 1982). It is possible that patients in DRG categories with a negligible profit margin may have trouble finding care. This profit-driven market has fostered the emergence of less costly outpatient rehabilitation and ambulatory facilities.

Federal Funding for Professional Education

Federal funding has affected not only the buildings that house patients but also the professionals who provide care. The federal role in the education of health professionals has been significant. As the government assumed responsibility for providing health-care services to the public, it made a simultaneous commitment to supply nurses and physicians.

HISTORICAL PERSPECTIVE

The government became briefly involved with funding for nursing education during World War II. In 1956, the Health Amendments Act authorized traineeships for advanced nursing education. The Health Professions Education Assistance Act of 1963 provided construction grants for teaching facilities. Student loans were made available to nurses, physicians, dentists, pharmacists and podiatrists. The Comprehensive Health Manpower Training Act of 1971 escalated the federal involvement in funding educational programs for health-care professionals. Capitation grants were made available to schools that could increase first-year enrollments. Grants were also extended to new schools of medicine, dentistry, and osteopathy. Loan provisions were extended so that students who, upon completion of their programs, practices for three years in health-shortage areas could cancel 85% of their loans. Scholarships were instituted for needy students. Family medicine programs received funding and medical programs in geographically underserved areas were established and promoted (Kronenfeld and Whicker, 1984).

Through the Nurse Training Act (1965–1981), the federal government appropriated $1.5 billion (Institute of Medicine, 1981). These monies were especially important to the development of collegiate and graduate level programs.

Federal Funding for Education and Research

Armed with data that predicted an overabundance of physicians by 1990, President Reagan reduced federal funds for medicine. Capitation grants for medical schools were eliminated in 1982; similar grants for schools of nursing had been eliminated in 1981. All nurse training funds were cut by 26% in fiscal 1983 (Kronenfeld and Whicker, 1984).

The reduction of educational grants to physicians and nurses had an immediate effect. Reduction of federal funds for research may have a more insidious influence.

HISTORICAL PERSPECTIVE

Funding for health research began in 1897 when the federal government provided monies for microbiology research. The government instituted a hygienic laboratory as part of the Marine and Hospital Service. The name was changed to the National Institute of Health in 1930 but remained focused on microbiology rather than health promotion. The 1935 Social Security Act included up to $2 million annually for the investigation of disease and problems of sanitation (Strickland, 1978).

The Randall Act of 1928 issued a national policy regarding health research. Today the nation's health policy is administered through the National Institutes of Health (NIH). Congress mandated the function of the institutes as well as the functions of the NIH director (Larson, 1984). The NIH is directed "to cover new knowledge that will lead to better health for everyone" (National Institutes of Health, 1983). The components of the NIH are outlined in Figure 13-4. Nursing has historically had difficulty securing grant money for nursing research because the NIH has tended to focus on curing rather than on the more nursing-directed focus of prevention (Culleton, 1983). In 1983 the Institute of Medicine brought the need for nursing research to the attention of the scientific community (Larson, 1984). The Institute of Medicine called for a federally funded center for nursing research.

> "A substantial share of the health care dollar is expended on direct nursing care, yet the professionals who deliver this care work without the benefit of a strong organizational base to stimulate and support scientific investigation in their field. The committee believes that a center of nursing research is needed at a high level in the federal government to be a focal point for promoting the growth of quality nursing research" (Institute of Medicine, 1983).

In 1984 nursing research received $9 million of the $3.6 billion allocated to the NIH. Congress recently sent the President a three-year reauthorization of the National Institutes of Health. In its package was provision for a National Center for Nursing research at NIH. The bill passed when both the House and Senate overrode the presidential veto.

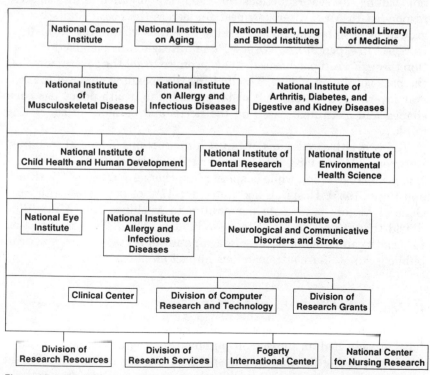

Figure 13-4 *Components of the National Institutes of Health.*

PRESIDENTIAL INFLUENCE

A national health policy is a composite of social consciousness, economic factors, the nature and history of existing institutions, popular opinion, behavioral characteristics of key political figures, and the general goals and values of society (Kronenfeld and Whicker, 1984).

Throughout history we have seen how economic development and social consciousness have dominated health policy formulation. We have seen how strong presidents view health care. We endured the Great Depression and saw the institution of Roosevelt's New Deal. The complexion of the nation was forever changed with Roosevelt's policy. We heard President John F. Kennedy deliver the first presidential address to Congress devoted entirely to the need for a health program. We heard him urge that hospital insurance for the aged be added to Social Security. The public heralded him as a great Democrat, Congress passed the necessary legislation and quickly instituted the program. Inflationary costs were predicted and ignored. President Carter's message to Congress was one of cost containment. The American people were not prepared to support his position and he saw his proposals for cost containment legislation defeated time and again by Congress. Taxpayers were not willing to see reductions in Medicare or Medicaid. Congress responded to Mr. Carter's request for across-the-board limits on the growth of hospital revenue by asking hospitals voluntarily to restrain increases in expenditures. We saw Ronald Reagan win a landslide reelection through a campaign based on his promise to get the government "off the backs of the people . . . ," by limiting the spending power of the federal government. Throughout history, American health policy has been shaped and instituted, based on the needs and opinions of the voting public.

Today health care is a major target for reductions in federal spending. Between 1967 and 1983, the Consumer Price Index rose 297%. Prescription prices rose 122%, while hospital room charges jumped 644% (Bloch and Pupp, 1985). Hospitals accounted for 47% of personal health care. General Motors pays more per annum to Michigan Blue Cross/Blue Shield than it does to U.S. Steel (McKinlay, 1981). The new direction for health care promulgated by Reagan and supported by the American public is sure to have a tremendous impact on nursing.

IMPACT ON NURSING PRACTICE

Changes in federal funding for health planning and plan construction have already had an impact on nursing. For the first time in history, nurses are facing the threat of hospital downsizing and layoffs. Recent nurse graduates are finding it difficult to secure positions in hospitals.

Nurses in hospitals are becoming involved in cost-saving strategies while serving a client population who is older and who presents with more complex health problems. There are fewer federally funded community resources and there is the every present pressure to reduce the length of hospital stay. Major leaders in health care are predicting that hospitals will be huge intensive care units by 1990 (Levine, 1980).

The reduction of funds for inner-city hospitals and the tendency for hospitals to control their patient mix to maximize reimbursement will compound the problem of uncompensated care. The Children's Defense Fund reported that almost 700,000 children lost Medicare coverage as a result of the Reagan administration's cuts in health spending. The rising infant mortality rate in some cities has been implicated in the federal cuts (Cimons, 1983). In an effort to control spiraling hospital costs, more and more care is being offered *away* from the central hospital. Nursing is being practiced in unconventional places, such as shopping malls and mobile vans.

With fewer monies available for nursing education, it is predicted that the already declining enrollments in schools will continue to fall. Graduate schools will not be able to provide the numbers of academically prepared leaders that health care will require. Health economists have reported that the labor market for nurses does not respond to changes in supply and demand (Altman 1971). There doesn't appear to be a direct association between the hospital vacancy rate and the number of nurses graduating from school. When nursing school graduates reached a record high in 1978 the hospital shortage was more severe than ever (Altman, 1971). It seems that nurses are driven into the hospital by forces other than sheer numbers and supply. If research monies become even tighter questions as to why nurses leave their profession may go unanswered.

When the funding for health care changes, so too must the delivery system. The focus of the American public and, consequently, its elected officials has changed from concern about access to care, to the excesses of health care. History has shown that legislation responds to the needs of the American public. Today's health care consumers are better educated and more interested in helping themselves than any other group in the history of health care.

With its profound commitment to restoration of health and prevention of disease, nursing is in a strong position to answer the country's need for quality, less expensive health care. Numerous studies have documented nursing's impact on the elderly (Master et al, 1980); teenage mothers (Corbett, 1976); post MI patients (Pozen, 1977); retarded adults (Haurl, 1979); patients with chronic disease (Runyan, 1975); dying children (Martinson, 1977); patients with psychiatric disturbances–neonates (Kleinman, 1978).

In all these cases, nursing provided quality care and positive patient outcomes at a reduced cost to the consumer. In some cases nursing intervention had better outcomes than medical intervention. Nursing must bring this information to the public. Nursing research is the critical element that could provide the impetus to change the way America defines health care. Studies of nursing impact on consumers, both in the hospital and at home, are essential at this time. The government must be persuaded to supply nurses with funds to conduct these studies.

Nursing Responsibility To Influence Health Policy

The concept of wellness has been a tenet of nursing since Florence Nightingale. Educating persons to care for themselves has always been the domain of nursing. Nursing deals with individuals in their totality. Nurses are the health-care providers who coordinate all aspects of care and assist the person to adapt to illness or strive for optimal restoration of health. Nursing must position itself so that the public has access to nursing care. The public must be made aware that it has a choice of health-care provider and that nursing is a viable alternative. Insurance policies need to be broadened to provide reimbursement for nursing care. Educational funding for advanced practice and leadership must be addressed if nursing is to meet the health-care needs of America.

Nursing can assist the public and elected official in redefining health care in America. Nursing is in a position to be a master of change (Moss–Kanter, 1983). We must redefine our own concept of health care and create innovative new models of care. We can no longer define nursing in the current sense of hospital care or home care. We must define it in terms of consumer need, without walls and stereotypical roles. Nursing has always been closest to the clients of health care. Successful companies have learned that increased profit margins are obtained by listening to the client. Nursing has been listening and now must speak for reform within in the system. There has never been a better time to put nursing in the forefront of change. Milo has outlined 14 strategies for nurses to influence public policy. She cites the following guidelines for influencing public policy:

1. Organize. Activists who work alone or sporadically in loose association almost inevitably suffer "burnout".

2. Do your home work. Know the formal political process, the legislative and executive units that shape and evaluate the policies that concern you. Know the interest groups involved in the process and those that stand to gain or lose from a change in policy.... Keep

abreast of related health policies and the linkages, spillovers, and tradeoffs being made as policy discussion moves forward. . . . Good sources are legislative newsletters, lobbyists, legislative staff, elected representatives, bureaucrats, secretaries, and reporters.

3. Frame your arguments to appeal to the specific audience you want to persuade. . . . Show how it would generate community or special-interest group support for the policymaker.

4. Support and help strengthen the position of already converted policymakers. For example, convey to legislators your approval of positions they take and support these positions publicly.

5. Concentrate your (finite) organization energies. Be sure to prioritize your policy goals and agree on how to frame the core issues to develop a strategy that will move them forward.

6. Stimulate public debate about your policy issue. Public debate almost always moderates decision making because it tends to widen the options and thereby fosters compromise.

7. Make your position visible in the mass media—newspapers, radio, television.

8. Your main strategy should be the one that is probably most effective. Create political value for your policy position by showing how policymakers will gain with important constituencies if they support it.

9. Act in timely fashion, at the right point in the policymaking process.

10. Maintain your activity. Sustained communication, monitoring, and mutual support with policymakers and liaison people is essential during noncritical periods in order to be effective when policy actions are imminent.

11. Keep your organizational format decentralized or "policy-centered"; grass roots, small local units linked to each other, such as district nursing groups, are more effective than pyramidlike organizations.

12. Always obtain or develop the best research data available on your policy position.

13. Always take time to learn from your experiences.

14. Never give up trying.

Affiliation with the state nurses' association is generally an effective way in which to keep abreast of health policy changes. It provides a good population through which coalitions can be built and strategies formulated to influence the legislative process.

IMPACT OF STATE MANDATES ON NURSING PRACTICE

Licensure

The American Nurses' Association Social Policy Statement describes the inter-relationship between the nursing profession and the society that it serves. The Statement contends that it is the needs and desires of the consumer that dictate the role of nursing. So that the profession may grow and flourish, the practice of nursing must be consistent with the goals of society in general. Public trust is observed as society grants authority, status, and control over practice issues to the profession. Licensure laws are an example of a social contract (Snyder & LaBar 1984). Licensure is a mechanism through which society grants to individual nurses the authority and responsibility to maintain professional standards, and practice according to ethical codes. Self-regulation is the mark of a mature profession (Donabedian, 1976). Self-regulation confers upon the profession the responsibility of

1. Establishing a code of ethics
2. Establishing standards of practice
3. Fostering development of nursing research
4. Establishing educational requirements for entry into professional practice
5. Developing certification processes for the profession
6. Pursuing developmental work directed toward making more specific nursing's accountability to society (ANA, Social Policy Statement, 1980).

Nurse practice acts are an example of licensure laws. Nurse practice acts are statutes established by state legislature. They describe the scope of nursing practice and establish educational requirements for practice. Practice acts generally name a regulatory authority that has responsibility for implementation of the statute.

Nurse Practice Act.   Each state and U.S. territory has a nurse practice act. The Constitution of the United States grants police power to individual states under the states rights provision of Article X. Police power was conferred upon the states in order to protect the individual rights of its citizens. Each state has the right and responsibility to formulate statutes that protect and safeguard the health and safety of its citizens.

Nurse practice acts are generally administered by a board of nursing that is an agency of the executive branch of state government (Snyder and LaBar, 1984). The boards are usually comprised of an all nurse panel but some states have physicians on the board and in some instances physicians sit in the majority. Some states require that consumers also sit on the board. The size of the board varies from three to 20 members. Board members are generally appointed by the governor and are charged with establishing rules that, when passed by the board become part of the state codes and have the authority of law (Snyder and LaBar, 1984). The board is generally responsible for:

- Determining the eligibility of applicants for licensure
- Administering examinations to applicants for licensure
- Issuing licenses to qualified applicants
- Establishing licensure procedures
- Establishing minimum standards for approving educational programs preparing persons for licensure
- Overseeing of mandatory continuing education in some jurisdictions
- Investigating complaints against licensees and taking disciplinary action when appropriate
- Promulgating rules that regulate nursing practice (Snyder and LaBar, 1984)

The nurse practice acts of most states define how each one of these responsibilities is interpreted and met. Copies of nurse practice acts are generally available from the state nurses' associations.

State of Board of Nursing.   There seems to be a trend to centralize the board of nursing and place it and other licensing boards under a central arm of the state government. Out of 50 states recently surveyed, 31 report some degree of centralization, 19 consider themselves to be totally autonomous (Snyder and LaBar, 1984). The degree of centralization varies from centralized boards that receive support services for administrative functions but continue to make primary decisions, to boards that have little control over personnel or funding. The majority of boards have retained power to make fundamental decisions over qualifications for licensure, regulation of practice, and disciplinary action. Licensing examinations are also under the auspices of the State Boards.

Licensing Exams.   The National Council of State Boards of Nursing offers two exams—the National Council Licensure Exam for Registered Nurses (NCLEX-RN) and the National Council Licensure Exam for Practical Nurses (NCLEX-PN).

The exams are designed to ensure that candidates who are licensed will demonstrate at least the minimal level of competency required for safe entry-level practice. Exam questions cover a range of practice-oriented situations. A job analysis is conducted to study the actual jobs that entry-level nurses perform nationally (*Issues*, 1985). Each exam question is put before a panel of judges and rated for its relevance to entry level practice.

The scale used to rate the NCLEX-RN examination ranges from 200 to 3200. A score of 1600 represents the score a candidate would achieve if she were minimally competent to practice entry level nursing. A score of 2000 corresponds to the demonstrated ability of the average person taking the exam (*Issues*, 1985). The test scores are presently reported as scaled number scores but there is consideration to rating the exam as pass-fail in the future.

Disciplinary Activities. The Board of Nursing is charged with investigating complaints against nurses and instituting disciplinary action when necessary. The Board of Nursing has quasijudicial authority to investigate a complaint and recommend disciplinary action. A complaint may be filed by anyone and the board is generally bound to investigate all complaints. Most boards define conduct for which disciplinary action may be taken. Fraud in obtaining a license, unprofessional conduct, conviction of a felony, drug or alcohol addiction that renders the nurse incapable, are often cited as areas in which disciplinary actions may be pursued. The precedent has been set and most courts defer to the determination of the nursing board in disciplinary hearings.

Requirements for Licensure. Statutory requirements for licensure of nurses vary slightly from state to state. All jurisdictions within the U.S. require that candidates for RN licensure complete a board-approved education program. Licensure may be granted by examination or by endorsement of other jurisdictions' licenses. Thirty-two jurisdictions issue temporary licenses for RNs. Temporary licenses are issued in order to allow candidates to work as RNs while awaiting results of licensure exams or completion of endorsement procedures. Some states make a distinction between permit and licensure. Temporary work permits are issued to new graduates awaiting examination results and temporary licenses are issued to RNs registered in another state awaiting endorsement (LaBar, 1984). Temporary work permits are valid for time periods of 60 days to one year. The temporary permit frequently becomes invalid upon receipt of exam results. Some states specify that the temporary permit is nonrenewable. A few states specify that persons working on a permit must function under the supervision of an RN. The frequency with which licenses must be renewed varies from every two years in some states to every four years in others. Persons applying for a permit or temporary license should be fully aware of the scope and limitations of practice in the state issuing the license. This information is contained in the practice act of the state and is available from the state nurses' association.

Statutory Definition of Nursing.   There is no universal definition of the practice of nursing throughout this country. Various processes, services, or acts are statutorily defined as nursing. Table 13-1 illustrates how various states approach the word "diagnosis" in their statutory definition of nursing practice. "Nursing diagnosis" is used by six states. Several states refer to the "diagnosis of human responses," other states substitute "nursing analysis" or "need identification" for nursing diagnosis. When one considers the composition of the state boards of nursing and the degree of individual autonomy of some boards, it becomes easier to understand why such different approaches have been undertaken. The term "diagnosis" in the context of nursing has historically been opposed by medical societies. The ANA Congress for Nursing Practice in the Nurse Practice Act suggested that state legislatures propose a model definition of nursing practice. The aim of the ANA work is to clearly define components of nursing practice.

Analysis of existing statutory definitions of nursing practice revealed four general components that are included to some degree in most acts:

1. The nursing function performed
2. Teaching, supervision, and delegation of nursing practice
3. The execution of medical regimen
4. The performance of additional acts by specially trained nurses. (Snyder and LaBar, 1984)

All nurses should understand clearly the statutory mandate governing their practice. Each separate component should be analyzed in terms of content, language, and intent of the law. The practice acts generally define terms and some definitions actually list activities that are deemed to be the province of nursing. Questions concerning the act should be

Table 13-1   References to the Process of Diagnosis in Statutory Definitions of Nursing Practice

IN CONTEXT OF THE NURSING PROCESS	"DIAGNOSIS OF HUMAN RESPONSES"	"NURSING DIAGNOSIS"	"PROBLEM" OR "NEED IDENTIFICATION"	"NURSING ANALYSIS"	"DIAGNOSIS OF DISEASE"
Florida	Alabama	Indiana	Rhode Island	Montana	Colorado
Kansas	Connecticut	Iowa	Utah		
Missouri	New Jersey	Maryland	Vermont		
Washington	New York	Missouri			
Wyoming	North Dakota	Nebraska			
	Oregon	South Dakota			
	Pennsylvania				

addressed to the state board of nursing. Most require that any inquiry be submitted to the board in writing.

Statutory Provision for Specialty Practice. Additional acts clauses address statutory provision for specialty practice in addition to the basic acts outlined in the original practice act. Four states have statutory definitions for additional acts by certain qualified nurses and 24 states have language that allows the board to promulgate future rules for these acts. Most of the clauses refer to acts recognized by the medical and nursing profession to be within the scope of advanced practice and others allow for the possibility of developing rules to regulate future advanced practice either by the board of nursing alone or in conjunction with the Board of Medicine. Table 13-2 illustrates conditions cited in additional acts clauses.

Table 13-2 Conditions Cited in Additional Acts Clauses

	ACTS RECOGNIZED BY MEDICINE AND NURSING	ACTS RECOGNIZED BY NURSING	RULES DEVELOPED BY BOARDS OF NURSING AND MEDICINE	RULES DEVELOPED BY BOARD OF NURSING	ACTS AUTHORIZED BY BOARD OF NURSING
Alabama	X				
Alaska		X			
Arizona	X		X		
Arkansas		X		X	
Indiana	X				X
Iowa	X				X
Kentucky					X
Louisiana		X			X
Maine*					
Maryland					X
Massachusetts	X			X	
Mississippi			X		
Nevada	X			X	
New Mexico*					
New Hampshire	X		X		
North Dakota	X			X	
Oregon		X			X
Pennsylvania			X		
South Carolina	X				X
South Dakota					X
Utah					X
Vermont	X				
Virgin Islands					X
Washington	X				X

*Not specified

Table 13-3   States that Require Protocols, Agreements, or Guidelines for Advanced Nursing Practice, by Specialty

NURSE MIDWIFE	NURSE ANESTHETIST	NURSE PRACTITIONER	CLINICAL NURSE SPECIALIST
Alabama	Alaska	Alaska	Florida
Arkansas	Arkansas	Arkansas	Massachusetts
Florida	Florida	California	New Hampshire
Massachusetts	Georgia	Florida	South Carolina
Mississippi	Maryland	Georgia	Texas
New Hampshire	Massachusetts	Idaho	Vermont
North Carolina	Mississippi	Maryland	
South Carolina	New Hampshire	Massachusetts	
South Dakota	South Carolina	Mississippi	
Texas	Texas	Nebraska	
Vermont	Utah	New Hampshire	
Virginia	Vermont	South Carolina	
Wisconsin	Virginia	South Dakota	
		Texas	
		Virginia	

The ANA has taken the position that upgrading practice above the minimum standards set by law should not be the function of state government but should be the jurisdiction of the professional association. Fixing advanced practice to law may, in the future, serve to constrict practice and hamper the evolution of practice arenas. There is also concern that physician involvement relinquishes legal control of professional nursing practice and establishes a situation in which another profession can define the scope of nursing practice. Twenty-four states include language in the statute or rules that requires medical protocols or written agreements between the nurse and physician. Table 13-3 lists states that require protocols, agreements, or guidelines as a practice requirement for advanced practice. Not infrequently, the scope of practice statement lists independent functions and those functions that must be performed under the direction and supervision of a physician.

Twenty-three states include statutory language that addresses the practice of nurse midwifery, 35 states speak to nurse practitioners, and 12 states make reference to clinical nurse specialists. The most common method used to authorize a nurse to engage in advanced practice is certification, although some states require specific academic credentials. Table 13-4 outlines academic requirements for advanced practice.

Table 13-4   Academic Degree Requirements for Advanced Practice

TYPE OF PRACTITIONER	BACHELOR'S DEGREE	YEAR*	MASTER'S DEGREE	YEAR*
Nurse Practitioner	Alabama	1983	Georgia	1990
	Idaho		Oregon†	1986
	Montana	1985	Utah	1987
	Oregon†			
	Utah			
Clinical Nurse Specialist			Louisiana	
			North Dakota	
			Utah	
Psychiatric/Mental Health Clinical Nurse Specialist			Florida	
			New Hampshire	
			South Carolina	
Community Health Clinical Nurse Specialist			New Hampshire	
			South Carolina	
Nurse Midwife	Montana	1985		
Nurse Anesthetist	Montana	1985		

*The year is listed only if the requirement is for a future year.
†Includes family, pediatric, adult, geriatric, psychiatric/mental health, nurse midwife, women's health, school health, and college health nurse practitioners.

Mandatory Continuing Education. Some states require that nurses wishing to become registered in their state must attend a pre-scribed number of educational programs and acquire a fixed number of contact hours. A contact hour is usually defined as *50 consecutive minutes of authorized instruction.* Proponents of this approach see it as an attempt to protect the public from nurses who practice under obsolete guidelines. Those opposed view continuing education as a professional responsibility, not something that should be mandated by law.

Fifteen jurisdictions have statutory language requiring continuing education for license renewal. Three of these states have not, as of this writing, implemented the programs. The number of contact hours required varies from 15 hours for a two-year period of renewal to 20 hours for a one-year period. Some states accept some hours in home study, and most will accept individualized learning activities (LaBar, 1984). Content acceptable to meet the requirements is outlined in the state rule governing continuing education. Eleven of the twelve states with functional continuing education requirements exempt new gradu-ate nurses from the requirement for one year.

Entry Into Practice. A number of jurisdictions are wrestling with entry into practice issues. The issue of entry into practice formally began

20 years ago when the ANA initiated a proposal to make the Bachelor of Science in Nursing degree an entry-level nursing requirement. The association hoped to have the proposition accepted and in place by 1985.

In 1984, the ANA House of Delegates modified the plan to have the BSN for entry into professional practice a requirement in 5% of the states by 1986, 15% by 1988, 50% by 1992, and 100% by 1995 (Hood, 1985). The most recent position speaks to two and only two categories of nurse, the BSN and the associate degree.

The current direction and position of the individual states regarding entry into practice can be obtained from the state nurses' association. Proponents of the BSN as entry level preparation see it as a method to ensure nursing's position in the mainstream of education and as a means of protecting the public. Those opposed to the BSN as an entry level requirement fear alienation of diploma and AD nurses and question the outcome of baccalaureate education.

Institutional Licensure.   Institutional licensure is another major issue facing nursing. The concept of institutional licensure has many facets that vary from plan to plan. In general, the concept of institutional licensure involves licensing health-care institutions rather than health care providers. Health-care personnel would be regulated by the institution within boundaries established by state institutional licensing boards. This approach would allow personnel to cross previously held boundaries. The licenses would recognize only general skills and allow individuals to upgrade into another category based upon the individual's ability to perform the activities in the new job category. Proponents of institutional licensure see it as a mechanism to enhance job mobility and reduce fragmentation of service. Critics of institutional licensure see other means of dealing with job mobility and fragmentation of care and caution that institutional licensure would lead to proliferation of unqualified practioners.

Summary

America has its roots firmly planted in a tradition of liberalism. It is a nation of fiercely independent persons who value free enterprise and a healthy profit margin. The prevailing winds are shifting Americans into a self-help model where participation and control are expected outcomes for individual health-care programs.

The state and federal governments have been established with checks and balances in order to guarantee a government responsive to the needs of the people. There is a growing realization that the national debt, strong pharmaceutical lobbies, and other special-interest groups may overshadow the health-care needs of the public.

Nursing must be sensitive to this political climate and use the political process to insure health access for all Americans. Nursing should be the pivotal arm to change the focus of government and the public from costly cures to less costly prevention.

Nursing should concern itself with issues of water and air pollution, hazardous waste, and food pollution. Policies consistent with the requirements for health protection and health promotion should be on the nursing agenda. Issues of family life in America and its impact on health should be the subject of nursing research and be brought to the attention of the public. Nursing has to broaden its definition of itself and view nursing, not exclusively as the profession that cares for the sick but the profession that promotes every facet of health.

On the state level nurses must examine their statutory mandates and how they contribute to free public access to nursing care. They must ensure that nurses are reimbursed for services essential to the public health. Research must be conducted to further examine the impact nursing has on the underserved, elderly, and emotionally troubled. It must establish a mechanism to bring these results into full public view. Each state's entry-into-practice position should be examined for its long-range effect on American health care. Once a position has been taken, legislators and their aides must be petitioned to endorse the wishes of nurses on entry-into-practice, mandatory continuing education, institutional licensure, and extended roles for nurses.

Social policy in this country has always been formulated in response to the wishes of a minority group. Nursing can have a tremendous impact on policy formulation when our elected officials realize that 1 in 44 women voters is a nurse!

Bibliography

Susan R. In Aiken LH, Gortner SR (eds): Nursing in the 1980's: Crisis, Opportunities, Challenges. Philadelphia, JB Lippincott, 1982

Agree BC: The threat of institutional licensure. Am J Nurs 73(10):1758–1762, 1973

Altman S; Present and future supply of registered nurses. Department of Health, Education, and Welfare Publication No. (NIH) 72–134, 1971

American Nurses Association: Nursing: A Social Policy Statement, pp 1–32, 1980

American Nurses Association: The Regulation of Advanced Nursing Practice as Provided for in Nursing Practice Acts and Administrative Rule. Kansas City, Mo, ANA, February 1984

Bloch H, Pupp R: Supply, demand, and rising health care costs. Nurs Econ 3:119–123, March–April, 1985

Bradham DD: Health policy formulation and analysis. Nurs Econ 3:167–171, May–June, 1985

Cimons M: U.S. child, maternity care cuts called life threatening. Los Angeles Times, p 1, January 12, 1983

Corbett MA, Burst HV: Nurse midwives and adolescents: The South Carolina experience. J Nurse Midwife 21:13–17, Winter, 1976

Culliton BJ: Nursing institute for NIH? Science 222:1310–1312, 1983

Davis CK: The federal role in changing health care financing. Nurs Econ I:98–146, September–October 1983

Dodd, LC, Scholt RL: Congress and Administrative State. New York, John Wiley & Sons, 1979

Donabedian A: Foreward. In Phaneuf M: The Nursing Audit and Self Regulation in Nursing Practice, 2nd ed. New York, Appleton-Century Crofts, 1976

Ertel PY, Aldridge GM (eds): Medical Peer Review: Theory and Practice, p 42. St. Louis, CV Mosby, 1977

Federation of American Hospitals: The 1983 Directory: Investor Owned Hospitals and Hospital Management Companies. Little Rock, FAH, 1982

Hauri CM et al: Cost effective primary care. Nurse Pract 4:54, September–October, 1979

Hood G: At issue: Titling and licensure. Am J Nurs 592–593, 1985

Iglehart JK: The administrator's assault on domestic spending and the threat to health care programs: Health policy report. New Eng J Med: 525–528, February 21, 1985

Institute of Medicine: Six Month Interim Report by the Committee of the Institute of Medicine for a Study of Nursing and Nursing Education. App. I. Washington, National Academy Press, 1981

Issues 6:2. Chicago, National Council of State Boards of Nursing, 1985

Johnson DL, Punch L: Multi-hospital systems survey. Mod Healthcare, 12(5):74–122, 1982

Klein LW: Passing NCLEX Issues 6(2):1–8, 1985

Kleinman JC et al: A comparison of 1960 and 1973–1974 early neonatal mortality and selective states. Am J Epidemiol, 108:454–469, December 1978

Kronenfeld JJ, Whicker ML: U.S. National Health Policy: An Analysis of the Federal Role. New York, Praeger, 1984

LaBar C: Statutory Requirements for Licensure of Nurses, pp 1–112. Kansas City, Mo, ANA Center for Research, September, 1984

Larson E: Health policy and NIH: Implications for nursing research. Nurs Res 33(6):352–356, November–December, 1984

Levine E: Hospital headlines. Hospitals 54:18–19. September 16, 1980

Martinson I: Taking the dying child home: What effect on patient family? Am Med Nurs 237:2591–2593, June 13, 1977

Master RJ et al: A continuum of care for the inner-city: Assessment of its benefits for Boston's elderly and high-risk populations. New Eng J Med 301:1434 1440, June 26, 1980

McKinlay JB (ed): Issues in health care policy. In Melbank Reader. Cambridge, MA MIT Press, 1981

Moss-Kanter R: The Change Master: Innovations for Productivity in the American Corporation. Greenville, NC, S & S, 1983

National Institutes of Health: NIH Almanac. NIH Publication No. 83–5. Bethesda, MD, U.S. Department of Health and Human Services, 1983

Peres JR: Update on federal regulatory trends.J Med Group Manag Assoc, January–February 1985.

Peters TJ, Waterman RH, Jr: In Search of Excellence. New York, Warner Books, 1984

Pozen NW et al: A nurse rehabilitator's impact on patients with myocardial infarction. Med Care 15:830–837, October 1977

Puetz BE: Legislating a continuing education requirement for licensure renewal. J Contin Ed Nurs 14(5):5–12, 1983

Ripley RB: American National Government and Public Policy. New York, Free Press, 1974

Runyan JW, Jr: The Memphis chronic disease program: Comparisons in outcome and the nurse's extended role. JAMA 231:264–267, January 20, 1975

Salmon WJ: Who benefits from competition in health care? Nurs Econ 1:129–134, September–October 1983

Santaiti BJ: The federal budget process. Nurs Econ 3:103–108, March–April 1985

Snyder M, LaBar C: Issues in Professional Nursing Practice. Nursing: Legal Authority for Practice, pp 1–21, Kansas City, MO, American Nurses Association, 1984

Somers AR, Somers HN: Health and Health Care: Policies in Perspective. Germantown, MD, Aspen Systems, 1977

Strickland S: Research and the Health of Americans: Improving the Policy Process. Lexington, MA: Lexington Books, 1978

Walholz M: Some hospitals are entering diverse businesses, often unrelated to medicine, to offset losses. Wall Street Journal, p 56, August 12, 1982

Warren KF: Administrative Law in the American Political System. St. Paul, West, 1982

Weber M: The Protestant Ethic and the Spirit of Capitalism, translated by Talcott Parsons. New York, Charles Scribner and Sons, 1958

Woll P: Public Policy. Cambridge, MA Winthrop Publishers, 1974

Chapter 14

Legal and ethical issues

RICHARD W. ASHTON

It is important for the new professional nurse to know about and under-stand the implications of laws that will affect her throughout the course of her employment in the health-care field. Such laws will directly influ-ence the conditions of employment and have an impact on nursing prac-tice and patient care. Federal and state laws regulate the relationships between management and employees, between management and unions, and between unions and their membership. Federal and state laws affect the employment process from pre-employment advertising, throughout the course of employment, and until retirement, to ensure equality in employment opportunities.

This chapter will enable you to

1. Determine specific Civil Rights laws that affect a nurse's course of employment.

2. Describe the legal rights, duties, and objectives of employees, employers, and unions as established by the National Labor Relations Act and the National Labor Relations Board.

3. Describe the prima facie case of negligence (malpractice).

4. Describe the elements of informed consent.

5. Identify recurring potential legal issues in the nursing role and environment.

6. Identify potential legal issues related to the withdrawal or refusal of medical treatment.

7. Identify the purpose and duties of the state agency regulating nursing practice.

8. Describe the functions of an institutional bioethics committee.

Sources of Law and the Judicial System

Law is a social institution evolved over time by a society and molded to reflect, maintain, and inculcate a society's culture, values, and mores. The basic purpose of a legal system is to establish and control human conduct and relationships to reduce the use of force and violence in resolving interpersonal conflicts and disputes. American law can be separated into two major divisions: private law and public law. The rights and duties of individuals and organizations are established and enforced by private law, which consists primarily of contract law, tort law, and property law. The relationship between the government and its citizens is regulated and enforced by public law. Public law includes such areas as criminal law, which protects the social order, and administrative law, which advances the general welfare of society through the activities of such agencies as the Environmental Protection Agency (EPA), and Health and Human Services (HHS), among many others.

SOURCES OF LAW

The law of the United States is derived from four sources: the federal and state constitutions, federal and state statutes, judicial decisions (case law), and administrative law. At its inception the federal government received a grant of powers from the several states and those powers are reflected in the Articles of the Constitution. All powers not granted to the federal government are reserved by the states and by individual citizens. Article VI of the United States Constitution clearly enunciates that the Constitution and the laws of the United States shall be the supreme law of the land.[1]

The United States Constitution establishes the principle of separation of powers, dividing government into three branches: the legislative, executive, and judicial branches. State constitutions establish similar structures of state government. Congress and the state legislatures perform the legislative function of enacting, amending, or repealing laws. Legislated laws are called statutes. The executive branch of government is charged with the administration and enforcement of laws enacted by the legislative branch. The Chief Executive is the president of the United States or the governors of the various states. The actions of the executive branch of government, which administers and enforces statutes and administrative regulations, are adjudicated by the judicial branch. The judiciary establishes the legal principles and procedures to resolve conflicts arising from private and public law.

Serving as a fourth branch of government and the source of a vast body of law is the administrative agencies. Both Congress and the state legislatures establish an administrative agency through the enactment of a statute and delegate to that administrative agency the traditional powers of government; that is, the power to legislate by promulgating rules and regulations, the power of the executive to administer and enforce rules and regulations, and the power to adjudicate by determining whether such rules and regulations were violated by the acts of individuals or organizations. Administrative agencies are established because Congress or the state legislatures cannot devote sufficient time or lack sufficient expertise to deal with the complex issues and multitude of details necessary to regulate properly certain societal and governmental activities. Examples of administrative agencies on the national level include the Department of Health and Human Services, Food and Drug Administration, Federal Trade Commission, and the National Labor Relations Board. On the state level nurses are more familiar with the example of the State Board of Nurse Examiners or similar agencies that regulate licensure activities of nursing and the various other professions.

Federal and state agencies can operate only within the scope of authority delegated to them by the legislative body. The rules and regulations promulgated by an administrative agency have the force of law unless they are subsequently overruled by a court because the agency exceeded the authority granted to it or because the proper procedures were not followed in promulgating the rules. The federal government and most states have an Administrative Procedures Act specifying the process that administrative agencies must follow when promulgating rules or regulations, or adjudicating disputes. The Administrative Procedures Act usually requires public notice of proposed rule making through publication to provide the public an opportunity to comment. For example, the agencies of the federal government are required to publish in the Federal Register all proposed and final rules and regulations.

In brief then, the sources of law in the United States originate from the federal and state constitutions, statutory law enacted by Congress or the state legislatures, administrative law consisting of the decisions of administrative agencies and the rules and regulations promulgated by such agencies and, finally, judicial decisions.

The body of law stemming from court decisions, frequently called case law or judge-made law, is the product of a court's decision in a specific case. If a legal issue is presented to a court with appropriate jurisdiction, the court, through the legal process, will hear facts pertaining to the case and apply statutory law or prior case-decision law, reach a verdict, and pass judgment. Case law is an evolving body of law based upon the ancient heritage of the common law of England and is constantly adjusted to reflect new court decisions in resolving, on a case-by-case basis, the multitude of legal conflicts presented to the federal and state courts on a daily basis. While case law is continually evolving and is dynamic, it is not unstable and chaotic due to the steadying influence of the doctrine of *stare decisis,* the doctrine of precedent. The application of this doctrine provides for stability and certainty in prognosticating legal outcomes by applying to similar cases with similar fact patterns the same legal rules and principles that were applied in cases previously decided, so that consistent legal conclusions and judgments can be reached in similar cases. Prior case decisions can be overruled, however, by a court to reflect changing social conditions, values, and mores.

THE JUDICIAL SYSTEM

The federal and state court systems are quite comparable: both have trial courts of original jurisdiction in which a suit is initiated, evidence is received to determine the facts of the case, and the applicable law is applied to reach a decision. In a trial court, the judge determines what the law is and the jury determines what the facts are, and applies the law as instructed by the judge. The trial court for the federal system is the United States District Court and the trial courts of the various states have various names, such as Court of Common Pleas. The federal system and most state systems have intermediate courts of appeal that consider and decide on appeals from trial court decisions. Appellate courts do not retry the case; they review the record of the trial court to determine whether proper legal procedures were followed and whether the trial court properly interpreted statutory or case laws when applying them to the case on appeal. Cases from the United States Federal District Court are appealed to a United States Court of Appeals.

The final level in most court systems is the Supreme Court. The Supreme Court of the United States is a court of limited jurisdiction that selectively takes cases for review and adjudication through the process of a writ of certiorari.

The Trial

The person who believes he has been injured by another and who begins a law suit is called the *plaintiff*. The person or organization who is sued is called the *defendant*. The suit is commenced when the plaintiff requests the court clerk to issue a writ for the sheriff to serve a summons or a complaint upon the defendant. The service of the summons or complaint places the defendant within the jurisdiction of the court, informs the defendant that a legal action has been initiated, and states the nature of the action. When the summons or complaint is served upon the defendant, the defendant should immediately notify his attorney or insurance representative. Often called a pleading, the complaint sets forth the plaintiff's facts of the case. The defendant responds to the complaint by filing an answer that either denies or admits to the facts and allegations contained in the complaint.

Once the suit has been filed and the summons or complaint is served upon the defendant, the discovery process can begin. The purpose of the discovery process is to provide both parties with sufficient information to determine the true facts of the case. Permitting them to assess the relative strengths and weaknesses of their legal positions encourages early settlement and provides for judicial economy. The two major forms of discovery are written questions called *interrogatories,* which are answered under oath, and *depositions,* which are oral questions answered orally, again under oath and recorded by a court stenographer. Other discovery devices include court orders requiring the parties to produce for examination records, papers, and other physical evidence. Through court order a party to the suit may be required to submit to a physical or mental examination if the physical or mental status of the party is at issue.

The progress and course of the trial is governed by court procedures and rules and enforced by the judge. This provides for the orderly presentation of evidence to demonstrate facts of the case. The facts are presented in the form of evidence consisting of oral testimony by witnesses and the entry into evidence of records and other documents, and other physical evidence such as equipment, instruments, x-rays and photographs, if they are pertinent to the case. Evidence may also include testimony of an expert witness.

Trial can be before a judge only, called a bench trial, or before a jury. The plaintiff presents his case first by calling and examining witnesses and introducing other evidence into the record. The plaintiff's witnesses may be cross-examined by the defense attorney. Following the presentation of the plaintiff's case, the defendant introduces the testimony of witnesses and other evidence to refute the plaintiff's case. The plaintiff's attorney may also cross-examine the defendant's witnesses. After both parties have presented their cases in a jury trial, the judge instructs the jury members with respect to the legal principles to be applied to the facts elicited through testimony and other evidence. The jury then considers the evidence presented at trial, applied the instructions of the judge and reaches its verdict. If there was not a jury the judge considers the evidence himself, applies the law, and renders the verdict. The losing party may then move for a retrial or file an appeal to the intermediate court of appeals. Once an appeal progresses to the highest appellate court the legal process is at an end.

Laws Affecting the Employment Relationship

The new professional nurse should be cognizant of the Federal Civil Rights Laws that exist to protect her as she seeks employment and during the course of her work career. While salient federal laws will be discussed in this chapter, it should be noted that most states have enacted similar laws that may also be used to address and remedy discrimination in employment.

TITLE VII

Title VII of the Civil Rights Act of 1964 is the major federal statute protecting employees from discriminatory practices by employers, employment agencies, and labor organizations.[2] Since 1972, this statute has covered the United States government and state and local governments, as well as private industry. The purpose of Title VII is to provide all persons equal opportunity in all aspects of employment. Title VII prohibits discrimination in employment on the basis of a person's race, color, religion, sex, or national origin, except where religion, sex, or natural origin is a bona fide occupational qualification (that is, a characteristic or attribute necessary to conduct a particular business). Sex, as a nondiscriminatory characteristic, also includes pregnancy, childbirth, and abortion.

Title VII is quite comprehensive in that it affects pre-employment practices related to advertising, recruiting, pre-employment inquiries, and hiring standards. Job advertisements or notices may not indicate any preference based on race, color, sex, religion, or natural origin, except where a bona fide occupational qualification can be substantiated. Hiring quotas based on these impermissible characteristics are prohibited and the referral sources used by an employer must recruit and refer applicants for employment in a nondiscriminatory fashion. Pre-employment inquiries by the employer concerning race, color, religion, sex, or natural origin are prohibited, including inquiries concerning arrests or conviction records, unless a business necessity can be demonstrated.

The employer's recruitment and hiring procedures should be standardized and objective and not result in a "disparate impact" on protected groups. "Disparate impact" means employment practices that are facially neutral in their treatment of different groups (such as blacks, females), when, in fact, they statistically affect one group more than another and cannot be justified by a business necessity. Tests used in selecting candidates for employment or for promotion must be nondiscriminatory in their impact and be validated by one of several procedures. Construct validity determines the psychological traits that underlie successful performance on the job and measures the presence or absence of the traits in applicants for the position. Criterion-based validity is established by demonstrating a statistical relationship between scores on a test and objective measures of job performance. The final test of validity pertains to the test content by proving that the test procedure represents significant examples of the job tasks and duties.

Title VII extends beyond the recruitment and hiring phase of the employment relationship and requires that the employer's personnel policies and practices and work policies and procedures that affect employees during the course of their employment be administered in a consistent, uniform, and nondiscriminatory manner to avoid "disparate treatment" of individuals. Disparate treatment occurs when one employee is treated less favorably in the employment relationship than other employees because of his race, color, religion, sex, or national origin.

Sexual Harassment

Title VII of the 1964 Civil Rights Act includes sexual harassment as a prohibited act. In 1980 the Equal Employment Opportunity Commission (EEOC) published an amendment to its guidelines on discrimination to define what it regards to be unlawful sexual harassment, to establish the employers' legal responsibility for the unlawful acts of its agents, supervisors, and other employees, and to recommend affirmative actions by the employer to prevent sexual harassment in the workplace.[3] Sexual harassment is defined by the EEOC to be sexual advances, requests for sexual favors, or other verbal or physical sexual conduct when: (1) submission to the conduct is either an explicit or implicit term or condition of employment; (2) submission to or rejection of the conduct is used as a basis for employment decisions affecting the person submitting or rejecting; (3) the conduct has a purpose or effect of substantially interfering with an individual's work performance or creating an intimidating, hostile, or offensive work environment. Applying this definition and its related criteria to specific conduct on a case-by-case basis, the EEOC will determine whether sexual harassment has occurred. Employers are responsible for the acts of their supervisory employees or their agents, regardless of whether or not the acts were authorized or forbidden by the employer. Employers are also responsible for the acts of other persons only when they, their agents, or their supervisory personnel know or should have known of the sexually harassing conduct and did not take immediate and appropriate corrective action. The amended guidelines recommended that employers take affirmative steps to prevent sexual harassment by discussing the subject with their employees, informing them of their right to raise the issue as a complaint, by stating a strong position or disapproval of such conduct, and taking appropriate sanctions against persons who perpetrate sexual harassment.

Administration of the Act is through the Equal Employment Opportunity Commission (EEOC), which is headquartered in Washington, D.C., with regional and district offices throughout the United States. An employee is required to file a charge with the local EEOC within 180 days of the discriminatory act and subsequently the EEOC, through field investigators, will investigate the charge by conducting a fact-finding conference. If "reasonable cause" is found to exist that Title VII was violated, the EEOC will conduct a conciliation meeting with the employer. If the conciliation effort does not lead to a redress and remedy, either the EEOC or the individual alleging discrimination may file suit in a Federal District Court.

ADEA

In 1967 Congress passed the Age Discrimination and Employment ACT (ADEA) to protect employees and job applicants who are between the ages of 40 and 70 years.[4] This act was subsequently extended by amendment in 1974 to public employees. The ADEA prohibits employment decisions based on age unless age can be demonstrated as a bona fide occupational qualification reasonably related to the normal operation of a particular business. The act covers all aspects of the employment relationship from pre-employment advertising through selection and hiring, promotion, and discharge. Mandatory retirement prior to age 70 is prohibited if the employee is otherwise capable of performing the tasks and duties of the job. The Equal Employment Opportunity Commission also administers this act. A protected individual may bring a civil suit after the EEOC has been given a 60 day notice of intent to file a legal action. When notice is received, the EEOC will attempt to resolve the issue through a conciliation meeting with the employer.

EQUAL PAY ACT

The Equal Pay Act of 1963 prohibits employers from discriminating on the basis of sex by paying one sex at a higher rate than employees of the opposite sex for equal work where the work requires equal skill, effort, and responsibility and is performed under similar working conditions.[5] A differential in pay may exist, except where it is based on a characteristic of sex; that is, a merit system is permissible as well as seniority system, and systems based upon productivity or quality of work performed. State and local governments are exempted from the Equal Pay Act. The Equal Employment Opportunity Commission administers this act and an employee may initiate a civil suit after giving notice to the EEOC.

COMPARABLE WORTH THEORY

The concept of comparable worth exceeds the scope of the Equal Pay Act of 1963 by contending that entire occupational fields historically employing women, such as nursing, elementary and secondary education, secretarial and library sciences are inappropriately undervalued and underpaid. Proponents of the comparable worth theory seek to establish an equitable compensation relationship between male- and female-dominated occupations or job clusters. It is assumed that appropriate unbiased job evaluation systems would demonstrate great similarities between jobs although the specific job may be in a male- or a female-dominated occupation or job category. Thus, certain jobs in education (a female-dominated occupation) and engineering (a male-dominated occupation) may be determined to be comparable in terms of substantially similar skills, knowledge, effort, educational requirements, experience, working conditions, and responsibility and, subsequently, in terms of compensation. Comparable worth theory is closely entwined with women's equality issues since there is perceived unfairness in existing job evaluation systems and promotion opportunities. On the average, employed women earn 60% less than males. It is argued that without the application of comparable worth theory, job segregation by sex will continue. It has also been noted by some theorists that job segregation on the basis of sex and the underevaluation and unfair compensation of work performed by females will accelerate the feminization of poverty as the numbers of women heading single-parent families increases.

Those opposing comparable worth advance the following arguments: that the disparity in wages between men and women is attributable to a multiplicity of factors such as education, work experience, individual choice, and the marketplace, and not just by sex segregation. Strong arguments are made that the free marketplace, that is, the law of supply and demand, should regulate salary levels and not comparable worth. Other arguments address the economic impact of increasing employment costs by possibly billions of dollars that would have a catastrophic affect upon our economy; that comparable worth would undermine collective bargaining and bring about the demise of unions; that there is appropriate legal redress for employees who are discriminated against in compensation because of their sex, such as Title VII or the Equal Pay Act; that existing job evaluations and wage and salary systems are reliable and fair and that the application of comparable worth will destroy the free market environment of employment.

To date, conflicting judicial decisions have been reached concerning comparable worth and the current administration (as of this writing) has voiced its opposition to the theory. The future of comparable worth is uncertain and must be played out over the next decade through the legal and legislative processes. The future of comparable worth as a viable and applicable theory within our social system and culture will parallel the fortunes of the women's movement since the issue and theme of comparable worth is sexual equality.

THE NLRA

The National Labor Relations Act (the "Act"), actually a series of federal statutes enacted and amended over the last 50 years, applies to all employers engaged in or affecting interstate commerce, including non-profit health institutions.[6] The United States government and state governments and their political subdivisions are exempted from the Act. The purpose of the Act is to decrease the possibility of obstructing interstate commerce caused by labor disputes by providing employees the right to self-organize; to engage in collective bargaining through representatives they select, and to participate in concerted activities for their mutual aid and protection. The Act also protects the right of employees to refrain from participation in such activities. These rights of employees are usually referred to as Section 7 rights.

Certain definitions of the Act are of particular importance. Health-care institutions, as defined, include any institution primarily involved in the care of the sick, infirm, or aged persons. As employer is any person, that is, one or more individuals, acting as the agent of an employer. A supervisor is any individual having the authority of the employer to direct and supervise employees, and who can hire, fire, reward, or discipline, or adjust employee grievances, or recommend such actions. Labor organizations are any organizations, including employee representation committees or similar arrangements, in which employees participate, that deal with employees concerning grievances, labor disputes, wages, rates of compensation, hours of work, and conditions of employment.

These definitions are interpreted by case application and demonstrate that the employer, that is, a hospital and its agents, such as a head nurse, are considered one legal entity. The acts of the head nurse in respect to employee-management matters are vicariously attributed to the hospital corporation. When the head nurse meets with a group of nursing personnel at their request to discuss work-related complaints, pay issues, or other conditions of employment she may be meeting with what will subsequently be construed as a labor organization by the National Labor Relations Board (NLRB), which administers the Act, particularly if the content and manner of discussion moves from a dialogue to a negotiation session.

"Concerted activities" is a technical definition (a word or phrase) and appears to be subject to various interpretations. So case-to-case comparability is made difficult because of the specific facts, circumstances, and events that vary greatly in each case. In essence, concerted activity is an employee activity which is: (1) a work-related complaint; (2) a concerted activity that furthers some group interest; (3) a specific result sought through such activity, and (4) an illegal activity (violence, work slow-down, etc.). Employees need not be represented by a union or be union members to receive protection of the Act when engaged in concerted activities.

The Act prohibits certain employer and union conduct and labels them as unfair labor practices. It is an unfair labor practice for an employer to interfere with, restrain, or coerce employees who are exercising their Section 7 rights. Employers cannot subject employees to surveillance to uncover union-related activities; interrogate employees as to their union affiliation or interest; discriminate against employees in respect to their condition of employment or tenure to affect their membership in a union; subject employees to economic threats (such as closing the facility if the union wins an election), or interfere with or dominate a labor organization (to organize a company union, to contribute financial support to a union).

Unions also are prohibited from interfering with employees' Section 7 rights. A union commits an unfair labor practice if it attempts to cause an employer to discriminate against a nonunion employee, coerce employees to join the union, and to extract excessive fees or dues to become union members. Labor organizations have a duty of fair representation that requires the certified or designated union to represent *all* employees in the bargaining union, whether or not they are members of the union.

Both employers and unions commit an unfair labor practice if they refuse to bargain in good faith once a union is certified or designated. Again, good faith bargaining is a phrase of art that requires certain mutually binding elements: (1) to meet at reasonable times; (2) to discuss in good faith matters related to wages, hours, and other conditions of employment; (3) to negotiate on such items; and, (4) to execute a written contract incorporating bargained-for agreements that have been reached under the negotiating process. The only mandatory subject matters of negotiations are wages, hours, and other terms and conditions of employment. All other subjects discussed or proposed during collective bargaining are permissive or discretionary. The Act does not compel either the employer or the union to agree to any offer or concession; that is, a mutual agreement in the form of a labor contract is not a legal requirement or outcome of the NLRA.

The reasons professional nurses seek a collective bargaining representative are varied, complex, and diverse. There is no one cause for the unionization of a health-care institution. Union organizing efforts are usually by invitation of the employees and occur where employee-management relationships are ambiguous or based on mutual distrust, suspicion, disrespect, and fear. Employees develop negative feelings and ultimately alienation from the employer when they are treated with disrespect by management personnel. Professional employees want to be treated as individuals with unique needs who seek opportunities to upgrade their skills and knowledge, and expand their scope of practice and accountability. All employees want to be treated equally and without discrimination based on factors unrelated to job performance. Professional nurses want to participate in and influence the decisions that affect them and their nursing practice. Unilateral management decisions and actions are objectionable to the professional. Employees want to work in a safe and attractive environment where the interpersonnel and employee-management relationships are friendly and relaxed, and demonstrate a mutual recognition of the inherent dignity of personhood.

When management is unenlightened and over-reaching and when employees are chronically dissatisfied and alienated, a union organizer will be invited in by a disgruntled group of employees. The purpose is to determine the level of interest the staff may have in being represented by a collective bargaining agent. A union organizing committee will be established with members coming from the ranks of employees to be unionized. The expression of interest in collective bargaining is usually determined by soliciting persons who would be members of the proposed bargaining unit. The solicitation is usually in the form of requesting interested staff members to sign an authorization card appointing a specific union to be the exclusive bargaining agent for them. In order to petition the NLRB for a representation election, the union must demonstrate a "showing of interest" requiring that 30% of the employees in the proposed bargaining unit sign a union authorization card. Unions commonly will not proceed to petition the NLRB unless at least 50% of the bargaining unit employees sign authorization cards.

Through the local organizing committee and sympathizers, unions will continue to increase bargaining unit awareness and interest in collective bargaining by solicitation and distribution efforts. Solicitation refers to those verbal discussions of the pros and cons of unionization, general oral persuasion concerning representation, and the dissemination of union authorization cards. Solicitation is permissable in employee cafeterias, lounges, and other public areas, including the corridors in patient units, elevator lobbies, and patient-visitor lounges.

Distribution refers to the passing out of printed union literature under rules determined by the NLRB and federal case law. Solicitation is permissible in health-care institutions if it occurs on nonwork time; that is, breaks, lunch, prior to or after work, and in areas not directly related to patient treatment. Employers may prohibit the distribution of union literature at all times in working areas and the distribution of such materials on company time in nonwork areas. Employees may distribute and receive union literature on nonwork time in nonwork areas; that is, during breaks, in the cafeteria, and entering and exiting the hospital.

Employers often establish a nonaccess policy to limit the opportunity for employees to solicit their fellow workers and distribute union literature. Such a work rule prohibits off-duty employees from remaining on the premises for any purpose after working hours or returning to work areas after the completion of work. All nonemployees may be prohibited from soliciting employees and distributing union literature on the hospital property.

The composition of the bargaining unit membership is of particular import to the employer, professional nurses, and the prospective collective bargaining agent. A controversy has existed since 1974 between the NLRB and the federal courts, with the federal courts holding that Congress intended to avoid unnecessary proliferation of bargaining units in the health-care industry while the NLRB repeatedly recognized seven separate bargaining units on the basis of a "community of interest." The seven units consist of physicians, registered nurses, other professional employees, technical employees, business office and clerical employees, service and maintenance employees, and skilled maintenance employees. The NLRB has now abandoned the "community of interest" standard of inclusion into a bargaining unit and has adapted a "disparity of interests" test. The board will now seek a broad inclusive group of job categories and exclude only those that can prove a significant scope of disparate interest. An all-RN bargaining unit may not be impermissible and RNs may be included within a bargaining unit that includes physical therapists, occupational therapists, dieticians, medical technologists, and others. Section 9 (b) (1) of the Act requires that nonprofessionals not be included within a bargaining unit of professionals unless the professionals vote in favor of such an inclusion. Supervisors and all other managerial personnel are not considered "employees" under the NLRA and consequently cannot be members of a bargaining unit or vote in union elections.

The Legal Concept of Professional Liability (Malpractice)

The new professional nurse should be aware of the scope of civil legal liability attached to the practice of nursing within a health-care institution. The nurse is personally liable for her acts and omissions that lead to the injury of a person or a person's property, or to the infringement of the legally recognized rights of individuals. As discussed below, the conduct of the nurse employed by a health-care institution can also be attributed to the employer through the legal doctrine of *respondent-superior* under which the employer is vicariously liable for the consequence of an employee's activities occurring within the scope of employment. The body of law addressing the legal consequences of a person's acts or omissions is referred to as the field-of-tort law. A tort is a civil wrong, excluding a breach of contract, that interferes with the legally recognized rights of an individual with respect to his person or property, for which the legal system will provide a remedy in the form of an action for damages. The law of torts is concerned with the allocation of losses arising out of human conduct: that is, the law attempts to strike a balance by distributing risks equitably throughout society and between individuals. The common thread in all tort actions is the unreasonable interference in the interests and rights of others.

Tort actions are usually classified as intentional torts; that is, those willful acts that violate a person's rights; for example, the tort of assault, which is placing another person in apprehension of being touched in an offensive and harmful manner without the person's consent; or negligence, which is discussed below. Other intentional torts include battery, defamation, false imprisonment, invasion of privacy and intentional infliction of emotional distress, all of which will be briefly discussed. The second major category of torts is the area of negligence, which occurs when the rights of a person are violated due the incorrect performance of a duty or when the duty to perform an act is ignored or overlooked. The basis of the negligent action involves committing or omitting an act, placing another in the position of assuming an unreasonable risk of injury, and the subsequent occurrence of the injury.

As noted above, an assault occurs when one places another person in apprehension of being touched in a harmful or offensive manner without that person's consent. It is not necessary that an actual touching occur; it is the apprehension of such an act that forms the basis of liability. When a touching actually occurs, the tort of battery is realized. The torts of assault and battery are the legal recognition that an individual has a right to be free from the unconsented infringement upon his person. Assault and battery situations frequently arise when medical and nursing care is attempted without the consent of the patient. Procedures performed upon a patient without his prior informed consent can be the basis of a suit for assault and battery.

A nurse's conduct giving rise to the torts of assault and battery may also be extended into the tort of false imprisonment. The latter is the unlawful restriction of a person's freedom. This may occur in the healthcare field when the patient is physically restrained or detained within an institution. In all cases where a patient is an adult and mentally competent, the nurse should not restrain or detain a patient unless specifically required by an appropriate policy or directly authorized by an appropriate supervisory person ar administrator. Mentally ill patients who are legally committed to the institution obviously can be restrained and detained; however, the nature and length of physical restraint must be limited to that which is reasonably necessary under the circumstances. Mentally ill patients can be detained if there is a danger that they will be harmful to themselves or others; however, such detention must be immediately followed by the initiation of commitment procedures required under the appropriate state statutes.

Defamation is a tort action addressing the wrongful injury to another person's reputation. Libel is the *written* form of defamation and slander is the *spoken* form. The law of defamation is extremely complex and technical and a full discussion of the topic is beyond the scope of this chapter. It is essential, however, to be sensitive to the situations in which allegations of defamation can arise. A patient may claim that he has been defamed because the inappropriate or inaccurate release of medical information concerning him has injured his reputation; or your nursing colleagues, medical staff, or other employees may claim that untruthful statements were made concerning them, which injured them in their employment or their profession. The nurse must then be very cautious and release medical information only with the consent of the patient and in accord with the established hospital policies and procedures. In respect to other employees, professional colleagues, and medical staff, the nurse should not utter unsubstantiated opinions or judgments, pass on rumor or gossip, or state untruths about others in respect to their personal or professional lives.

The fear of a defamation suit should not preclude nurses from communicating truthful matters concerning medical staff or employee performance that affect patient safety and welfare. Such communication is necessary for the orderly management of a safe and therapeutic patient-care environment and is recognized by the courts by the granting of a "qualified privilege" to such communication. To be so privileged, the communication must be made within the established channels or organizational authority and communicated to a person who has a legitimate organizational right to receive and act upon such information.

Correlative to the avoidance of a possible claim of defamation by a patient for releasing medical information is the concern to avoid the allegation of the unlawful invasion of a patient's privacy. The courts recognize a person's right to be free from unwarranted publicity and exposure to public scrutiny without their consent—the right to be left alone. This right extends to a patient's name, photograph, and other reproductions of his physical likeness. In the course of providing health care, nurses legitimately learn much about a patient's private life and personal affairs. The nurse must be particularly careful in divulging any information from a medical record or about the patient's personal life unless the patient consents to such disclosure to a third person.

A growing body of case law provides remedy for the tort of intentionally inflicting emotional distress upon another person. This action is often initiated by insensitive interpersonal relationships and acts that border on outrageous conduct and cause severe emotional trauma to the patient or immediate members of the patient's family. Although the majority of jurisdictions require actual physical injury caused by the outrageous act to find the intentional infliction of emotional distress, a growing number of courts have held that recovery may be allowed where there is no demonstrable physical injuries. A minority of courts also recognizes this tort when the emotional distress is suffered by a third person, that is, a close immediate member of the family, such as a spouse, a parent, or a child, when the third party is present at the time and the mental stress on that person was forseeable. Thus, the nurse is not only required to be professionally competent, but should be courteous, compassionate, and concerned about the feelings of others.

NEGLIGENCE

The greatest exposure to civil legal liability faced by the nurse is in the area of negligence. Negligence in providing professional services is termed *malpractice*. The plaintiff in a malpractice suit must establish a *prima facie* case by proving four elements: (1) that the defendant had a duty to the plaintiff; (2) that the defendant breached the duty; (3) that the plaintiff was injured by the defendant's breach of duty, and (4) that the injury was caused by the breach of duty.

When a patient is admitted to a health-care institution the duty of due care is immediately established between the patient and the hospital, and when the registered nurse is assigned to provide care for the patient, the duty of due care is established between the individual professional nurse and the patient. Once the duty of due care is established, the question of the scope and nature of that duty is raised. The scope and nature of the duty is referred to as the standard of care. The hospital as the employer and the registered nurse personally have a legal obligation to meet the standard of care and both will be liable if they fail to meet the standard. The standard of care for registered nurses is the degree of care that would ordinarily be exercised by a reasonably prudent nurse with similar training acting under similar circumstances. The appropriate standard of care will be determined through expert testimony, licensure regulations, standards developed by professional organizations, standards of accreditation agencies, and institutional policies and procedures. In certain malpractice cases the use of expert testimony is not required because the standard of care is nontechnical and within the common knowledge of the general public.

The second element of the *prima facie* case is to prove that the duty of due care (the standard of care) was not met, that a breach of duty occurred. The plaintiff must prove the breach of duty by showing that what should have been done in the care of the patient was done improperly or was omitted. Proof of the breach duty, that is, the deviation from the standard of care, is provided by testimony or witnesses and through documentation contained in the patient's medical record that is entered into evidence at the trial.

Proof of injury, the third element required to prove negligence, requires the plaintiff to demonstrate physical, mental, or monetary injury. The final element required to establish a malpractice case is to prove the relationship between the breach of duty and the injury; this element is called *causation*. Causation is often established by the application of the rule that "the patient would not have incurred this injury *but for* the act of this nurse." If the acts of more than one defendant are involved in the injury to the plaintiff, and it appears that the action of either one of the defendants alone would have been sufficient to cause the injury, all of the defendants will be found liable since each defendant's act was a *material factor* in causing the injury.

Occasionally it is difficult to prove all four elements required to establish a *prima facie* case of negligence. One legal concept attempts to assist the plaintiff in proving the breach of duty and certain elements of causation. The assistance is provided by the doctrine of *res ipsa loquitur,* "the act speaks for itself." In the fact situation where *res ipsa loquitur* is applicable, the fact that the act occurred at all tends to establish the breach of duty owed to the plaintiff if the following factors exist: first, that the incident is of a type that does not normally occur except for someone's negligence; secondly, that the cause of the injury was within the exclusive control of the defendant, and third, that neither the plaintiff nor any other third party contributed in any way to the plaintiff's injuries. An example of a typical *res ipsa loquitur*-type case is the hemostat that is left in the abdomen of a patient undergoing surgery and subsequently discovered months or years postoperatively.

INFORMED CONSENT

The right of persons to be free from unauthorized harmful or offensive touching has been recognized and supported in American case law through the common law action of the tort of battery. Health-care providers, particularly physicians, may be liable for battery if they perform medical treatment without prior consent of the patient, even though such treatment may be done in a non-negligent manner and benefit the patient. Liability is specific to the unauthorized touching of the person's body. Over the last two decades the concept of authorization for medical treatment has evolved from the common law concept of a tort of battery to the concept of informed consent with the legal action based on the tort of negligence when informed consent is not obtained.

Informed consent requires a full explanation by the health-care provider to the patient concerning the patient's medical condition, the nature and goals of the proposed treatment and diagnostic test, the risks attendant with the treatment or test, other appropriate alternatives for treatment or diagnosis, and the expected outcomes if no treatment or diagnosis is initiated. Full, in the sense of complete, disclosure of information relating to a person's medical condition and the risks related to treatment, testing, or non-treatment is impractical, if indeed possible; thus the scope of disclosure to gain informed consent should be focused upon what is pertinent and material to the patient in reaching the decision to forego or accept the proposed treatment or test.

Consent can be conveyed orally or in writing and will be legally binding in either mode unless state or federal statutes or institutional policies require written consent. In order to meet the Joint Commission on Accreditation of Hospitals (JCAH) standards, most health-care institutions require written documentation of informed consent for specific types of diagnostic tests or treatments. Consent may be implied by the patient's behavior when he voluntarily submits to a medical examination and treatment, or consent may be explicit through direct words or written assent to offered treatment or diagnostic testing.

Depending upon the state, the courts use one of two standards to determine whether the adequacy of the information shared with the patient was sufficient to gain informed consent. In some jurisdictions, the professional standard is used: the physician has the duty to disclose any information that the reasonable medical practitioner would disclose to the patient under similar circumstances. Determining what the reasonable physician would disclose requires the entry of expert testimony at trial. The courts of other states rely upon a reasonable patient standard of disclosure. This standard rejects the standard of professional practice and seeks to determine what a reasonable person would think is "material" and requires the physician to place himself in the patient's position to determine what risks, alternatives, or outcomes are significant in reaching the decision to accept or reject proposed treatment.

There are certain exceptions to the disclosure and consent requirements compelled by various circumstances, such as emergencies, patient waiver, and the grant of therapeutic privilege. In some emergency situations, time is of the essence in providing diagnosis and treatment in order to preclude increased morbidity, permanent physical impairment, or perhaps death. Thus consent is implied. A mentally competent adult may expressly waive the right of disclosure of medically pertinent material information and consent for treatment foregoing the scope of disclosure required for informed consent.

The concept of therapeutic privilege has been recognized by the courts of a majority of states and permits the physician or other independent health practitioners from disclosing information that, in their professional opinion, would be harmful to the patient. The courts are particularly cautious in applying this doctrine to prevent the undermining of the opposing doctrine of informed consent. The courts will not apply the therapeutic privilege to those situations where the professional fails to disclose pertinent and material information to the patient solely on the basis that such disclosure would discourage the patient from consenting to the proposed treatment. The exercise of therapeutic privilege is only recognized in those circumstances in which disclosure would lead to pathological anxiety and stress or severe mental anguish and suffering.

Within the health-care institution, it is only the physician or other independent practitioner who can gain informed consent from the patient to perform a surgical procedure, a diagnostic technique, or provide a specific therapy. The legal duty of gaining informed consent is based on the patient-physician relationship. Health-care institutions have a duty to establish and supervise mechanisms, such as policies and procedures, to ensure the public they serve that informed consent will be obtained. Although hospitals will generally not be liable for diagnostic and therapeutic procedures performed by nonemployee physicians, some hospitals have been found liable for failing to intervene when they were deemed to have knowledge or had actual knowledge that surgery was being performed without the patient's consent. In order to meet their legal duties in respect to informed consent, hospitals frequently require patients to sign a consent form for a specific diagnostic or therapeutic procedure indicating that the person signing the form has received information and that all questions raised by the patient have been answered satisfactorily.

In practice, nursing personnel often complete the form by writing in appropriate blanks the name of the physician or physicians who will perform the procedure, the name of the specific procedure, and request the patient to sign the consent form. Frequently the nurse also signs the form as a witness. When acting in this capacity, the nurse is performing a ministerial duty and is not gaining informed consent or attesting to the fact that the patient has received sufficient information to grant an informed consent. The legal implication of this ministerial act is that the informed consent process has occurred between the patient and the patient's physician prior to the patient's signing of the consent form. The nurse as witness only indicates that it is the patient's signature that has been affixed to the consent form. However, in performing these ministerial duties, the nurse should inform the patient's physician and, if necessary, the hospital administration, if the patient raises further questions concerning the procedure. These questions might indicate that the patient does not fully understand the nature of the procedure and its risks or that the patient has expressed hesitation and concern in authorizing the treatment. Hospitals, as employers of nurses, and nurses themselves should be wary of accepting delegated responsibility from the physician to provide information to the patient necessary to gain informed consent. Since the essential element in informed consent is the scope and nature of pertinent and material facts related to proposed treatment, the nurse and the hospital would be assuming additional liability for accepting this delegated task.

The is no legal magic to the signed consent form. As a document signed by the patient it does raise the presumption that the patient has consented to treatment. However, that presumption can be defeated by evidence to the contrary. For example, the patient could claim that there was inadequate disclosure of material information, that the consent was signed under duress, that he did not understand the technical language of the explanation, or that he was mentally incompetent, or impaired by the effects of medication.

Just who *can* consent for diagnostic or therapeutic services is often questioned in respect to certain classes of patients such as incompetent adults and minors. State statutes should be referred to if the age of majority is questioned. Mental competency is legally presumed unless a court of appropriate jurisdiction has declared the adult to be incompetent. Although physicians and other health professionals often assess patients as to their competency, it is only a court of proper jurisdiction that can declare a person to be mentally incompetent. As a matter of practice, physicians and other independent practitioners who believe the patient to be incompetent should seek consultation of a psychiatrist and, if necessary, petition a court for a declaration of incompetence and the appointment of a guardian before a nonemergency treatment is initiated. The guardian of an incompetent has the legal authority to make an informed decision and provide consent for the care of the patient. If the incompetent patient had expressed a choice concerning treatment prior to the period of incompetency, such desires or opinions should be seriously considered by the guardian in determining the course of treatment.

It is not an unusual practice, often supported by subsequent case decisions, for the close relatives (a spouse, a parent, a brother, or sister) to provide authorization for treatment for patients who are incompetent but who have not been determined to be incompetent by a court and who do not have a court appointed guardian. This practice is usually supported in those medical situations deemed to be emergent in nature or in which action is required within a short time period to prevent increased morbidity, permanent physical impairment, or death. If an incompetent patient objects to an elective-type procedure that has been approved by a close family member, it would be prudent to defer the procedure until a guardian could be appointed by the court.

The treatment of minors should not be undertaken without parental consent unless treatment is necessitated by an emergency, or a court of proper jurisdiction authorizes such treatment, or in cases in which the minor is emancipated. With minors, as with adults, consent for treatment is implied under emergency circumstances where lack of treatment would cause serious impairment to the patient's health or place his life in jeopardy. In certain situations, parental refusal to give consent for the treatment of a minor is considered child abuse, abandonment, or neglect and a court order can be obtained to treat the minor. Some courts recognize a "mature minor" status and permit minors age 15 or above to consent to medical treatment even though parents refuse consent for such treatment. In many states statutes exist that permit minors to consent to medical care related to venereal disease, drug abuse, and pregnancy without parental knowledge and consent. Minors are considered emancipated if they provide their own support, are living out of the parental home, free from the direction and control of their parents; in such situations, they can consent to their own medical treatment.

REFUSAL AND WITHDRAWAL OF TREATMENT

The right of competent adults to refuse medical treatment is limited only by compelling state interests. The right of the competent individual to refuse care is based on the common law right to be free of unauthorized violations of bodily integrity. The patient's right to make decisions concerning his own body and life necessarily extends to medical care and includes the right to decline medical attention. The constitutional right of privacy is also a basis for refusing treatment by the competent adult. These common law and constitutional rights can be subordinated to compelling state interests such as preserving life, preventing suicide, protecting third parties, protecting the public health, and maintaining the ethical integrity of the health professions.

The state has a compelling and enduring duty to preserve life that, under certain circumstances, may outweigh the right of an individual to refuse medical care. One boundary line of the states' interest to preserve life has been established by the Quinlan decision, which stated that:

> We think that the State's interest contra weakens and the individual's right to privacy grows as the degree of bodily invasion increases and the prognosis dims.[7]

Thus the courts generally recognize that the terminally ill have a common law and constitutional right to decline medical treatment.

This right extends to the nonterminally ill competent adult who is not pregnant and who does not have minor children. Courts will intervene where the competent adult is pregnant to maintain the life of the fetus and where minor children are involved to protect the children from emotional trauma and financial injury. While the state has a compelling interest to prevent suicide, the courts have firmly decided that refusal or withdrawal of treatment by the terminally ill is not irrational self-destruction (suicide). Again, a competent adult has the common law and constitutional right to decline medical treatment that may prolong life although refusal of such treatment is contrary to medical advice.

The police powers of the state to protect the health, welfare and safety of the public will override the right of a competent adult to refuse medical treatment if such refusal is a threat to the public health. A weak and controversial state interest of protecting the ethical integrity of the medical profession has been expressed in case law. The rationale of this interest is that physicians and hospitals should be permitted to provide care that is consistent with ethical and clinical standards of medical practice. Other decisions hold that this state interest in supporting the medical profession is superceded by the constitutional right of privacy.

If competent adult persons have the right to refuse or withdraw from medical treatments, those rights must be extended to incompetents who have no less a measure of personhood. The Quinlan court stated that all patients have a right of choice, and for the incompetent

> The only practical way to prevent destruction of the right is to permit the guardian and family of Karen to render their best judgment. . . . [7]

The Quinlan position provided guidelines for the Saikewicz and Severns decisions, which followed the Quinlan court holdings and expanded upon them.[8,9]

Subsequent court decisions indicate that the courts need not be involved in every case where there is a refusal or withdrawing of treatment from the terminally ill, incompetent patient. Court involvement is usually required only in those circumstances where there is disagreement among those involved in the decision-making process, such as disagreement between the attending physician and family members or disagreement among family members concerning withholding or withdrawing treatment. If such a situation exists, a court of proper jurisdiction should be petitioned for guidance.

When no guardian has been appointed by the court, it is common practice to accept treatment decisions made by the spouse or close family members if the patient is incompetent. It is generally recognized by society and the courts that spouses, parents, and siblings will act in the best interests of the incompetent patient. Courts do not discourage family members from making decisions for incompetents since it serves the purpose of judicial economy. Decision making by close family members is also practical because it expedites diagnosis and treatment that could be delayed by the lengthy time it takes to appoint a guardian. In the typical case of familial decision making, the attending physician exerts considerable control since the physician's primary duty is to the incompetent patient and he can accept or reject the family's treatment decision.

DNR ORDERS

Nurses frequently voice concern about practices related to "do not resuscitate" (DNR) orders. In the recent past, and with the tacit approval of hospital administrators, physicians frequently did not actually *write* into the patient's medical record the order not to resuscitate. Rather, they communicated the order *verbally* to the nursing staff, because of an unsubstantiated fear of legal liability. During this last decade, the courts have determined that it is within acceptable medical practice for physicians to limit medical treatment to those therapeutic measures appropriate for the patient's condition and prognosis, including or excluding cardiopulmonary resuscitation (CPR). It is well understood that the purpose of CPR is the prevention of sudden unexpected death and is not medically indicated in cases of terminal irreversible illness. The decision to withhold CPR should be determined through the patient-physician relationship, that is, with the consent of the patient in those situations in which the patient is alert and competent and participating in the management of his care. When the patient is incompetent or comatose, the DNR decision should be made after full consultation with the patient's family members such as a spouse, children, parents, or siblings. To meet JCAH standards, and for proper and prudent recordkeeping, the physician should record the DNR order in the medical record. A written order identifies the authority and authenticity of the health-care provider issuing the order, and ensures that the critical decision is clearly communicated to other health disciplines providing patient care. A written order will prevent the occurrence of CPR being provided inappropriately when DNR was medically desirable. Defense attorneys have advised their clients that the risk of liability from a failure to resuscitate is greatly reduced when there is a written DNR order, rather than when such documentation is lacking.

ADVANCE DIRECTIVES

In anticipation of the inability to communicate and when the potential of incompetency during a terminal illness and prior to death may exist, some patients attempt to express their determination to limit treatment by creating a "living will." Living wills initially had no common law or statutory foundation. Consequently, many health-care providers refused to carry out the patient's instructions for fear of potential legal liability. Building upon the concept of the living will, a number of states have legislated natural death acts that expressly authorize health-care personnel to honor the patient's directives concerning treatment and provide immunity to health-care providers for carrying out the directives in a non-negligent manner. Usually the natural death acts permit competent adults to state the scope of treatment they wish to receive, or to exclude particular treatments when they are terminally ill. The acts vary according to each state. Some indicate that the directive will be binding only when executed after the patient is diagnosed as having a terminal illness. Some states provide sanctions for health-care providers who do not follow the directive, while other states do not. Under some statutes the attending physician who declines to act upon the patient's directive has a duty to transfer the patient to another physician who will act according to the patient's wishes. Most statutes identify the manner in which the patient's directive is to be revoked, usually requiring a written revocation, although verbal revocation is also recognized by several states. Although the formal requirements of revocation may be contained in the statute, it is legally prudent not to carry out the directive if there is any reason to suspect that the patient has changed his mind concerning treatment. Natural death acts are cumulative to the common law and constitutional rights that patients have to refuse or withdraw from medical treatment (as described above). Thus patients who have not signed a directive under a natural death act can still decline or withdraw from treatment. A variation of the natural death act approach is a statute that provides for a durable power of attorney. This permits a person designated by the patient to make decisions concerning treatment if the patient should become incapable of communicating his treatment desires or becomes mentally incompetent.

Regulation of Nursing Practice

Mandatory licensure of Registered (professional) Nurses and Licensed Practical Nurses is required in most states. The regulation of nursing practice by the various state governments is an exercise of the police powers of a state to legislate laws in the interest of maintaining public health, safety, and welfare. The purpose of licensure for the nursing profession is to prevent unqualified nurses from engaging in the practice of nursing. Licensure identifies qualified nurses who have demonstrated a satisfactory level of competence and expertise in the nursing arts by completing an approved educational program and successfully passing a licensing examination. The nurse practice acts of the various states establish the authority of the state board of nursing, with the state delegating power to the state board to approve nursing education programs, to promulgate rules and regulations pertaining to nursing practice, and to carry out disciplinary procedures in accord with the administrative procedure of the respective states. Most nurse practice acts establish criminal and civil penalties for persons practicing nursing without a license. The criminal penalties include a fine and/or imprisonment.

The nurse practice acts define the composition of the licensing board. As do most administrative agencies, the board has the power to legislate by promulgating rules and regulations that pertain to nursing practice; to exercise quasijudicial powers by hearing and deciding cases involving alleged violations of professional standards, rules, and regulations, and to exercise the executive powers necessary to control the licensure function. The state board of nursing established the requirements for licensure by defining the standards of academic and clinical training that must be successfully completed before an applicant can take the licensing examination. The state board also has the authority to determine the content and nature of the licensing examination and the requirements for successfully passing the test. The board determines the licensing requirements for nurses who have been qualified to practice in other states by providing for licensure by reciprocity, endorsement, examination, or waiver.

The nurse practice acts usually define the scope of nursing practice by indicating the content and nature of the duties, and the authority that collectively constitutes the nursing role and function. The scope of practice is controversial in many states ". . . focusing on two broad issues: (1) who may make the judgment that certain procedures may be performed?; (2) who may perform the procedures?"[10] The definition of nursing practice varies by state statute and the common definition of nursing does not include "diagnosis" as a part of nursing practice. In some states the 1955 American Nurses Association definition of practice is incorporated in the statute. Other states expand this traditional definition of nursing by enabling the nurse to practice under standing orders or protocols authorized by physicians or under the direct supervision of physicians. Finally, some states do not define the practice of professional nursing in their nursing acts, but rather permit the state board of nursing to promulgate administrative rules and regulations that define and evolve the scope of nursing practice. In most states, the boundaries to the scope of nursing practice cannot be identified without reference to the medical practice act, the pharmacy act, and similar licensing statutes for other health professionals. Further limits to the scope of nursing practice are established by published opinions of the state attorney general that identify permissible or prohibited nursing practices. Further boundaries are established by judicial decisions (case law), promulgated rules and regulations of the state agencies regulating medical practice, nursing practice, and the practices of other health professions.

Of particular importance to the new nurse are the disciplinary powers of the state board of nursing. The state board of nursing has the power to conduct investigations and to make judicial decisions in response to complaints pertaining to specific nursing practitioners. The investigative and judicial functions of the board are established by the nurse practice act and the administrative procedures act of the respective state. The board's disciplinary authority is limited to the specific areas defined by the statute that established the board. The disciplinary authority of the board generally pertains to fraud and misrepresentation in obtaining a license; illegal, immoral, or unprofessional conduct; conduct that violates the nurse practice act or rules and regulations promulgated by the state board of nursing; conviction of a felony, and alcohol and substance abuse.

In the conduct of this judicial power, the board must be careful to comply with the due process requirements necessary to protect the legal rights of the licensed professional nurse. Due process requires that the nurse be informed of the nature of the complaint and the alleged wrongful conduct, and be given the opportunity to present information to defend herself against the complaint. Failure to provide due process prior to enforcing a disciplinary judgment can cause a court to reverse the decision of the state board.

The new professional nurse should become familiar with the various circumstances and conduct that could lead to disciplinary action and subsequent suspension or revocation of her nursing license. Particular attention should be paid to the definition of "unprofessional conduct" since this definition varies from state to state and is vague if one does not read the nurse practice act; the rules and regulations promulgated by the state board of nursing; the disciplinary decisions of the board, or judicial decisions of the state court.

In most states, the decision of the state board in respect to disciplinary actions can be reviewed by state courts. However, the courts often defer to the administrative agency that has expertise and experience in administering the licensing law, and will overrule the action of the state board only if the decision is arbitrary, capricious, or unreasonable.

Major issues to be faced and solved by state boards of nursing in the future will be

1. Broadening of the definition of nursing to accommodate expanded roles and practice

2. Competency assessment to be required for license renewal
3. Development of standards of nursing practice and professional conduct
4. Development of separate testing and licensing for the three types of educational programs graduating nurses
5. Need to have the licensure examination job-related
6. Development of qualifications for specialty practice

Hospital Bioethics Committees

Advances in medical science and biomedical technology have far exceeded the common ethical understandings of the various health professionals. Ethical dilemmas arise frequently within the hospital environment and overtax the ability of the interdisciplinary team to make clear noncontroversial ethical judgments. Consequently, ethical confusion and doubts generate disharmony, conflict, intolerance, and anxiety among team members, which is unfortunately conveyed to the patient or the patient's family and friends. The hospital bioethics committee is a forum developed to assist and guide health-care professionals in examining ethical principles and precepts applicable to clinical decision making, with regard to individual patients, classes of patients, and institutional policies. Professional nurses are often members of the interdisciplinary bioethics committee.

Statutory or case law does not legally require a hospital to establish a bioethics committee. However, the existence of such a committee can assure the courts and general public that bioethical dilemmas receive thoughtful and careful deliberation by members of the medical, nursing, and allied health professions. Most bioethic committees are organized to

1. Provide educational programs pertinent to bioethical issues
2. Increase professional awareness concerning ethical dilemmas through interdisciplinary discussions
3. Serve as a resource to professionals involved in bioethical decision making
4. Provide guidance and advice to the governing body of the hospital in regard to institutional policies of bioethical import, such as the allocation of health resources; recognition and support of patient's rights; the patient's right to refuse treatment, right to withhold or discontinue treatment, and do-not-resuscitate orders

The bioethics committee should not have the authority to function in a manner that would interfere with the legally and professionally recognized authority and accountability inherent in the professional roles of the physician, nurse, or other allied health disciplines. Further, the ethics committee should not function as a professional ethics review board retrospectively to review and judge the ethical dimensions of prior decision making by physicians and other health professionals. Above all, the bioethics committee should not function as a decision maker when presented with bioethical dilemmas. In respect to the individual case, the role of the bioethics committee is to provide a forum for the full discussion and exploration of ethical alternatives to patient care, diagnosis, and treatment.

The committee functions best when it is a hospital committee, that is, a committee established by the governing board and composed of members representing the board, the organized medical staff, other health disciplines, and hospital administration. The committee function should be available to patients, patients' family members, physicians, other health-care professionals, the hospital administration, and the board itself. The bioethics committee is often assisted in its deliberations by an ethicist, a person specifically educated in the field of ethical and morale decision making, and by legal counsel, since ethical decisions are often constrained or supported by legal considerations. Throughout its deliberations, the bioethics committee must be concerned with the confidentiality of patient information and the right of the patient to have his privacy respected.

Members of the bioethics committee must be carefully selected to prevent bias or narrowness in considering and exploring ethical alternatives to patient treatment and care. Committee membership should include appropriate representation of the various health professions and, if possible, clergy representing the predominant religious groups constituting the hospital's patient population. Members should accept appointment to the committee only if they are willing to dedicate the necessary time, effort, and intellect to develop a thorough knowledge and understanding of the ethical theories, systems, and precepts necessary to assist others in formulating ethical judgments and to guide them in ethical decision making. Continuous self-education through readings, discussions, and attendance at continuing education activities is necessary if the bioethics committee member is to perform effectively his role for the benefit of the patients, the health professions, and the public.

Comments on Professional Codes

Professional duties and obligations between the profession and the greater society, among members within the profession, and between the professional and the client are represented by the Hippocratic Oath, which originated more than 2300 years ago on the Greek island of Cos.

The ethical principles, customs, and practices articulated by the various professions were continually codified and incorporated into the professional body of knowledge. They were taught to new practitioners as guides to practice within the profession and to direct the relationship between professionals and the public they serve. Ancient codes of ethics have been modernized and codes have developed for professions that did not previously exist. As a profession nursing, too, has articulated an ethical code of practice.

As with other professional codes, the American Nurses Association Code For Nurses With Interpretive Statements raises several questions: 1. Are the ethical statements related to general ethical principles that are universally valid? and 2. What is the relationship between the professional code and law? The value of a professional code is greatly diminished if the code establishes professional duties and obligations solely upon the basis of definition by the profession of its duties and obligations, and if the code is merely self-imposed. To be meaningful and effective, a professional code must be based upon ethical principles held in common by lay persons as well as by professional members, that is, universal ethical principles. Such principles may be theological in nature or be secular principles such as beneficence and justice. While the professional code may be given a special meaning within the membership of the profession, such codes have no legal significance since they do not originate from the legislative branch of government and have not been established through judicial decision making. Thus, professional codes do not have the power of law. However, the professional code for nurses does function as a guide to the highest standards of ethical practice for nurses and fulfills an inspirational purpose. The code of ethics promulgated by the ANA should serve as a substantial and meaningful guide for ethical behavior in nursing practice.

References

1. U.S. Constitution, article VI, section 2
2. Title VII, Civil Rights Act of 1964, 42 U.S.C. section 2000(e) et seq
3. 29 CFR, Chapter XIV, Part 1604.11
4. Age Discrimination in Employment Act of 1967, 29 U.S.C. section 621 et seq.
5. Equal Pay Act of 1963, 29 U.S.C. section 206(d)
6. Labor Management Relations Act; National Labor Relations Act; Taft-Hartley Act, 29 U. S. C. section 151 et seq
7. Matter of Quinlan, 70 N.J. 10, 355 A.2d 647, 664 (1976)
8. Superintendent of Belchertown V. Saikewicz, 373 Mass. 728, 370 N.E. 2d 417, 426 (1977)
9. In re Severns, 125 A.2d 156, 158 (Del. Ch. 1980)

10. Rhodes AM, Miller RD: Nursing and The Law, p 22. Rockville, MD, Aspen Systems, 1984

Bibliography

American Hospital Association, Office of Legal and Regulatory Affairs: Legal Memorandum Number One: Legal issues and guidance for hospital biomedical ethics committees. Chicago, American Hospital Association, January 1985.

Annas GJ et al: The Rights of Doctors, Nurses and Allied Health Professionals. New York, Avon Books, 1981.

Ashton R: Wrongful discharge suits. Aspen's Advisor for Nurse Executives 1(4): January 1986

Ashton R: Strikes: What the nurse executive must know. Aspen's Advisor for Nurse Executives 1(6): March 1986

Beauchamp TL, Walters L: Contemporary Issues in Bioethics. Belmont, CA, Wadsworth Publishing, 1978

Burdea D: Comparable worth battle spreads to new fronts. Hospitals 60(5):42–46, March 5, 1986

Drucker PF: Management: Tasks, Responsibilities and Practices. New York, Harper & Row, 1973

Gorman RA: Labor Law: Unionization And Collective Bargaining. St. Paul, West Publishing, 1976

Maida AJ (ed): Labor-Management Dialogue: Church Perspectives. St. Louis, Catholic Health Association Of The United States, 1982

Pozgav GD: Legal Aspects Of Health Care Administration. Rockville, MD, Aspen Systems, 1979

President's Commission for the Study of Ethical Problems in Medicine and Biomedical and Behavioral Research: Deciding to Forego Life-Sustaining Treatment. U.S. Government Printing Office, March 1983

Prosser WL: The Law of Torts. St Paul, West Publishing, 1971

Ramsey P: The Patient As Person. New Haven, Yale University Press, 1970

Randal J. Are ethics committees alive and well. The Hastings Center Report, December, 1983

Rhodes AM, Miller RD: Nursing and the Law. Rockville, MD, Aspen Systems, 1984

Shepard IM, Doudera AE (eds): Health Care Labor Law. Washington, AUPHA Press, 1981

Stevens BJ: The Nurse As Executive. Wakefield, MA, Nursing Resources, 1980

Strickler MM, Ballard FL, Jr: Representing Health Care Facilities. New York, Practicing Law Institute, 1981

Veatch RM: A Theory of Medical Ethics. New York, Basic Books, 1981

Youngkin Q: Comparable worth: Alternatives to litigation and legislation. Nurs Econ 3:38–43, January–February, 1985

Younger SJ et al: A national survey of hospital ethics committees. Crit Care Med 11(11):902–905, 1983

Chapter 15

Labor relations in union and nonunion environments

J. ELIZABETH OTHMAN AND
HARRIETT S. CHANEY

Labor relations refers to the relationship between management and employees (labor) within the work environment. This relationship is dependent upon the extent to which labor and management can agree on the conditions required for meeting each other's needs and wants. The goals of management will reflect the desire to produce a profitable product or service through the efforts of employed workers. Labor desires safe working conditions, reasonable tangible and intangible remuneration, job security, and opportunities for growth and advancement. The most desirable circumstance is for labor and management to dialogue, conference, problem-solve and compromise in achieving mutual agreement. When this is not possible, our democratic society acknowledges and provides for the employees' right to organize and bargain collectively with management. The power of an organized collective group is inherently stronger than the cries and outrage of an individual when dealing with unacceptable employee working conditions. In fact, management that is not competent, responsive, and economically strong would be a sorry match for organized employees. Conversely, a union will never be successful in an organization where management is strong, understands the employees and provides for the responsible fulfillment of employee needs and wants.

This chapter will enable you to

1. Distinguish between the characteristics of a union and nonunion environment.
2. Describe the evolution of the labor movement in nursing.
3. List the steps in the collective bargaining process.
4. Understand the negotiation process.

The presence of unions in the health-care industry and professional nursing in particular has had an interesting and recent evolution. The unionization process (collective bargaining) is inherently complex because a wide range of both appropriate and inappropriate behaviors is specified by law. Further, the unionization process is highly charged emotionally because collective bargaining issues always relate to one's work and security. These considerations are further compounded in health care by the following: the nature of providing care, the extreme interdependence between the care provider and the client and the moral and ethical ramifications of the unionization and collective bargaining processes. Each staff nurse will have to make judgments and decisions about collective bargaining from a knowledge base regarding the process and careful consideration of the circumstances of each individual situation.

Our Labor Relations Heritage

The American labor movement began in the nineteenth century. Extremely poor working conditions existed for workers who were uneducated and helpless in the face of the power of state and economic capital. Early craftsmen's unions experienced limited success although these unions still exist. Industrial unions did not become a practical powerful reality until long after the rise of factory systems and the development of mass production (Beal, and Begin, 1982). Even then the size and successes of unions fluctuated with economic conditions and the world wars. Specific laws and precipitating events can be reviewed in Chapter 13.

Details regarding the working conditions for nurses in America are of particular interest. Prior to 1930, student nurses provided most of the nursing care for patients in the hospital. "Graduate nurses" practiced independently as private duty nurses in homes, community agencies, and other health-care organizations. The depression of 1929 brought a reduction in personal health expenditures including the hiring of private duty nurses. Coupled with the decline in nursing school enrollment during the period, hospitals found it economically feasible to hire "graduate nurses" for little more than room and board. Thus, hospitals became the nurses' primary work place (Bullough, 1971).

Hospital employees were permitted to engage in collective bargaining under the National Labor Relations Act (Wagner Act) of 1935. Two years later, the American Nurses' Association (ANA) drafted its charter, which included provisions for improving "every phase of (nurses') working and professional lives" (Pointer, 1972). However, it was not until 1946 that the ANA officially initiated its Economic Security Program (Berneys, 1946). The ANA received a mandate from its membership to act as the bargaining agent for nurses to improve the economic conditions and status of the profession.

The "Brown Report" titled *Nursing for the Future* was published in 1948 and it described the working conditions at that time. Essentially, staff nurses had little freedom in making clinical nursing judgments and had no participation in solving the simplest of problems. The environment was highly authoritarian and unrewarding (Alexander, 1978).

The U.S. Department of Labor's Survey of the Economic Status of Nurses (1946–1947) found that nurses worked longer hours, did more shift work, and received less pay and fringe benefits than most workers in industry or in comparable occupations. The average annual salary was $2,100, well below the level of female industrial workers, teachers, secretaries, and social workers.

Wide-scale attempts at collective bargaining were further complicated by the Labor-Management Act of 1947 (Taft-Hartley Act), which excluded not-for-profit hospitals from its jurisdiction and protection. During congressional debate on exclusion of not-for-profit hospitals from the protection of the act, Senator Taylor of Idaho expressed concern that the amendment would bar nurses from organizing. " . . . I have in mind that nursing is one of the most poorly paid professions in America . . . it is perhaps the poorest paid, in proportion to the service rendered to humanity. I do not want to place the nursing profession under any handicap in their efforts to obtain an improved standard of living." The senator withdrew his objection when he was assured that the amendment ". . . will (not) affect them in the slightest way . . . they can still protest, they can still walk out" (Gershenfeld, 170).

Finally, during the 1960's, the collective voices of professional nurses began to ring out. Federal and state employees were protected in collective bargaining by several statutes, including President John F. Kennedy's Executive Order #10988 of 1960. Nurses participated in demonstrations, picketing, sit-ins, call-ins, and slow-downs. Typical of the era, Cook County Hospital in Chicago, for example, lacked basic resources such as toilet paper and suction machines in addition to having inadequate staffing ratios. The nurses attempted to make the seriousness of these problems known without results and therefore resorted to stronger tactics and a unionization drive. The nurses emphatically stated that their main goal was the improvement of nursing care through improved working conditions and increased salaries (Mauksch, 1971).

The Taft-Hartley Amendments of 1974 extended the legal protection of nurses for collective bargaining to 2 million employees in 3300 nonprofit hospitals. These amendments were eagerly supported by unions because of the decline in union membership in the traditional manufacturing industries. The Service Employees International Union, for example, designated the 1980's as the decade in which every nonunion healthcare worker would be the focus of an organizing drive (Rectz & Rectz, 1984). While the Taft-Hartley Amendments opened the possibility for many nurses to bargain collectively, it should be noted that some states prohibit the unionization of employees in the public sector.

Current Status of Labor Relations

The majority of nurses (1,120,000) in the United States work in non-unionized environments (Ballman, 1985). Many staff nurses are quite satisfied with the way their organization is managing labor relations and they do not feel the need for union representation. Some nurses do not believe that union representation reflects the professional level of representation they prefer. Still another group of nurses may not recognize that union representation is an alternative method for problem resolution when management and labor relationships are fractured. The American Nurses' Association's economic and general welfare program and numerous other competing unions represent approximately 180,000 nurses (Ballman, 1985). The geographical distribution of union activity is currently concentrated in the northeastern States: New York, New Jersey, Massachusetts, and Pennsylvania along with California and Michigan (Kilgour, 1984). This reflects the fact that collective bargaining is not a national phenomenon.

The general economic environment of health care influences the issues important to nurses. It has been suggested that in collective bargaining, the settlement with regard to wages has a 99% correlation with the inflation rate (Abelow, 1985). Wages were an important issue during the early period of collective bargaining; however, by the mid-1980's nurses were concerned with job security, crosstraining for clinical and job diversity, shift rotations, health-care benefits and the general organizational wage structure (Yanish, 1985). Additionally, because of the deep concern regarding escalating health-care costs, many unions elected to form health-care coalitions to control costs (Powills, 1985).

The nonunion organization met the economic environment demands of the mid-1980's by maintaining open communications with employees during periods of fiscal belt-tightening. Careful and sensitive planning for strategic downsizing, forewarning of impending employee cutbacks, providing counseling services and assisting employees with job placement efforts eased the challenge of streamlining staff levels to fit decreased client census and utilization patterns.

The current labor relation practices within health-care organizations have emanated from the 1974 Taft-Hartley amendments. Since that time, health care administrators have examined their approaches to employees and have attempted to establish successful employee relation programs in order to maintain their nonunion designation status. Along with attitude changes, most administrators routinely examine compensation packages for equity, both within the organization and the marketplace. Thus, the enhancement of labor relations in the health-care work environment during the past decade is directly attributable to the unionization of a portion of health-care workers.

Professionalism and Collectivism

Nursing for many decades promoted the service and "calling" ideals of Florence Nightingale. She described the professional nurse as one who possessed physical, intellectual, and spiritual motives to serve the informed (Cook, 1942). Further, Miss Nightingale recognized the need for adequate and organized educational processes for professional nursing. Historically humanitarianism and self-sacrifice on behalf of the patient have been more highly valued than the nurses' own economic and social welfare. This ideology has been described as "Nightingalism" and was prominent until the 1960's (Grand, 1971).

Contemporary concepts related to the professional nature of nursing focus on the academic preparation, roles and functions, and the increasing autonomy of nurses. It should be noted that the concept of professionalism in nursing has received considerable attention and analyses. A distinction is emerging between *professionalism,* which emphasizes the composite character of the position, and *professionhood,* which focuses on the characteristics of the individual who is a member of a profession (Styles, 1982). Achieving consensus among nurses about these issues would certainly impact the practice of nursing and the labor relations environment where nursing is practiced. Questioning whether nursing is a true profession is appropriate in the context of collective bargaining; most professions have shown little interest in collective action because it is viewed as unprofessional (Werther and Lockhart, 1976). Nursing, however, may merit separate consideration because of its unique characteristics.

Most practicing professional nurses are women who face the realities of working in a job category called a "women's ghetto." Traditionally, jobs in this category have low status, low pay, difficult hours, and little or no control on the job (O'Rourke and Barton, 1981). These conditions in combination with the power differential between nurses and administration have made collective bargaining a viable alternative for problem solving in spite of the professionalism issue.

"Professional collectivism" has become an acceptable term for those who wish to participate in collective bargaining without the stigma of being unprofessional (Bloom, 1977). "Professional collectivism" embraces the idea that the quality of patient care is inherently related to working conditions and that collective action is a professional responsibility. Certainly collective action is one way to accommodate the dilemma that arises between professional norms and values and organizational demands and constraints.

The Collective Bargaining Process

The work of a staff nurse is highly demanding. It requires physical stamina, emotional commitment, and psychological health and robustness. Therefore, the environment and conditions under which the staff nurse works must be supportive and in concert with her activities. If they are not, problems and conflict will emerge that can escalate, fester and lead to unionization efforts. Usually a number of problems exist that are not resolved through normal procedures when the staff nurse embarks on unionization. (See the listing of possible reasons on the opposite page.)

Under the provisions of the Taft-Hartley amendments not-for-profit hospital workers have the right to choose a representative (union) who will speak on their behalf in negotiations with their employer. The process of unionizing is initiated by the employees and proceeds as follows:

1. Thirty (30%) to fifty (50%) of employees sign a petition or cards demanding an election for union representation.
2. A preliminary hearing is held to determine if the employees are

REASONS EMPLOYEES JOIN UNIONS

Management fails to fulfill employee's needs.

A. Security

Fair treatment of all employees is lacking
Favoritism is shown to specific employees
Opportunity for advancement is not available
Recognition as a person is rarely extended
Unsafe working conditions
Training is not provided
Economic security is not perceived by employees

B. Benefits are not measurable, adequate and/or competitive

Hours of work
Wages
Opportunity for overtime
Rate of overtime pay
Vacations
Sick pay
Retirement coverage
Medical insurance
Hospitalization insurance
Life insurance
Holidays
Severance pay
Funeral pay
Jury duty
Educational/training subsidies

C. Poor Leadership

Poor top and line supervision
Ineffective grievance adjustments
Communications are poor
Opportunity for self-expression is not present
Toleration of poor quality performance
Inconsistent treatment of all

under the jurisdiction of the National Labor Relations Board (NLRB) and to set the date, hours, and place of the election.

3. Appropriate employee placement into bargaining units is achieved. Employees are grouped as indicated in Chapter 14—technical, service and maintenance, business and clinical, professional employees, and registered nurses.

4. Preelection behaviors are observed to assure compliance with the law. (A summary of unlawful activities is outlined below.)

5. The election is conducted by the NLRB in the workplace with the outcome being determined by the simple majority of those who vote.

6. Appealing the election results may be attempted and exhausted and if the election is won by the employees, the NLRB issues a certificate to the labor organization reflecting its right to represent the employees.

7. Both parties, management and union, prepare to negotiate the collective bargaining agreement. Subjects to be negotiated include: wages, hours, and other terms and conditions of employment (Henry, 1984).

The above unionization process proceeds swiftly and is usually completed within 45 days. The general atmosphere of the process is one of

UNLAWFUL ACTIVITIES DURING THE UNION CERTIFICATION PROCESS

MANAGEMENT

1. Management cannot promise pay increases, promotion, improved benefits, betterment, or special favor for voting against a union.

2. Management cannot say the organization will close if unionized.

3. Employees cannot be fired, laid off, given a less favorable job, or otherwise discriminated against because of union activities.

4. Employees cannot be interrogated about union activities or encouraged to withdraw from the union.

UNION

1. The union cannot use threats or actual violence against employees who refuse to participate or cooperate with the union.

2. Union members cannot interfere with, restrain, or coerce employees in forming, joining, or assisting labor organizations.

3. The union cannot use surveillance or questioning concerning employee interest or activities related to unions.

confusion and turmoil as the opposing forces, management and union, jockey for the employees' vote and support.

The Union Contract

The collective bargaining agreement is known as the contract. It defines rights, responsibilities, and benefits to both management and the union. The agreement usually gives the union rights related to a grievance procedure, dues check-off and access to a bulletin board. Most agreements grant the hospital a Management Rights provision and a no-strike clause for the duration of contract. The Management Rights provision allows management residual rights, that is, control of any issue not in the contract. The contract is valid for an agreed-upon number of years, although specific portions of the contract may be negotiated within the life of the original agreement. For example, there may be a three-year contract with the wages portion to be reopened for negotiations after the first year.

A contract for unionized health-care organizations usually contains a clause stating that management shall not discharge or take other disciplinary action without just cause. This clause effectively limits the organization's authority to discipline and fire employees. "Just cause" may be defined as "substantial reasons to justify the actions taken" and is open to interpretation and often arbitration for a final decision. This forces the organization to adopt and uniformly administer personnel policies.

Each collective bargaining agreement seeks to establish an effective grievance procedure outlining the method for handling employee complaints and providing for a continuous relationship between the parties. It is meant to cover the gaps and ambiguities in the contract. Thus, the contract becomes a living document in that the parties continue to bargain through the grievance procedure. Usually the grievance procedure consists of three steps or stages of appeal. Such procedures are also usually outlined in personnel manuals.

The first step is usually a presentation of the grievance or alleged wrong to the immediate supervisor. If the manager at this level is unable to resolve the conflict or right the alleged wrong, the employee may take the grievance to the next step, which is usually a review by a higher level manager who can overturn the previous decision. In a unionized organization the contract defines the time parameters for reviews at each step and the employee is represented by a union steward. Both parties are usually eager to settle the conflict since the final step of arbitration can be costly and may mean adherence to a decision that neither party desires (Fay and Morill, 1985).

One of the most important aspects of unionization is the adherence to the concept of seniority. Seniority defines each individual employee's longevity or length of continuous service in an organization. As a concept, seniority is deeply ingrained in our society and long service means benefits and security; however, a nonunionized organization is under no obligation to consider employee seniority. The seniority clause in a contract offers protection against untimely layoff and may create a preferred status for vacation periods, shift assignments, overtime opportunities, and promotions.

Negotiations of a new contract occur at the end of the life of the present contract. Both parties send representatives to the bargaining table with demands for changes in the contract. The changes will reflect the current national and industrial economic status, the maneuvers required to match the organization's competition, and changes in the professional practice and care for patients. The negotiation period can be very brief or can go on for many months, as long as it is deemed that the parties are negotiating in good faith.

The costs of unionization are incurred by both management and labor. Management loses flexibility relative to job assignment and promotion. The salary and benefit packages may result in higher costs to the organization as well as diminished flexibility in quoting salaries or adjusting them to maintain a competitive position. Finally, management is forced to work through a third party (the union) to resolve problems and initiate some types of changes. This can cause unwanted delays and complexity.

The unionized employee pays dues and fees to the union for the maintenance and activities of the union. The employee, like management, utilizes the union as a third party to resolve conflict and grievances. In the event of a strike, participation is required and at times advancement can be constrained by seniority.

While the above conditions are described as costs, it is clear that an individual may choose to view the conditions as gains. This typifies the nature of collective bargaining and the divergence it can engender.

Negotiation Difficulties

The law specifies that the contract negotiations must proceed in a timely manner with substantive results. This obligation to negotiate in good faith is actually a state of mind that is difficult to measure (Henry, 1984). Behaviors (listed at the top of the opposite page) have been identified, however, that characterize surface bargaining.

CHARACTERISTICS OF FAILURE TO BARGAIN IN GOOD FAITH

1. Failure to participate meaningfully
2. Issuing unreasonable demands or conditions
3. Postponing negotiating sessions repeatedly
4. Rejecting proposals without reason
5. Engaging in dilatory conduct
6. Making no real effort to reconcile differences

Strikes are not a desirable way of resolving labor disputes but they can and do occur with varying success. The various types of strikes (outlined below) include economic, unfair labor practices, sympathy, jurisdictional, and recognition. The union must provide ten days' notice to management prior to striking. The purpose of this is to ensure the continuity of client care, or at the very least to lessen the impact of the work stoppage on continuity of care.

TYPES OF UNION STRIKES

TYPE	DESCRIPTION
Economic Strikes	Employees are attempting to compel their employer to accept their demands by withdrawing their services.
Unfair Labor Practice Strikes	A strike that is caused or prolonged by the unfair labor practices of an employer or a union.
Sympathy Strikes	Employees of one employer or craft strike in support of workers of another. Employees can also refuse to cross the picket line of another.
Jurisdictional Strikes	A work stoppage because of a dispute between two or more unions over the assignment of work. Unions will strike because the employer will assign a particular job to another union.

continued

TYPES OF UNION STRIKES *Continued*

TYPE	DESCRIPTION
Recognition Strikes	Work stoppages to force an employer to bargain with a particular organization.
Illegal Strikes	Examples of illegal strikes include violent strikes, secondary or boycott strikes, wildcat or unauthorized strikes.

A total of 43 major strikes occurred at a health care institution between June 1954 and March 1982, each involving 1,000 or more employees (Metzger, Ferentino, and Kruger, 1984). These strikes averaged 18.8 days and ranged from 1 day to 95 days. Strikes occur less frequently when the unemployment rate is up and inflation is down. Southern states experience less strike activity, and nursing home strikes last longer.

Striking is costly to both parties. The organization loses patient revenues and incurs costs related to overtime, security, legal council and also incurs a loss of public confidence. Striking workers lose pay and can be replaced (Metzger, Ferentino, and Kruger, 1984). Striking causes considerable stress to all involved. It is not easy for the staff nurse to face the ethical dilemmas associated with striking. However, when one or both parties are unable or unwilling to reach agreement, striking has a definite effect on the positions of both labor and management.

Summary

Labor relations in optimal form ensures that the needs and wants of the organization and the employee are met responsibly. A match between the values and behaviors of the employer and employee promotes job satisfaction and organizational profitability.

A number of specific factors contribute to the optimization of organizational labor relations. Employees expect and should receive competent supervision, equitable and consistent treatment, adequate compensation and benefits, written rules, policies, and procedures, personal recognition, and a reasonable amount of job security. Professional nurses should be able to practice nursing with autonomy and participation in the administrative process. Organizational management expects and should receive the best performance an employee can offer, professional conduct, compliance with the rules, policies, and procedures, loyalty, and a commitment to fiscal constraint and profitability in the delivery of quality client services.

Occasionally irreconcilable differences between management and labor will result in the unionization of employees. This creates an environment where management and employees are in a more balanced power posture; however, their positions tend to be adversarial.

The new staff nurse has a dual role with regard to labor relations. The first role is that of a consumer of management's programs and style. Associated with this is the responsibility to provide direct feedback to management of the union representative. The other role is that of extender of labor relations when working with nonprofessional personnel. Each staff nurse must commit considerable personal effort to positive labor relations if quality patient care is to be provided.

Bibliography

Abelow KB. Quotation. In Yanish D: Nurses' unions lower sights on wages to make gains in non-economic areas. Mod Health Care, p 76, November 8, 1985

Alexander E: Nursing Administration in the Hospital Health Care System. St. Louis, CV Mosby, 1978

Ballman C: Union busters. Am J Nurs 9:963–966, 1985

Beal E, Begin J: The Practice of Collective Bargaining. Homewood, IL, Richard D. Irwin, 1982

Berneys EL: How to influence your own future. RN 12:42–44, 1946

Bloom B: Collective action by professionals poses problems for administrators. Hospitals 174:167–168, March 16, 1977

Bullough B: New militancy in nursing. Nurs Forum 11:273–288, 1971

Cook E: The Life of Florence Nightingale. New York, MacMillan, 1942

Fay MS, Morril AK: The grievance-arbitration process: The experience of one nursing administrator. J Nurs Adm 6:11–16, 1985

Gershenfeld W: Hospitals. In Wolfbein AL (ed): Emerging Sectors of Collective Bargaining. Braintree, MA, DH Mark, 1970

Grand N: Nightingalism. Employeeism and professional collectivism. Nursing Forum 11:289–299, 1971

Henry K: The Health Care Supervisor's Legal Guide. Rockville, MD, Aspen Systems, 1984

Kilgour J: Union organizing activity in the hospital industry. Hosp Health Serv Adm 29:6, 79–90, November/December, 1984

Mauksch IG: Attainment of control over practice. Nursing Forum 11:232–238, 1971

Metzger N, Ferentino J, Kruger K: When Health Care Employees Strike. Rockville, MD, Aspen Systems, 1984

O'Rourke K, Barton S: The politics of nursing. In Shepard I, Doudera A (eds):

Health Care Labor Law. Ann Arbor, Health Administration Press, 1981

Pointer D: Organizing of professionals: Associations serve union functions. Hospitals 46(5): 70–73, March 16, 1972

Powills S: Labor: A growing force in controlling health costs. Hospitals: 82–85, November 16, 1985

Rectz R, Rectz J: Collective bargaining in the health care industry: Implications for the long term care administration. J Long-Term Care Adm: 11–19, Spring 1984

Styles M: On Nursing: Toward a New Endowment. St. Louis, CV Mosby, 1982

Werther W, Lockhart C: Labor Relations in the Health Profession. Boston, Little, Brown and Co, 1976

Yanish D: Nurses' unions lower sights on wages to make gains in non-economic areas. Mod Health Care: 76, November 8, 1985

Chapter 16

Overcoming sex-role stereotyping in nursing

LINDA CARRICK TOROSIAN AND MARIANNE DIETRICK-GALLAGHER

From the moment of birth, each of us is labeled as male or female. This sex-role identity has far-reaching consequences. Our identity as male or female impacts upon our self-esteem, interpersonal relationships, and career choices. Many professions are influenced by the sex-role characteristics held by the majority of their workers. The purposes of this chapter are to explore sex-role development and to analyze the effects of traditional sex-role characteristics on the nursing profession. Problematic areas in the profession that have been influenced by traditional sex-role characteristics will be delineated and strategies to modify these problems in personal practice will be explored. The majority of nurses have been and continue to be women. Thus, many of the concerns of the nursing profession can be viewed as women's issues. Men in nursing face unique problems and bring different assets to the profession. The problems encountered by men in nursing are also discussed.

This chapter will enable you to:

1. Describe sex-role characteristics in the profession of nursing.
2. Identify areas that are problematic in the profession as they relate to sex stereotyping.
3. Explore strategies to modify these problems in clinical practice.

Sex Role

Many scientists have studied sex-role development. The results of these investigations are divergent theories about how one develops maleness and femaleness. While it is beyond the scope of this chapter to explore theoretical explanations of sex-role development, three major theories have been proposed. These theories are based on psychoanalytic, social learning, and cognitive learning development and are outlined briefly below.

THEORIES OF SEX-ROLE DEVELOPMENT

THEORY	BASIC IDEA	PROBLEMS ASSOCIATED WITH:
Psycho-analytic	Desire for mother (Oedipal complex)	Does not adequately explain female development
	Fear of father's retaliation (castration anxiety)	Does not verify events that occur in a young child's unconscious mind
	Identification with father (Oedipus resolution and masculine sex-role identity)	
Social Learning Learning process based on reinforcement and imitation	Attachment to same-sexed parent as major rewarder/punisher. "I want rewards."	Little evidence exists to substantiate that differential reinforcement occurs at a level mandated by this theory
	Identification and modeling of same sexed parent. "I am rewarded for doing girl/boy things."	

continued

THEORIES OF SEX-ROLE DEVELOPMENT *Continued*

THEORY	BASIC IDEA	PROBLEMS ASSOCI-ATED WITH:
	Sex-typed behaviors and attitudes. "Therefore I want to be a boy/girl."	Little evidence to support that imitation of same-sexed parent accounts for sexed typed behaviors
Cognitive Learning (developmental)	Sex-typed identity (gender self-labeling) "I am a boy/girl"	Little evidence to support that imitation of same-sexed parent accounts for sex-typed behaviors
	Modeling of same-sexed parent. "I want to do boy/girl things."	Little support for major thesis
	Attachment to same-sexed parent	

Factors Influencing Gender Development

BIOLOGICAL FACTORS

Compare the average 5′5″ male to the average 5′4″ female. Certainly the sexes are different. Are these biological differences responsible for the sex-role preferences attributed to males (strong, aggressive) and females (dependent, nurturing)? Is anatomy destiny? The evidence that biology and hormonal environment affect behavior is inconclusive.

Testosterone has often been linked to aggression. Macoby and Jacklin reviewed more than 50 studies of human aggression and concluded that "aggression is related to levels of sex hormones and can be changed by experimental administration of these hormones."[1] Other researchers dispute this relationship. Androgenized girls have demonstrated more tomboy behaviors and fewer nurturing behaviors than a control group. However, males exposed to excessive amounts of androgens have shown more interest in caring for infants than their normal brothers.[2] Conclusive answers to the question of hormonal and chromosomal influences on sex-role development must come from additional study.

SOCIAL FACTORS

As a child is born, the first words uttered by the obstetrician are, "You have a bouncing baby boy/girl." From that moment on, every interaction is colored and influenced by gender identity. Parents in the first 24 hours after birth describe infant boys as strong and hardy, girls as pretty and soft, despite no difference in size or Apgar score. Later, female infants are touched and spoken to more often than males.[3] Such early interactions contribute to the development of gender identity. As early as 13 months, females demonstrate less exploratory and more dependent behaviors than do males.[4] Boys are encouraged to achieve, compete, and control their feelings whereas girls are rewarded for dependent, caring, and verbal behaviors. Toys provided by parents parallel traditional sex-role characteristics. Female children nurture dolls while male offspring enjoy cars and trucks. Thus, unwittingly and perhaps unknowingly, parents treat female and male children disparately.

Parents are not the sole influencing factors in the development of gender identity. School systems, teachers, peers, and the media are strong socializing agents. School systems and teachers reinforce gender identity by tolerating aggressive behavior in male students more readily than in females. Females are encouraged to achieve scholastically and perform consistently better than boys until reaching the high school level. What is responsible for this performance decline in the teenage years? Are girls encouraged at this age to change their focus from achievement to affiliation (competing for the attention of males) or do standard achievement tests house a strong male bias? Organized team sports have long been the realm of the male in school. Within this arena, they learn the needed skills of collaboration, cooperation, and team work—skills mandatory for survival in the corporate business world (and hospitals are businesses). When career planning occurs females continue to be "tracked" into traditional female-oriented jobs rather than being given the opportunity to explore the realm of career potentials. Males, too, are influenced by the school system. They are labeled "hyperactive" more frequently than females and may be penalized for exhibiting their sex-role characteristics of independence and high levels of activity. The setting of many classrooms is one in which conformity, orderliness, and self-discipline are needed to maintain order.

In American society, values, beliefs, and behaviors are strongly influenced by the media. Take time to analyze sex roles portrayed in television commercials, prime time programming, and children's shows. Sex-role differences, often traditional and anachronistic, are blatantly portrayed. With children spending an average of 7 hours a day being entertained by television, it is no surprise that they perceive and incorporate portrayed sex-role differences. Childrens' books, texts, comic books, and magazines contribute to the development of perceived sex-role differences. A number of studies document a very traditional portrayal of men and women in written materials.[5,6,7] Table 16-1 compares common sex role stereotypes.

One of the strongest socializing forces is the peer group. Among peers, individuals practice learned behaviors and roles relatively free from adult scrutiny. As children age and separate from their parents, the peer group takes on additional importance. Boys are more harshly chastised by their same-sexed peers for sex role indiscretions than are girls (no boy wants to be a sissy). Young female "tomboys" may not receive the same negative pressures from their peer groups. In fact, they may benefit from "boyish" behaviors. As females become teenagers, appropriate sex-role behaviors become more paramount. Adolescent girls learn that popularity (in itself a measure of success) is indirectly proportional to perceived intelligence. Young women learn that popularity—especially with the opposite sex—is attained by masking one's intelligence. Perhaps this is responsible for the decline in female scholastic achievement in the high school years.

Thus, many factors influence sex-role development. In the spectrum of sex-role development, keep in mind that no individual is socialized into strictly male or strictly female behaviors. Many females demonstrate so-called male behaviors while males can be nurturing and compassionate.

Table 16-1   Common Sex-Role Stereotypes

MALE	FEMALE
Achievement Orientation	Affective Orientation
Initiative taker	Nurturant
Ambitious	Emotional
Worldly-wise	Expressive
Competitive	Warm
Level Headed	Noncareer Orientation
Unemotional	Home-centered
Unexpressive	Modest
Cold	
Dominant	Dependent
Independent	Submissive
Strong	Weak
Aggressive	Undecisive
Leader	Passive
	Follower

Influence of Traditional Sex Roles on Nursing Practice

In 1860, the Nightengale School and Home for Nurses was founded. Thus, nursing education was born in the midst of the Victorian climate of the mid-nineteenth century. The profession has undergone significant change since its beginning; however, the flavor of the Victorian era and traditional sex roles continues to be evident. A number of these influences impact positively upon the profession; others may impair nursing's growth and development. By identifying and analyzing these factors, we, as nurses, can understand their influence on our profession and take steps necessary to alter negative aspects in our practices. "Hold over" influences on the profession of nursing can be categorized into two areas: altruism and paternalism.

ALTRUISM

Altruism is the practice of putting others before oneself. Victorian ideology stressed the essence of being female as living for others. Women were well suited for this life work. They were seen as compassionate, nurturant, and empathetic. Altruism is a contemporary force in nursing. Nurses effectively respond to psychosocial needs because they are empathetic and compassionate. Nurses nurture patients to health. Nurses are routinely asked to place others (patients, administration, physicians) first by a supervisor who repeatedly requests overtime from a nurse who has stated her reluctance, adding, "but the patients need you!"; by the physician who interrupts a nursing admission interview to perform a physical, asserting: "but I'm busy! . . . I can't wait!"; by administration and society who often do not financially reimburse nurses commensurate with their responsibilities.

PATERNALISM

In Victorian England, women were viewed as wives and mothers *only*. As men's inferior (less rational and weaker), they were placed under the control of their husbands. Some suggest this patriarchal philosophy pervades nursing today. In past years, nurses were defined as handmaidens to physicians and in many settings this subservience remains. How many nurses continue to locate charts for physicians? Physicians still request and receive help from nurses during procedures they could perform alone, that is, instances not requiring the nurse's presence for patient support. Paternalistic influences are manifested by nonassertive deference to physicians or others in authority roles. Until recently, nurses were not seen as decision makers but simply those who followed orders prescribed by others. Implementation of the nursing process, including nursing care plans, and the clinical nursing specialist/practitioner movement have contributed to changing in a more positive way this perception of the nursing profession.

Nurses against nurse behavior demonstrates another aspect of paternalism. In a system where one group (the M.D.'s) dominate and are viewed as more powerful, members of another perhaps oppressed group (nurses) may identify with the dominant group. An aspect of this identification is intragroup conflict within the second group, pitting nurse against nurse.[8] Nurses may find themselves in the midst of unhealthy nurse-against-nurse competition rather than collaboration for the benefit of the patient. Divisiveness and a lack of cohesiveness are evident not only between individuals but among groups (shift versus shift, unit versus unit, diploma versus baccalaureate).

As the women's movement becomes more firmly engrained in American society, sex-role socialization and secondary education will evolve in ways that promote collaborative skills in women. In recent years, nursing education has stressed conflict resolution skills and promoted strong nursing identification. Certainly these changes will effectively impact upon unhealthy competition among nurses.

Men in Nursing

Nursing remains a sex-typed occupation. In fact, expressed interest in entering nursing is often identified as a feminine indicator on masculinity-femininity scales. Monnigerode, Kayser-Jones, and Garcia surveyed nursing students to conceptualize the "ideal nurse."[9] This nurse rated high on both masculine and feminine traits, evidencing a need for both males and females in the profession. While the number of men in nursing has increased, they continue to be a minority. Concerns of the male in nursing that have been anecdotally reported are listed on page 324.

A sample of ten male nurses of varying ages, experiences, and educational backgrounds was interviewed to assess the validity of these concerns. No male felt incapable of nurturing. Differences in empathetic or nurturing qualities were considered individual differences. Nurses may nurture differently (touch versus listening) but not along sex-based lines.

All male nurses interviewed were frequently identified as physicians and explained their choice of nursing to patients repeatedly. Females in nonstaff nurse positions also deal with this on a regular basis although not to the same extent as men. The males interviewed were pleased with their choice of nursing, often entering the profession after working in

CONCERNS OF MALE IN NURSING

- Masculine sex role not lending itself to nurturance
- Patient preference for female care-givers
- More rapid advancement of men in nursing
- Disproportionate amounts of physical labor (lifting or moving patients)
- Differential treatment by patients and physicians
- Uncomprehension by patients that men would choose nursing as opposed to medicine.

other fields. Reasons for selecting nursing varied from feeling too old to enter medicine to enjoying the goals of nursing—"doctors cure patients, while nurses make them better." Patients did not state a preference for caregivers based on sex. Perhaps this is attributable to the professional and respectful approaches of the men.

Half the men saw themselves being treated with more respect by physicians than females feeling they could make the same request as a female without being labeled "bitchy." Sex difference may not be the underlying reason. Men, seeing themselves treated with more respect, were better educated, were older, and taller than those who felt equally respected. Patients were seen as treating some males with more respect; perhaps these were the patients who saw the men as physicians. One nurse felt subjected to more harsh criticism from his coworkers.

All men identified physical labor as an issue. Resolutions varied from openly confronting and resolving the problem to making trade-offs. Some did nothing about the disparity.

The majority of men did not support the premise that men advance more rapidly than women, based on sex. The issue was career orientation—that men were more conscious of their careers and planned strategies to meet their goals. Two thirds of those interviewed has specific career paths planned. Noncareer orientation was viewed as a significant problem for the profession.

Overwhelmingly, the men interviewed identified differences in the interpersonal interactions of males and females. They saw women as taking criticisms personally to the point of interfering with their responsibilities and as being more inflexible in "bending the rules." This created some difficulties for men in the profession.

In summary, it appears that men in nursing are well adjusted in this predominantly female profession. Identified areas of concern were not supported by the men interviewed. Those who identified problems tended to be younger, newer, less experienced nurses. Males in nursing deal with reality shock and role development as do females. Perhaps as these men grow professionally and develop, anecdotally described concerns are resolved. Their sample was selected from a progressive teaching institution. Findings may be different in other health care settings.

Sex Role Orientation: Nursing Issues and Strategies

All professions are influenced by the sex-role orientation of their workers and nursing is no exception. Difficulty in interpersonal communication, assertion, collaboration, decision making, and career commitment can be linked to traditional sex-role orientations.

CAREER COMMITMENT

In the 1980's, teenage girls continue to be tracked into traditionally female jobs without internalizing a career orientation. Boys mature with the understanding that they will embark upon a career after completing formal education. For some women, jobs are seen as "stopgaps" to marriage or something to fall back upon—an ideology which affects women's views of themselves and their jobs. Women's traditional responsibilities for the home and family have inhibited many nurses' professional commitments. Working women continue to assume a majority of these responsibilities.

It has been hypothesized that women are afraid of success—that the independence and achievement necessary for success are unconsciously seen as sex-inappropriate activities. Achievement sets the stage for internal conflict between traditional sex role orientation and characteristics needed for success. This conflict serves to inhibit career orientation.

ASSERTIVENESS

As nurses have evolved from "handmaidens" to physicians, simply following orders, to autonomous decision makers, assertiveness has become a necessary technique. The act of making one's own choices and of standing up for one's self, assertiveness is a difficult skill for women when sex-role orientation has followed traditional patterns. Assertive communication improves self-confidence and esteem and can impact upon patient care and collaboration when properly used within the health care system.

Assertive behavior is frequently confused with aggression. In reality, the two are diametrically opposed. Aggressive behavior minimizes the worth of others. Assertiveness involves presenting one's views without impinging on another individual. Table 16-2 summarizes the differences between aggressive, assertive, and nonassertive behavior. Assertive behavior has three prerequisites. First, one must WANT to change from a nonassertive or aggressive style of communication to an assertive one. Second, an assertive individual must be confident of the message she plans to project. Third, an assertive person must have specific techniques to ensure that an accurate message is being projected.

Assertiveness Techniques:
Nonverbal Behaviors
Assertiveness encompasses nonverbal and verbal behaviors. In every interpersonal interaction a strong message is given by nonverbal behavior (posture, distance, voice, and eye contact). Behaviors specific to styles of communication are summarized in Table 16-3.

In assertive encounters, facial expressions must be consistent with the spoken message. When pointing out a potentially serious mistake made by an aide or colleague, smiling is in direct opposition to the intended verbal message. Other nonassertive behaviors include lateral or downward head tilts. Submission may be portrayed by looking up to another person. Most nurses are women, shorter than predominantly male physicians and, therefore, may project submission in this subtle way.

Assertiveness Techniques:
Verbal Behaviors
Generally assertive encounters involve the use of "I" statements. For example, when a colleague does not follow through on the plan of care

Table 16-2 Differences in Aggressive, Assertive, and Nonassertive Behavior

NONASSERTIVE	AGGRESSIVE	ASSERTIVE
Self-denying	Self-enhancing at others' expense	Self-enhancing
Inhibited	Expressive	Expressive
Hurt, anxious	Deprecates others	Feels good about self
Allows others to choose	Chooses for others	Chooses for self
Does not achieve desired good	Achieves desired goals by hurting others	May achieve desired goal

Adapted from Curry J: Assertiveness training for supervision nurses. Superv Nurse 9(8): 43, 1978.

Table 16-3   Behaviors Specific to Communication Styles

	NONASSERTIVE	AGGRESSIVE	ASSERTIVE
POSTURE	Not facing person Nonerect posture (slouching)	Facing person Defensive stance (i.e. hands on hips; clenched fists)	Directly facing person Erect posture
VOICE	Soft, hesitant	Loud, accusing	Firm, audible, confident
DISTANCE	Yields space Leans backward Moves away	Invades space	Respects individual's personal space
EYE CONTACT	Downward gaze Looks away	Direct contact Staring	Direct contact Steady gaze

for a patient, an assertive response is "I am upset that . . . ". Alternative responses include the aggressive statement that "You caused Mr. Smith an extra day's stay because . . . ", or the nonassertive response of saying nothing. "I" statements are less threatening and allow you to assume responsibility for your own feelings.

Assertive verbal statements are direct and specific to a particular incident. Assertive statements do not begin "You always . . . ", but focus on the behavior in question only. An example of an assertive statement is, "I am concerned about your late arrival this morning"; in contrast, a nonassertive response is, "You always come in ten minutes late."

Assertive responses are honest and sensitive to the occasion. It is inappropriate to discuss problematic behavior in a crowded nursing station. Assertive nurses contemplate the timing of their message to optimize its impact while considering the feelings of the other person.

The following specific assertive techniques may seem awkward and mechanical. Through practice (perhaps role playing) they can comfortably become part of your verbal repertoire.

The broken record technique is useful for individuals who have difficulty saying "no." Without becoming irritated, the verbal message is persistently repeated again and again. This technique allows one to state her position without addressing side issues raised by the other person.

Negative assertion, negative inquiry, and fogging are three assertive techniques for handling criticism. Negative assertion is accepting and assuming responsibility for aspects about oneself that are negative. This is useful when valid criticisms are made. A negative assertion would be "Yes, I did forget to complete the public health referral. What can we do to make certain the patient is seen?" Negative inquiry requests additional information about critical statements. It encourages the constructive use and analytic examination of criticisms. Fogging implies that one accepts the criticism in general without anxiety or defensiveness. It eliminates counter attacking. Examples of fogging statements are: "You may have a point"; "That's probably right"; "That's true."

The process of learning assertive behavior is long and difficult. Start on a small scale and persist. Practice assertive techniques with friends. Use role playing, audiotapes, videotapes, or mirrors to help evaluate assertive skills.

Decision Making

Traditionally, nurses have seen themselves as nondecision makers. They have not perceived themselves as an integral part in overall hospital decision or policy making. Because of the service component of nursing and female dominance in this discipline, nursing historically has not recognized or capitalized on its important role in decision making.

Although this perception may still exist at the present time, it is generally not accurate. Nursing practice centers on problem solving and decision making. The nursing process itself represents a decision making framework. Beginning nurses learn to assess, plan, intervene and evaluate early in their training. Patient care management requires continual decision making and evaluation. According to Levey and Loomba, "a decision is the conclusion of a process by which one chooses among available alternatives for the purpose of achieving a set of desired objectives. Decision making involves all the thinking and activities that are required to produce a choice among alternative courses of action."[10] It is clear that the process of decision making is an essential component of professional practice.

There have been several major changes in health care management that have facilitated nursing involvement in institutional decision making. The first change has been an increased number of decentralized nursing departments. The philosophy of decentralization is to allow and encourage decision making at all levels within the department. This allows staff nurses to become more actively involved in nursing and organizational policy development and decision making. The second change is increasing acceptance of a joint practice approach to patient care. This approach utilizes the physician and nurse as collaborative decision makers for patient care.

If nurses are educated in problem solving and decision making and if many organizations are now encouraging and facilitating nursing involvement in decision making, why then do nurses perceive themselves as nondecision makers? Certainly, organizational constraints in many hospitals hamper nursing's decision making to a degree that depends on the strength and position of the nursing department within the organization. However, the more important issue is that nurses are not always comfortable with decision making and often perceive themselves as followers rather than leaders. To be comfortable in a decision-making role, one must have self-confidence, a comprehensive knowledge base and a level of independence. Many nurses do not see themselves as having these traits. This may be due to the sexual-role development and stereotyping that occurs in predominantly female groups. Nurses, however, must overcome this attitude as the decision-making process is essential to their professional practice.

Collaboration

According to Marriner, "Collaborating is assertive and cooperative. It is a win-win strategy. It contributes to effective problem solving because both parties try to find mutually satisfying solutions."[11] Collaboration facilitates the utilization of unique strengths and skills found in each person. Competition, however, is a win-lose method of interaction and may create a great deal of conflict.

For any interaction to be effective and rewarding, communication and collaboration are essential. Successful relationships are often defined as being shared or joint or collaborative. An individual cannot enter into a mutual collaboration without having a strong sense of self-concept. Collaboration is not effective if either party is inflexible, defensive, or narrow-minded.

In health care, interdisciplinary collaboration should be the framework for determining and implementing patient care. Unfortunately, not everyone develops effective communication and collaborative skills during their adolescence. Men and women both may have difficulty collaborating. Men can interpret it as competitive and women may perceive it as uncomfortable and confrontational. Given that physicians are predominantly male and nurses predominantly female, their attempt at collaboration is somewhat fraught with these innate difficulties.

Over the past decade there has been growing recognition of the importance of nurse/physician collaboration in improving health care services and facilitating improved continuity.[12] Everyone agrees that nurses, physicians, and other health-care workers should be working as a team. The vital elements of collaboration include open communication, role clarification, and trust in the performance of others. One major problem in physician/nurse collaboration is a lack of knowledge concerning each other's role. Without an understanding of roles, one is not able to trust another's performance. In addition, when professional roles are not clearly articulated and understood, it is much easier to fall into a pattern of sexual stereotyping. Marketing nursing both internally and externally is one mechanism to educate other disciplines about nursing. Another mechanism is to informally educate physicians and other health-care team members through group and one-to-one interaction. Nurses must also keep an open mind when learning about the roles and issues of other professions. Health care providers must avoid intellectual or professional ethnocentrism in the sharing of knowledge. The mixing of professional perspectives and skills is necessary in solving these complex problems.[13]

The second issue concerns the efficacy of nursing communication. The nurse, functioning as the advocate for the patient, communicates with numerous people every day. The purposes of these many communications may differ. "Common purposes include to inform, to entertain, to inquire, to persuade, to command. The goal may be to evoke a particular attitude or a particular behavior, verbal or actional."[14] The most difficult communication is usually one in which individuals must agree on the goal and the process for achieving that goal. This type of communication typically exemplifies a collaborative effort.

Nurses learn a great deal about effective communication through their educational and daily operations in the health-care system. However, learning communication skills to achieve an intended goal is a never-ending process. Various strategies need to be employed, depending on the desired goals and the individuals involved. Female nurses can often use female stereotyping to their advantage when combined with knowledge. When dealing with individuals who are much older, it is sometimes effective to begin a collaborative approach by asking for help. With physicians, a well-structured, empathetic, nondefensive, but persistent and assertive approach may be desired. When attending group meetings one should be conscious of body language and indirect as well as direct communications.

It is essential that nurses become more knowledgeable about communication strategies. Nurses must be aware of the stereotype associated with their role and sex and should combat stereotyping with knowledge, skill, and effective communication. It is not deceptive to use different approaches; it is the key to successful interaction and collaboration.

Nursing leaders need to assist nurses in learning and implementing effective communication strategies. Mentors or role models should be identified to facilitate this growth process. Interactions with physicians, health-care members and patients/consumers should be viewed as opportunities to educate others about nursing. Nurses and physicians working together as colleagues toward improved patient outcomes represent the framework for health-care delivery. In addition, interdisciplinary collaboration and support is vital to the growth and development of professional nursing.

Conclusion

Although traditional sex role stereotyping has affected the profession of nursing, times are changing. Nursing continues to attract intelligent and motivated individuals both males and females, who are committed to professional goals and objectives. Nurses must be aware of sex-role stereotyping and not allow this to interfere with professional growth.

The image of nursing must be built on competence, commitment, knowledge, and the continuous pursuit of professional growth and development.

References

1. Macoby E and Jacklin C: The Psychology of Sex Differences. Stanford, Stanford University Press, 1974
2. Money J, Ehrhardt A: Man and Woman/Boy and Girl. Baltimore, John Hopkins University Press, 1972
3. Rubin J, Provenzano F, Luria A: The eye of the beholder: Parent's views on sex of newborns. Am J *Orthopsychiatry* 44:516–17, 1974
4. Goldberg S, Lewis M: Play behavior in the year old infant: Early sex differences. Child Dev 40:21–31, 1969
5. Sternglanz S, Serbin L: Sex role stereotyping in childrens' television programs. Dev Psychol 10:710–15, 1974
6. Long M, Simon R: The roles and status of women on children and family TV programs. Journalism 51:107–10, 1974
7. Tedesco M: Patterns in prime time. J. Communication 24:119–24, 1974
8. Roberts S: Oppressed group behavior: Implications for nursing. Adv Nurs Sci 5(4):21–30, 1982
9. Monnigerode F, Kayser-Jones J, Garcia G: Masculinity and femininity in nursing. Nurs Res 27(5):299–301, 1978
10. Levey S, and Loomba NP: *Health Care Administration: A Managerial Perspective,* p 169. Philadelphia, JB Lippincott, 1973
11. Marriner H: Guide to Nursing Management, 2nd ed, p 183. CV Mosby, 1984
12. Joiner C, VanServellen G: Job Enrichment in Nursing: A Guide to Improving Morale, Productivity, and Retention, p 72. Rockville, MD, Aspen Systems, 1984
13. Fuszard B: Self-actualization for nurses: Issues, trends and strategies for job enrichment, p 123. Rockville, MD, Aspen Systems, 1984
14. Stevens B: The Nurse as Executive, 3rd ed, p 185. Rockville, MD, Aspen Systems, 1985

Chapter 17

Professional organizations

DEBORAH J. TEASLEY

The complexity and rapid change in nursing is more manageable when joining with others who have common goals, problems, and needs. Professional organizations were developed for this reason. Some organizations are comprised of nurses with a wide variety of backgrounds and practice settings while others focus on nurses who share one major interest. Some organizations are so large that they have international affiliations, while others have only a few hundred members. Regardless of the size or focus of the organization, they all share two common goals. The first goal is the promotion of quality nursing care. The second goal is the development of nurses and the nursing profession.

This chapter will enable you to

1. Describe the benefits available to nurses as members of professional organizations.

2. Identify major nursing organizations of interest to the new nurse.

Benefits of Membership

Unfortunately, many nurses do not participate in a professional organization. The common reasons for nonparticipation are cost, lack of time, and inability to identify with the issues addressed by the organizations. The membership dues for many organizations are quite modest. The American Nurses' Association is the most expensive organization to join, but it offers the widest variety of benefits.

A lack of time is always a concern; however, a small amount of time spent in a professional organization can result in significant benefits. These benefits in turn may help one operate more efficiently and effectively at work. Thus the time invested is worth the return received. If a nurse chooses not to commit time to active participation in a professional organization, monetary support of the organization through membership can still be money well spent.

In the past 20 years the number of nursing organizations has increased dramatically. Almost every area of nursing practice has an associated organization. It is not difficult to find one whose interests match your own. Professional organizations not only make major contributions to nursing, but give many individual benefits to their members.

CONTINUING EDUCATION

The opportunity for continuing education is a major individual benefit from organizational membership. The half life of nursing knowledge is only a few years. This means that approximately one half of today's nursing knowledge will be obsolete within the next 2 to 5 years. This makes it imperative that nurses continually update their knowledge and skills throughout their careers.

Many professional organizations offer their membership a variety of means for obtaining these vital knowledge updates.

Local Meetings. Many organizations have local chapters that meet on a regular basis. The format is often a short business meeting, followed by a speaker. The speaker presents information on a topic of interest to the members. Sales representatives may demonstrate new equipment or bring product samples for members to try at work. These meetings are without additional cost to members.

Regional or National Meetings.   These meetings are usually held annually and last for several days. A portion of the time is spent in the operational process of the organization. Board meetings are held and national officers elected. Members are invited to attend forums where issues of organizational governance are discussed. This frequently includes information on the development and function of local chapters. However, the majority of the time spent at these annual meetings is for the purpose of continuing education. National leaders are available to discuss timely topics on both a formal and informal basis. Participants have the opportunity to choose from a variety of presentations in order to best meet their individual needs. Although the educational portions of these meetings are available to nonmembers, members attend for reduced fees.

PUBLICATIONS

Access to professional publications is another benefit of organizational membership. Many organizations include professional publications as a membership benefit. The simplest of these are usually developed at the local level. They are often photocopied "newsletters" that inform members about upcoming meetings, financial reports of the organization, member activities, and so forth. Newsletters frequently include research abstracts and information about new products or programs.

At the national level, organizations frequently publish professional journals. Some organizations publish two or more publications. These journals are edited with the needs of various member groups in mind. Some publications are restricted to the organization's membership while others may be obtained by nonmembers as well. Nonmembers must pay a subscription fee for the publications while they are included in the membership dues for those who belong to the organization.

PROFESSIONAL NETWORKING

Professionals must learn to work with others to attain goals. When trying to accomplish a task, it is helpful to get input from others. For this reason, the development of a network of professional contacts is important at all career stages. Learning to effectively develop and utilize a professional network is an important skill.

A professional network consists of contacts who work in nursing or allied professions. It is not necessary that they be able to immediately impact your career in order to be identified as a network member. Membership in professional organizations is a valuable means for developing these contacts.

While those whom the nurse contacts frequently at work may form the network nucleus, this is not adequate for the development of a strong professional network. Contacts made at professional association meetings are an important network expansion. The optimum situation for network building is membership in at least two professional organizations. The first of these should be an organization that affords the individual nurse an opportunity to interact with many different nurses at all levels of practice. The American Nurses' Association is an example of this type of organization. The second organization chosen for membership should be a specialty organization in your chosen area of practice. Some examples of specialty organizations are listed in the "Resources" section at the end of this chapter.

As the need to expand a network grows, a third organization should be a broad based organization with both professional and lay members. Only one aspect of this organization may be health-related. Some examples of such groups are women's organizations, environmental concern groups, or organizations such as the American Red Cross.

Once a member of an organization, it is important to participate in its activities in order to meet and interact with network contacts. The cliche of getting out what one puts in applies to professional networking. Active participation on committees and task forces requires a time investment but the return is an opportunity to develop and expand your network of contacts.

PROFESSIONAL RECOGNITION

Recognition for individual accomplishments is another benefit of membership in professional organizations. The opportunity to obtain specialty certification is a benefit being offered by an increasing number of organizations.

As nursing knowledge has expanded many nurses have become proficient in delivering high quality nursing care to a specific group of patients. These nurses have sought a means of formal recognition of this additional expertise. Professional organizations have offered a means for attaining this recognition through the certification process. Certification differs from licensure in two main ways:

1. Registered Nurse licensure provides evidence of at least a minimal acceptable level of knowledge in all major areas of nursing practice.
   Certification is a way of recognizing outstanding knowledge in a specific area of practice. Licensure is required for all nurses. Certi-

fication is generally not required for practice in a nursing specialty. Instead, many certifying agencies require evidence of practice in a specialty area for several years before one becomes eligible for certification.

2. Once one attains licensure, it may be maintained as long as the required renewal fees are paid and the practice codes are not violated. This is true even if the R.N. is not employed as a nurse. Certification lasts a specified number of years (usually 2 to 5 years). At the end of this time one is required to show evidence of current practice and a specified number of continuing education credits in the specialty area. (Some certification programs offer the option of reexamination in lieu of continuing education credits). The purpose of these requirements is to ensure that nurses holding certification in a specific area possess knowledge of current developments in that area.

At present, there are over 30 certification programs in nursing offered by 16 professional organizations (listed below and on page 338). Several others will become available in the near future. Certification is obtained through the organization's certification board. This board administers testing and verifies credentials for certification and renewals. Certification fees range from $100 to $345. While membership in the sponsoring organization is not required for certification, members receive a reduction in fees charged. Certification has grown rapidly in popularity. Predictions are that this trend will continue since it is a valuable mechanism for assuring current knowledge and standardization of specialty practice.

AREA OF SPECIALTY CERTIFICATION

Adult Nurse Practitioner

Advanced Nursing Administration

Clinical Specialist in Adult Psychiatric-Mental Health Nursing

Clinical Specialist in Child/Adolescent Psychiatric-Mental Health Nursing

Clinical Specialist in Medical Surgical Nursing

Child and Adolescent Nurse

Community Health

Critical Care Nursing

continued

AREA OF SPECIALTY CERTIFICATION *Continued*

Emergency Room Nursing

Enterostomal Therapy

Family Nurse Practitioner

Gerontological Nurse

Gerontological Nurse Practitioner

Hemodialysis Nursing

High Risk Perinatal

Infection Control

Inpatient Obstetric Nurse

Maternal Child Health

Medical-Surgical Nurse

Neonatal Nurse Clinician

Neonatal Intensive Care Nurse

Neurosurgical Nursing

Nurse Anesthetist

Nurse-midwife

Nursing Administration

Nursing Home Administration

OB/Gyn Practitioner

Occupational Health Nursing

Operating Room Nursing

Pediatric Nurse Practitioner (2 programs)

Psychiatric and Mental Health Nurse

Rehabilitation Nurse Practitioner

Urological Nursing

In addition to offering certification as a means of professional recognition, organizations offer yearly awards to outstanding members. These awards recognize contributions made by members who have promoted the goals of the organization. Awards may be offered that recognize outstanding contributions to the organization, research, clinical practice, or other areas of professional practice. These awards are highly prized since they represent excellence recognized by one's peers.

FINANCIAL BENEFITS

Although not usually a sole purpose for membership in an organization, many organizations offer the possibility of financial benefits to members. These benefits are in the form of scholarships or grants. Scholarships are usually awarded to member-applicants on the basis of merit. Many nurses have taken advantage of these scholarships to further their education.

Organizations may offer grants to support members' research. This research, in turn, helps to further the attainment of the organization's goals.

POLITICAL BENEFITS

The opportunity to impact the nursing profession is a benefit of organizational membership. One person acting alone can rarely make changes of the magnitude that many persons acting cooperatively can achieve. The current health care environment requires that methods for high quality, cost effective care be devised. This will require many changes in the health-care system. These changes will strongly impact nursing practice. Nurses who have a voice in these changes can be excited by them rather than threatened by them. Professional organizations offer a means for creating changes that will have a positive effect for nurses and their patients.

An important way that organizations are actively influencing change is participation in politics. The American Nurses' Association is the most active organization in this area. Lobbyists can be hired by the organization to provide legislators with the nursing perspective on health-care-related issues. Nursing organizations act to keep members informed about important legislative issues and may organize activities such as letter-writing campaigns. They may sponsor open forum discussions where nurses can voice their opinions on important issues.

Another way in which organizations are influencing change is in public education. These efforts are toward informing the public about nurses and their contributions to health care. Many approaches are being used. These range from elaborate media productions to community based one-on-one activities such as health screening programs.

An additional way that organizations influence change is to define and clarify the practice of nursing. Nursing organizations have been instrumental in developing standards for nursing practice. Organizational representatives may act as consultants when practice issues are being analyzed.

The ability of professional organizations to influence change is indisputable. For this reason, it is important that nurses participate in professional organizations. Otherwise, decisions that impact the entire profession will be made by only a few persons. Nurses who choose not to participate should not then criticize the organizations for not representing their interests.

GROWTH OF LEADERSHIP POTENTIAL

A final individual benefit to membership in a professional organization is the opportunity to develop group participation and leadership skills. Most activities in health care today require the cooperation of a group of persons. Many times it will be the nurse who must facilitate this cooperation. As a member of a professional organization one learns how to participate in group discussions, to present ideas in a professional manner, accept compromise, and work together with individuals who have varied opinions and values. These skills can be transferred to work settings with great success. The value of these skills in attaining career goals is significant.

Nurses who would like to develop leadership skills may do this by assuming progressive leadership positions in their professional organization, particularly at the local level. The atmosphere in local organizations is generally supportive. This offers the novice leader the opportunity to develop skills in a nonthreatening environment. Many organizations offer leadership seminars or workshops for local officers to help them become more proficient in managing their chapters. These same management and leadership skills may be useful in other areas of practice.

ATTAINING MEMBERSHIP

Membership in professional organizations is attained in two ways. The most common way is through individual application for membership. Each organization has eligibility rules that may be obtained from the organization. Many require only that the prospective member be a registered nurse. Once potential members ascertain that they meet the eligibility requirements, they need only to complete an application form and pay the required membership dues. The organization may require that additional proof of eligibility, such as a license number, be submitted at the time of application. Upon receipt of the application, the organization will verify eligibility requirements and notify the new member of acceptance.

A less common method of attaining membership to an organization is through an invitation to join. This usually occurs when the organization is highly selective and requires that members show evidence of outstanding contributions prior to offering membership. Two examples of this type of organization are Sigma Theta Tau (nursing's professional honor society) and the American Academy of Nursing (discussed later in this chapter). An invitation to join such an organization is an honor and is rarely declined by the honoree.

Some organizations offer "associate" membership. These are available to interested persons who may not meet the eligibility requirements for full membership (such as student nurses). Information about the availability of such memberships can be obtained from the individual organization.

Professional Organizations

THE ALUMNAE ASSOCIATION

Alumnae associations were the first professional organizations for nurses. Each alumnae association is comprised of faculty and former students of a particular school of nursing. The associations serve a vital link between nursing education and practicing professionals. The alumnae association maintains close contact with the School of Nursing. Association activities often center around public relations efforts for the School or fund raising for scholarships. Alumnae association members may participate in school committees and act as advisors to faculty and administration on current practice issues.

Graduates become lifetime members of the school's alumnae association. The organization supports itself from contributions by the members rather than from annual membership dues. Active membership in one's alumnae association provides the same individual benefits as other professional organizations; however, the ability to maintain contact with others who shared nursing school experiences offers a dimension of friendship usually not present in other organizations.

This added benefit makes membership in this organization a social as well as professional experience. Even so, alumnae associations should not be viewed as primarily social organizations.

Alumnae associations offer a rich tradition as professional organizations. In 1897 several schools of nursing had alumnae associations. Representatives from ten schools prepared a constitution and bylaws establishing the National Associated Alumnae of the United States and Canada. This organization became the American Nurses' Association in 1911.

THE AMERICAN NURSES' ASSOCIATION

The American Nurses' Association (ANA) is the professional organization for all nurses. Its stated purposes are to work to improve health care and its availability for all people, to foster high standards of nursing practice, and to promote the professional development and economic and general welfare of nurses. This commitment to the economic welfare of nurses distinguishes the ANA from other professional nursing organizations. Although only a fraction of the total number of nurses belong to ANA, it represents nursing to many other health-care groups, governmental agencies and the public. Membership is available to all registered nurses. Individual nurses join the state nurses' association in the state where they are registered to practice. The national association is composed of state organizations. State organizations are divided into local organizations called districts. District membership is included with state membership.

The organizational structure of the ANA is complex and may be somewhat difficult to understand initially. At the national level the organization is run by the board of directors and the house of delegates. The board is elected biennially by the house of delegates (representatives from the state association). The board has an advisory council made up of two representatives from each state association.

The house of delegates meets annually and is the top policy making body of the ANA. The policies and programs of the ANA are set by the house of delegates.

The ANA also has committees, cabinets, and councils. Committees may be special or standing. Special committees are temporary and appointed for a specific purpose. Standing committees are permanent and help with the ongoing functions of the organization. Current standing committees are bylaws, nominating, ethics, and reference.

Cabinets report to the house of delegates and are assigned specific responsibilities for aspects of ANA, such as education, practice, and research. They evaluate and monitor trends pertinent to their area of responsibility. They make recommendations to the house of delegates for policies and standards.

Councils are established for major areas of nursing practice (medical-surgical nursing, administration, maternal-child nursing, and so forth). Councils are responsible for setting standards of practice, continuing education, and consultation on nursing practice.

Functions

Throughout this century the ANA has been active in all aspects of nursing practice. The functions of the organization have been adapted as the needs of the profession changed. Some of the major functions of today's ANA will be outlined here.

Publishing.   The official journal of the ANA is the *American Journal of Nursing.* It is published monthly. ANA also publishes a monthly newspaper, *The American Nurse.* The ANA owns the American Journal of Nursing publishing company that publishes other journals, such as *Nursing Outlook* and *Nursing Research.* The ANA also publishes non-print media such as films used for nursing education.

Collective Bargaining.   One of the most controversial activities of the ANA is its role in collective bargaining for nurses. Many state nurses' associations serve as collective bargaining agents for nurses. The ANA has provided support for these activities as part of its goal of promoting economic welfare for nurses. The focus of these negotiations is not only financial gains but also the improvement of patient care and the ability of nurses to have a part in determining their working conditions.

Politics.   The ANA maintains an office in Washington, D.C., through which registered lobbyists work with legislators on nursing-related issues. These activities offer the ability to keep members informed about crucial legislative matters.

The Nurses' Coalition for Action in Politics (N-CAP) is the ANA's political arm. It is a voluntary, nonpartisan organization that works to meet the ANA's legislative objectives. Its two major functions are education and political support. Educational efforts are aimed at helping nurses learn to function actively in the political environment. Support of political candidates may be financial or through endorsement. Candidates who are favorable toward nursing issues may receive this support regardless of their political affiliation.

Other Activities.   The ANA is involved in many other activities. It offers certification in 17 specialty areas of practice. It has a long history of support for nursing research and is active in continuing education. The ANA works cooperatively with other nursing and health-care organizations on common issues. Some of these organizations have a special relationship with the ANA. Among them are the American Academy of Nursing, the International Congress of Nursing, the National Student Nurses' Association, and the American Nurses' Foundation.

The American Academy of Nursing (AAN) was established to recognize professional achievement and excellence. Its members are called Fellows and use the initials F.A.A.N. after their name. The number of active Fellows is limited to 500. Membership in the AAN comes through nomination by active Fellows. The AAN is responsible to the board of directors of the ANA.

The International Congress of Nursing (ICN) is an international organization of nurses. The ANA is the United States representative to the

ICN. ANA delegates actively participate in ICN activities. These activities focus on the improvement of health care worldwide.

The National Student Nurses' Association (NSNA) is the association for nursing students. NSNA members address the ANA house of delegates on issues relating to nursing education and students. NSNA members may serve on ANA special committees. The NSNA is organized into state organizations like the ANA structure. Many schools of nursing have local chapters of the state SNA.

The American Nurses' Foundation (ANF) is a tax-exempt, non profit organization that supports nursing research. Members of the ANA board of directors sit on the ANF board of trustees. The ANF supports nursing research by administering grants, conducting policy analysis, and facilitates the educational and research efforts of the ANA. The foundation is funded by contributions from individuals and other organizations.

THE NATIONAL LEAGUE FOR NURSING

The National League for Nursing (NLN) was established in 1952. Its purpose is to work toward the enhancement of nursing service and nursing education. It has both individual and agency memberships. Nurses and nonnurses may belong.

Individual members may join through local "constituent leagues" or, if a local league is not available, may join the National League directly. A constituent membership gives one an automatic national membership. The presidents of the constituent leagues meet annually at the National Assembly of Constituent Leagues for Nursing. Here they discuss implementation of national programs, common concerns, and possible approaches for dealing with them, as well as to recommend actions to the national board of directors.

Agencies (hospitals, schools of nursing, and community health services) work through councils. There are six councils. They are associate degree programs, diploma programs, baccalaureate and higher degree programs, practical nursing programs, community health services and nursing services for hospitals and related facilities. Each council has committees that work in the areas of continuing education, consultation, and other activities identified by the council. The NLN carries out a variety of services and activities for the nursing profession.

Testing. The NLN offers three main testing services. Placement testing allows credit to be given to nursing students who may already have gained nursing knowledge that might exempt them from some nursing courses, such as an associate degreed nurse returning to school for a baccalaureate degree. Graduates of foreign nursing schools are given tests prior to immigration to the United States to ensure an acceptable level of nursing knowledge. Perhaps the best known NLN testing activity is achievement testing. Achievement tests provide information about the level of knowledge attained by nursing students while in school. These tests are developed and graded by the NLN. They give students information that compares them to other students throughout the nation for a particular nursing practice topic. This testing helps a school of nursing keep its curriculum broad-based rather than regionalized.

Accreditation.   The NLN is recognized by the National Commission on Accreditation as the official accrediting body for nursing programs. The NLN sets standards for nursing programs and upon request reviews programs to determine if they are meeting these standards. If the program meets the standards, it becomes accredited by the NLN. The standards are published and available from the League. Most nursing schools seek accreditation by the NLN. A list of accredited schools is published yearly and is available from the NLN.

Research.   The NLN conducts ongoing research on nursing school enrollments and students and faculty members. It also undertakes research projects on nursing service issues, such as availability of nurses and nursing needs.

Publications.   The NLN publishes a proliferation of books and pamphlets. They cover a variety of topics ranging from educational standards to statements on current practice issues. A catalog listing these publications is available from the NLN headquarters and is updated yearly. *Nursing and Health Care* is the official journal of the NLN.

Other Activities.   The NLN offers consultation to agencies on a wide variety of topics. It informs members on legislative issues pertinent to nursing, and sponsors workshops, conferences, and seminars.

Summary

Through membership in professional organizations each nurse has the opportunity to influence the nursing profession and to gain individual benefits. Among the individual benefits to be gained are opportunities for continuing education, building a professional network, professional recognition, financial and political benefits, and growth of leadership potential.

The American Nurses' Association (ANA) and the National League for Nursing (NLN) are the largest nursing organizations. The ANA represents nurses in every aspect of nursing. Its actions influence both members and nonmembers. For this reason, it should be of interest to all nurses. The NLN plays an important role in nursing education. In addition to these two associations, there are specialty organizations in almost every area of interest.

Bibliography

Duespohl TA: Nursing in Transition. Rockville, MD, Aspen Systems, 1983

Fickeissen JL: Getting Certified. Am J Nurs 85:265–269, 1985

Kelly LY: Dimensions of Professional Nursing. New York, Macmillan Company, 1985

Notter LE, Spalding EK: Professional Nursing Foundations, Perspectives and Relationships. Philadelphia, JB Lippincott, 1976

Persons CB, Wieck L: Networking: A Power Strategy. Nurs Econom 3:53–57, 1985

Puetz BE: Networking for Nurses. Rockville, MD, Aspen Systems, 1983

Resources

PROFESSIONAL NURSING ORGANIZATIONS

Alpha Tau Delta
489 Serento Dr.
Thousand Oaks, CA 91360

American Assembly for Men in
Nursing
c/o College of Nursing
Rush University
600 S. Pauline, 474-H
Chicago, IL 60612

American Association of
Critical-Care Nurses
One Civic Plaza
Newport Beach, CA 92660

American Association of
Neuroscience Nurses
Suite 203
22 S. Washington
Park Ridge, IL 60068

American Association of Nurse
Anesthetists
216-a Higgins Road
Park Ridge, IL 60068

American Association of Nurse
Attorneys
113 W. Franklin Street
Baltimore, MD 21201

American Burn Association
Box 3056
Duke University Medical
Center
Durham, NC 27710

American College of Nurse-
Midwives
Suite 1120
1522 K Street, N.W.
Washington, DC 20005

American Holistic Nurses'
Association
P.O. Box 116
Telluride, CO 81435

American Nephrology Nurses'
Association
North Woodbury Road
Box 56
Pitman, NJ 08071

American Nurses' Association
2420 Pershing Rd.
Kansas City, MO 64108

American Society for Parenteral
and Enteral Nutrition
Suite 500
8605 Cameron St.
Silver Spring, MD 20910

American Society of
  Ophthalmic Registered
  Nurses, Inc.
P.O. Box 3030
San Francisco, CA 94119

American Society of Plastic and
  Reconstructive Surgical
  Nurses, Inc.
North Woodbury Rd., Box 56
Pitman, NJ 08071

American Society of Post-
  Anesthesia Nurses
P.O. Box 11083
Richmond, VA 23230

American Allied Urological
  Association
6845 Lake Shore Dr.
P.O. Box 9397
Raytown, MO 64133

Association for Practitioners in
  Infection Control
505 East Hawley St.
Mundelein, IL 60060

Association of Operating Room
  Nurses, Inc.
10170 East Mississippi Ave.
Denver, CO 80231

Association of Pediatric
  Oncology Nurses (APON)
Pacific Medical Center
P.O. Box 7999
San Francisco, CA 94120

Association of Rehabilitation
  Nurses
2506 Gross Point Rd.
Evanston, IL 60201

Chi Eta Phi Sorority, Inc.
2247 Glendale Dr.
Decatur, GA 30032

Drug and Alcohol Nursing
  Association, Inc.
P.O. Box 6216
Annapolis, MD 21401

National Association of
  Pediatric Nurse Associates
  and Practitioners
1000 Maplewood Dr., Suite 104
Maple Shade, NJ 08052

National Association of
  Physician Nurses (NAPN)
3837 Plaza Dr.
Fairfax, VA 22030

National Black Nurses'
  Association, Inc.
P.O. Box 18358
Boston, MA 02118

National Intravenous Therapy
  Association, Inc.
87 Blanchard Rd.
Cambridge, MA 02138

National League for Nursing
10 Columbus Circle
New York City 10019

National Male Nurse
  Association
23309 State St.
Saginaw, MI 48602

Nurse Consultants' Association
P.O. Box 258765
Colorado Springs, CO 80936

NAACOG: The Organization for
  Obstetric, Gynecologic,
  Neonatal Nurses
600 Maryland Ave. S.W.
Washington, DC 20024

Nurses Alliance for the
  Prevention of Nuclear War
P.O. Box 319
Chestnut Hill, ME 02164

Nurses Christian Fellowship
233 Langdon
Madison, WI 53703

Nurses Coalition for Action in
   Politics (N-CAP)
Suite 408
1101 14th St. N.W.
Washington, DC 20005

Nurses' Environmental Health
   Watch
P.O. Box 811
Nassawadox, VA 23413

Nurses Organization of the
   Veterans Administration
505 W. Hawley St.
Mundelein, IL 60060

Oncology Nursing Society
Suite 200
3111 Banksville Rd.
Pittsburgh, PA 15216

Sigma Theta Tau, Inc.
1100 Waterway Blvd.
Indianapolis, IN 46202

Society of Gastrointestinal
   Assistants, Inc.
1070 Sibley Tower
Rochester, NY 14604

Society for Nursing History
Box 150
Teacher's College
Columbia University
New York City 10027

Society of Otorhinolaryngology
   and Head-Neck Nurses, Inc.
3893 East Market St.
Warren, OH 44484

Society for Parenteral and
   Enteral Nutrition
1025 Vermont Ave. N.W.
Suite 8110
Dept. N 81
Washington, DC 20005

Chapter 18

The future of nursing

GAYE W. POTEET AND
LINDA C. HODGES

Status of American Society

The 1980 election of Ronald Reagan as president of the United States represented a fundamental shift in the nature of the country's social, political, and economic thought. In the two decades that preceded Mr. Reagan, the Congress had enacted more health legislation than in all of its previous history. The optimism and faith of the 1960s and the 1970s however, ultimately changed to suspicion, distrust, and disillusionment with government and culminated in the Reagan election of 1980. Through the use of skillful budgetary processes Reagan succeeded in gaining approval of budgetary cuts reversing the expansion of the federal government that had occurred over the past 50 years. As president, Reagan negotiated and streamlined much of the budgetary process, and enlisted popular support for budget cuts designed to decelerate the expansion of the federal government.

More recent trends and the 1984 election results indicate that governmental policies, including health-care policy will be increasingly based on economic reality. For the past two years since 1984, American hospitals have been forced by the advent of diagnostic related groupings and surrounding economic circumstances to reexamine their foundations. Old health-care economic assumptions must be examined and changed. New structures and processes must be devised to guide the resulting changes throughout the health-care industry and within our own individual institutions. The desired outcome of the changes is a decrease in the cost of health care for all Americans. The percentage of the nation's gross national product (GNP) devoted to payment for health care is presently approaching 11%. The GNP refers to the value of an economy's annual output of goods and services. Resources devoted to health care are services that cannot be used for any other purpose—food, shelter, or recreation. There is a growing sense within our society that even if there is some benefit to be derived from the high levels of care available in the industry, these benefits are costing more than they are worth.

This chapter will enable you to

1. Describe the changing health-care arena.
2. Identify social trends that play a major role in shaping the future of nursing.
3. Describe nursing as it is evolving in a technological age.
4. Identify the practice roles to be played by a nurse in the future.

The Changing Scene of Health-Care Delivery

The process of change that is occurring in hospitals will result in a reshaping of these institutions. Nursing managers have traditionally held responsibility for an essentially closed and separate department of nursing. Increasingly nursing managers are finding that networks comprised of nursing and other disciplines both within the institution and at the local, state, and national level are essential to the problem-solving process. Changing institutional patterns, structures, financial exigencies, and other problems of retrenchment are combining to change the working environment. The desired outcome of these changes is increased organizational effectiveness resulting in a decrease in the cost of health care for all Americans.

Changes in the health-care delivery system were heralded by Public Law #97-248, creating the first second-order change in years. The health-care delivery system is presently experiencing more change than at any time in its recent history. One of the provisions of this law was aimed at curbing the rapid increase in Medicare hospital costs through the establishment of a Prospective Payment System for hospitals certified by the federal government to provide Medicare (Part A) services to the more than 30 million eligible American citizens.

Prospective payment has changed the way hospitals conduct their business. In the past, an increase in patient length of stay, use of multiple diagnostic tests, and increase in use of supplies, produced more income and higher profits. Since hospitals were reimbursed by third-party payees for services rendered, thus allowing price discrimination among hospitals, the incentive to compete based on one cost of services to all was absent. Today hospitals have been placed at significant financial risk when utilization of resources exceeds the expected demand for a specific diagnostic category. The emphasis on cost has forced nurses and physicians to practice within the framework of efficiency mandated by prospective payment. Under prospective payment, hospitals are increasingly being forced to choose a mission and to deliver only those services that are efficient and cost-effective for the institution.

This period of accelerated change in America's health-care industry is being hastened by increasing third-party demands that the costs of health care be reduced while maintaining a high quality of care. The federal government, the largest third-party payer, along with big business and major health care insurers such as Blue Cross and Blue Shield, is now demanding accountability for dollars spent. New sources and alternatives for health-care delivery are being explored, including an emphasis on primary care provided by nurse practitioners in areas such as gerontology and school health.

The increase in the number of physicians is also contributing to changes in the health-care industry, as more practicing physicians abort private practice and become paid employees of alternative health-care delivery systems. In the future, new physicians entering the labor market will find private practice less appealing as competition increases between those in practice and those providing care in health maintenance organizations (HMO's), independent practice associations, and preferred provider organizations (PPS's). For physicians, the future will offer less opportunity to achieve high incomes as prepaid services become the order of the day rather than the luxury of price discrimination. In response to Medicare's new payment scheme, the number and type of alternative health care systems are expected to expand. Physicians, like the graduate nurses following World War II, will find themselves part of the staff of an organized agency or bureaucracy.

SOCIAL TRENDS: THEIR IMPACT ON HEALTH CARE

A number of social trends (enumerated on the following page) are likely to play a major role in influencing the future of nursing. Of these, perhaps the greatest change is declining financial support for health-care programs. The decrease in funding can be attributed to multiple factors. Health care must compete under the Reagan administration with national defense. In the climate of an unprecedented federal deficit, health-care costs growing at a rate higher than any other commodity, a growing imbalance in trade ($148 billion in 1985), and the Federal Hospital Insurance Fund now estimated to be bankrupt by the year 2000, social policy has merged with economic policy. Those making decisions about health-care financing are being forced to consider critically the price tag of ongoing and new programs developed to meet the increasing demands of a citizenry that is getting older and poorer.

The American society today is experiencing a fundamental change in the composition of its citizens. The tides of spirited youth that were once the stereotypical Americans are giving way as the ratio of the aged increases. The number of 65-year-olds and over is growing at approximately twice the rate of the general population. Today those over 65 comprise about 11% of the population and generate 31% of national health expenditures (3% of the (GNP). By the year 2000, it is estimated that 13.1% of the population will be 65 or older. In the year 2030, if current statistics hold, there will be more retired workers than those working to contribute to the tax base. Assuming that federal financing for health care remains about 20% of the GNP and program funding continues at the present level, programs for the elderly in 2030 may consume up to 50% of the federal budget.[1] Not only will we have many more elderly, but within this group, there will be more women than men. Traditionally, elderly women have been among the poorest in our society, requiring more financial support than their male counterparts. With federal agencies currently paying 60% of all health-care costs for the elderly, in the future we can expect a sharp increase in cost for the core of this group.

In addition to declining health-care funding and an increase in the elderly population, we are also experiencing rapid change in the minority population. The Hispanic population is projected to outnumber the Black population by 1990, making Hispanics the largest minority group in America. While traditionally immigrants to America have come from western Europe, in most recent years, immigrants are more likely to be

SOCIAL TRENDS THAT INFLUENCE NURSING'S FUTURE

1. Decreased financial support for health care
2. Demographic changes in population
3. Increased cultural diversity in citizens
4. Changing family structure
5. Proliferation of knowledge and computer information systems

from Asia or Central America. Nurses face challenges in serving the client or patient needs of these new groups of Americans and nurses also face special problems and challenges in working alongside these new Americans.

An analysis of the shift in demographics points to a future of poverty for more Americans. As the numbers of elderly increase, together with the rapid expansion of minorities, and the growing number of immigrants, those persons in need of governmental assistance will surely increase. The number of dependent poor will present a major challenge in a climate many fear will be characterized by health-care rationing. The American family is also experiencing rapid change. The number of single parent families has risen to 19.2% of all families.[2] In 1981, births to unwed mothers numbered 18.9% of all births.[2] More than 52% of all women are employed in the work force, outside the home, a figure that has continued to rise since 1983.[3] The changes in health care have resulted in earlier discharge for acutely ill patients, including elderly family members. Increasingly more complicated procedures and treatments are being done on an outpatient basis. These changes have widespread ramifications for all areas of American society, but especially for women, including nurses. The shifting of care responsibilities to the home will place even greater demands on the American family and especially on its female family members.

Perhaps one of the major social trends we are now experiencing is the explosion of knowledge added by the ever increasing sophistication of knowledge. It is estimated by the year 2000 we will have instant obsolescence of knowledge. The utilization and management of knowledge production will be aided by an advanced technological system that will permeate all institutions, even the home. With the aid of computer information systems, we will move from the industrialized age to the information age. The major characteristics of both knowledge and technology will change.

In this climate of constant change, nursing as a profession has the opportunity to take giant steps forward. The standardization of nursing education into two levels as proposed by the American Nurses' Association has the potential to do for nursing what the Flexner Report did for medicine. Being a nurse will finally stand for something the public can clearly understand. For years, nursing educators, nursing service administrators, and others have debated the pros and cons of the various educational pathways to becoming a registered nurse. Those supportive of hospital-based diploma education have fought a valiant fight, yet the reality of the situation is that with a stroke of the pen, congress has the potential to eliminate pass-throughs for medical and nursing education. Hospitals are not likely to continue their support of diploma nursing education when the costs of such programs can not be passed on to Medicare and other third-party payors. The implementation of two levels of nursing, professional and technical, will collapse the Associate degree and the practical nurse role into one, thus eliminating the confusion surrounding three avenues to registered nursing licensure.

Tremendous time and energy will be freed up within the profession to devote to improving the quality of patient care. Many of the intraprofessional issues will be rendered moot by the demands and requirements of the marketplace. For example, the rapidly increasing acuity level of hospitalized patients is necessitating better educated and trained professional nurses. Thus the debates concerning the appropriate use of nurses' aides and licensed practical nurses become purely academic. There simply is no place for such workers in a complex care center. Based on these societal influences and changes in the health-care system, one can expect the following changes to occur in the nursing profession.

REWARDS FOR INNOVATION

In this period of rapid change, there will emerge a renewed recognition of the importance of individual employees, their ideas, and their contributions. According to Kanter, people seem to matter in direct proportion to an awareness of crisis. During the preceding years of growth and economic plenty for health care, individuals, including nurses, were largely taken for granted. When the health-care system was in the driver's seat and had admission waiting lists for patients, employers were expected to fit into the "system" and to assume that the "system," not the persons involved, was responsible for any success.[4] However, the rules for doing business in the health-care industry have changed. With that change have come opportunities for innovation and for entrepreneurs.

Because of the educational changes in the work force, supervisors in American industry are being forced to alter their approaches to management. More and more American workers fall into the category known as knowledge workers. Close supervision and controlling tactics, a management style known as "knocking heads together," is not effective with this group of workers. The organization is dependent on the knowledge and the individual commitment of these workers to their jobs. The key to managing knowledge workers is to leave them alone to use their knowledge on behalf of the organization.[4]

Since 1965, the number of college graduates in the American labor force has increased from 5% to 25% of all workers.[4] Similar changes have taken place in nursing. In 1966, 10.4% of all employed nurses held the Baccalaureate degree;[5] in 1983, 24.7% held the Baccalaureate.[6] Nurses educated in a college or university and even in a community or junior college acquire attitudes about rights, dignity, and entitlements.

These nurses, who are college graduates, do not respond favorably to supervision that consists of issuing orders and monitoring behavior. Instead, they prefer to be informed of the work that must be accomplished, the objectives and the goals, and then be free to do the work as they see fit.

There exists in the health-care industry tremendous potential for innovation. Employees, including nurses, have traditionally had little opportunity to bring new ideas into the system. Because of the state of the industry, problem-solving ideas such as those for cutting costs, reorganizing, or new budgeting and patient classification systems are likely to gain acceptance and recognition for the nurse-innovator.

According to Kanter, in the past entrepreneurs and the entrepreneurial spirit have, for the most part, existed outside our corporations and institutions. The necessity for innovations within the health-care industry requires intellectual efforts by nurses. If the industry is to respond to society's mandate for less costly, but quality, health care for all Americans, innovation must also take place within our institutions. Creative and imaginative nurses have the opportunity to serve their institutions and society in much the same way as Kanter describes "corporate entrepreneurs" in the following: "These 'corporate entrepreneurs' can help their organizations to experiment on uncharted territories and to move beyond what is known into the realm of innovation—if the power to do this is available, and if the organization knows how to take advantage of their enterprise."[4]

NURSING AND THE TECHNOLOGICAL AGE

The accelerating rate of change will necessitate emphasis on training and retraining within the health-care industry. Much opportunity will exist for the development and marketing of products designed to keep the nurse's knowledge current. Nurse executives will increasingly face the challenge of documenting the competency of their nurses. Thus, education as a product of the health-care system will become more entrenched than ever.

The computerized decision-making and monitoring support systems will allow/permit tracking of patient care outcomes of the individual care-giver, including the individual nurse. In the late 1960s and early 1970s, hospitals for the first time were able to participate in statistical reporting systems. These systems provided comparison data on a wide array of patient and institutional statistics including such things as the number of medications administered per patient, mortality rates for patient groups with specific clinical diagnoses, along with infection rates and length of stay. The feedback from these reporting services for the first time allowed individual hospital personnel to compare their data with that of other participating hospitals. An example of the effectiveness of these systems was the discovery of a problem in the coronary care unit of one community hospital. The observation eventually led to the arrest and conviction for murder of a hospital employee.

Computerized information support systems now have the capacity to allow nursing and other hospital managers to track individual patient outcomes for nurses. Imagine the following scenario. The nurse manager schedules the annual performance appraisal for all staff nurses. As part of the interview, the nurse manager shares with the individual staff nurse summary data on all the patients she has cared for during the past year. Based on the data, the nursing administrator and the nurse formulate mutual goals for the coming year. If the individual nurse's patients had a higher than average rate of postsurgical infections, goal statements might include a statement of the nurse's objective to reduce by 10% postsurgical infections in her patients. Again, rhetoric concerning performance based on criteria appraisals gives way to meaningful responses to quality of work performed.

Computerized systems will also free up more time for patient care and eliminate such practices as pouring drugs, writing nurses' notes, and manually checking vital signs. Individual patient drugs will be poured and provided on time according to a computerized system. Observations will be punched into the computer and vital signs will be recorded automatically through electronic computerized systems that include alarms. As more tasks that, in the past, required psychomotor nursing skills become computerized and managed electronically, the major function of nursing will become *thinking*. Nurses will be responsible for processing data and making sound judgments needed to activate systems and thus alter care delivered. A greater emphasis on human communication and touch will be needed as the era of technology grows. Nurses will be the guardians of humanistic care in a world of wires, alarms, and electronics.

The health-care industry is rapidly changing from a closely regulated industry to an industry characterized by technology and intense competition. For the nurse, this focus translates into the necessity of providing quality humanistic nursing care and customer service. This emphasis on pleasing the consumer involves a fundamental shift in the nursing approach. Previously nurses have focused, to a large degree, on pleasing the physician. The emerging emphasis on pleasing the consumer seems a more reasonable focus for nurses as a professional model of care becomes the norm.

ROLE OF THE STAFF NURSE

The health-care industry will increasingly value the competent, highly skilled staff nurse. In an industry characterized by intense competition among the various providers, hospital administrators will quickly recognize that the key to patient satisfaction is quality nursing care.

The prestige and status associated with staff nursing will increase for several reasons. The rising acuity of patients is essentially transforming our tertiary hospitals and health-science center hospitals into giant intensive care units. The status and prestige of intensive care nurses has always been higher than that of general duty nurses and this higher status will be transferred to all staff nurses in such situations.

As decisions at the bedside become clearly linked to profits lost and gained, the emphasis on the intellectual acumen of the staff nurse will take on a new meaning (see the outline on page 358). These nurses will be recognized as the key to efficient problem solving and decision making. The higher acuity level and increasing complexity of patient care, coupled with the demands of higher technology, will necessitate better preparation for professional nurses. Patient care-givers will increasingly be nurses prepared at the baccalaureate level who possess the knowledge and intellectual skills needed to solve problems quickly and accurately. Master's-prepared leaders will work beside these B.S.N nurses in such roles as head nurse and clinical nurse specialist. Within 20 years, patient complexity and the demands of a highly technological environment will necessitate Master's-prepared direct care-givers in the role of staff nurse.

The availability of computerized information systems that can track the patient care outcomes of individual nurses will provide us with the data that supports the effectiveness of both the Master's-prepared nurse and staff nurse. Nursing leaders and educators have long voiced the view that education *does* make a difference; always before, however, the data to support such a position was lacking. Such systems will remove any doubt about the effectiveness or ineffectiveness of care provided by all nursing personnel. Because of the change in financial incentives, hospitals can no longer afford patient complications. Since nursing personnel with lesser levels of education and skill are not likely to be as effective in preventing complications, the need for a higher ratio of professional nurses in the staff mix can be expected in the future.

As hospitals become more competitive, staff nurses of the future will be called upon to serve as hosts to their patients, visitors, and family members. Naisbitt has predicted that the increasing high technological nature of our society will cause consumers to place greater value on humanistic care or "high touch."[7] Persons are expected to seek the humanistic dimension in their care. Staff nurses will be the first line of defense in professional nursing, providing the humanistic dimension of care.

Provision of what some might call hotel services will be an increasingly important function of staff nurses. Health-care consumers, patients, and their families will expect to find in the hospital environ-

NURSING COMPETENCIES OF THE FUTURE

Interpersonal

Computer

Financial

Patient teaching

Ambulatory care

Health policy and economics

Organizational savvy

ment the comfort and cleanliness of any fine hotel. The staff nurse is in the position of coordinating and monitoring such services. At one time, hospital employees were permitted to respond with a sneer and the question, "what do you think this is—a hotel?" to patient requests for a bed change or for food. Rooms were policed to ensure that strict visiting hours were observed and family members in violation were asked to leave without protest. The reality of the situation is that our hospitals will of necessity need to cater to the patient and family in the same ways as a hotel, and patients and their families will increasingly demand the same level of environmental comfort, services, and respect.

As the agency becomes more and more aware of nursing's key position in making the organization attractive to patients, nurses at all levels will realize the benefits. As the agency recognizes nursing's shift as a financial cost center to that of a major revenue source, the nursing department can anticipate increased status and benefits. Hospital administrators can be expected to safeguard that which is linked to the institution's survival. Since in large measure quality nursing care is what patients have entered the hospital to receive, the hospital administration will move to protect the "goose (nurse) that lays the golden egg (quality nursing care)." Those benefits will take many forms and can be expected to include, in addition to better salaries, improved environmental conditions such as lounges, restrooms, cafeterias as well as employee health clubs and spas, and medical and retirement programs.

EDUCATION AND TRAINING

Women are abandoning the fantasy of the Cinderella syndrome. The Labor Department reports that in 1983, 52.9% of all women over the age of 16 are employed. In only 7% of all families in the United States does the wife stay home while the husband and two children go off to school.[3]

Fewer and fewer young women are growing up with the idealized Cinderella notion that some man will take care, in fact, take very good care of them. The abandonment of this fantasy will lead to greater career commitment on the part of young women. Although nursing as a profession is having a difficult time competing with medicine, business, and other professions for the best and brightest young women, the enhancement of the staff nurse role has the potential to place nursing in a more competitive stance.

Professional role-modeling is shaping the career commitments of young nurses. In the past the staff nurse was stereotyped as a young nurse; however, in the future, one will see the graying of the average staff nurse as staff nursing becomes an attractive lifetime career opportunity. It will be possible for these nurses to enjoy a long, successful career. Only then will our profession succeed in moving from the ranks of the semi- or quasi-profession to that of a true profession.

Another factor that will serve to make staff nursing attractive to nurses will be the emergence of the Master's-prepared head nurse or unit coordinator. The nursing profession, like most health and technical professions, has traditionally chosen its managers/administrators based on their demonstrated clinical and technical competence. Very few of these persons had any prior managerial experience or formal study of management science. The position of head nurse is an extremely complex and difficult one. Traditionally the position has not been one that found favor with Master's-prepared nurses. Early graduate nursing programs prepared students as nursing educators and as nursing administrators. The focus of most administrative programs was the preparation of what we now term the nurse executive position. So few nurses enrolled in graduate education that it was impractical to envision this level of education for any except those in top leadership and faculty positions.[8]

Today, however, the situation is changing. More and more nurses are enrolling in graduate education and, after two decades of neglect, administration or managerial specialization at the Master's level has become an appropriate area of study.[9] Education, coupled with institutional needs for competent nursing managers, provides another bright opportunity for nursing to move ahead.

Not all nurses who complete graduate education at the Master's level will qualify for or be successful in obtaining a nurse executive position. For an increasing number of these Master's-prepared nurses with managerial interests and expertise, opportunities for employment will be in first-line managerial positions. These Master's-prepared head nurses will possess the potential to manage their work units effectively and efficiently. Their previous study of human resource management, legal and ethical issues in nursing, organizational behavior, and financial management will prepare them to represent and manage nurses more confidently and expertly. For most employees, the single most important aspect of a job is who and what kind of supervisor they have. These Master's-prepared nurses will have the potential to be "good bosses."

In the future, nurse executives in complex health-care institutions will be prepared at the doctoral level. Their advanced education and knowledge will for the first time in nursing history bring to the managerial role in nursing prior study and preparation. These changes in educational preparation for assigned roles will be needed as practice patterns also change.

CHANGING PATTERNS OF PRACTICE

Of the total number of nurses in 1980 who held a license to practice as a registered nurse, only 76.67% were employed in nursing; 23.4% or 388,537 licensed registered nurses were not employed in nursing.[10] Such a model does not exemplify professional practice. Refrigerator or couch nurses, those who drop in and out of the work force as major household purchases are required, will disappear from the ranks of professional nursing. The advent of a professional practice model will support only those nurses with competence and career commitment. Those nurses who desire only to be involved in an occupation are not likely to fare well in a professional practice model of care delivery.

In the future, staff nursing will no longer be confined to the hospital. Staff nurses will move across lines following patients in and out of the hospital to the community. In fact, in some settings, staff nursing may move entirely out of the hospital. Agencies may then contract for 'round-the-clock nursing services and individual nurses may be employed by an agency. In fact, some health-care leaders are predicting that a smaller percentage of nurses will be employed by hospitals, that will employ a greater percentage of physicians. More nurses, but fewer physicians, will be self-employed. In the future the gap between the salaries of professional nurses and the salaries of physicians can be expected to decrease as the nurse becomes more valued by the system and the physician becomes an employee.[11]

As increasing numbers of nurses become self-employed or work for nurse-owned and nurse-run nursing care enterprises, nurse executives will become even more cognizant of the necessity for protecting nursing jobs. Support positions in nursing, such as budget officer or business manager, will increasingly be reserved for nurses who have acquired the additional financial skills necessary to succeed in such positions. Having competent nurses in these positions will strengthen the position of nursing departments and better promote the interests of the entire profession.

Presently, employers such as home health care agencies and public health departments routinely require 1 to 2 years of hospital nursing experience before they will consider hiring a nurse. If the number of nursing positions in hospitals decreases, as expected, where will new graduates obtain the requisite hospital experience to qualify for out-of-hospital nursing positions? Nursing educators and nursing administrators should begin now to work together to map out some alternatives for ensuring the success of newly graduated nurses in the profession. One idea is to advance the concept of nursing residencies and to make the concept attractive to all parties. Perhaps the new nurse will receive a reduced salary to make her attractive to employers.[8] Access to the institution and the opportunity to gain experience could offset the negatives of a reduced salary for a specified time appropriate for completing a nursing residency. Other alternatives and proposals can certainly be generated by resourceful educators, administrators, and new nurses.

Summary

Hospital admissions serve only one purpose. Patients come to the hospital for round-the-clock nursing care. If medical care is needed or if diagnostic tests are required, the patient can obtain these services without becoming a hospital in-patient. As this point becomes clearer to hospital managers and policy makers, nursing's status and the accompanying rewards, salaries, and benefits can only increase. A shift in the employment of nurses is expected to occur. Increasing numbers of nurses will launch privately owned entrepreneurial nursing agencies. Hospitals and other employers will negotiate and purchase round-the-clock and specialty nursing care from these private companies much as hospitals in the past have contracted with physicians for x-ray, laboratory, and emergency room services.

When the dust settles, the staff nurse role will emerge as a key position in the nursing profession of the future. Because that position is likely to be more valued and rewarded, nurses will increasingly see staff nursing as a career option, not simply an undesirable stop-off on the route to a more desirable or better position. Staff nurses of the future will have a higher intellectual level, and possess greater cognitive skills than they do presently. To paraphrase Eliza Doolittle's dad in *My Fair Lady*, "With a little bit of luck I'll make it to the church on time." Our profession, nursing, with just a little bit of luck has the potential to finally achieve for all its members the respect and professional status it deserves.

References

1. Noyes EJ: Children: A priority? Nurs Econom 3:136–139, May–June, 1985
2. Baldridge M, Brown C, Jones S, Keane J: National Data Book and Guide to Sources Statistical Abstract of the United States, 105th ed. U.S. Department of Commerce; Bureau of the Census, 1985
3. U.S. Bureau of Labor Statistics: Employment and Earnings and Monthly Labor Review. November 1983
4. Kanter RM: The Change Masters: Innovation and Entrepreneurship in the American Corporation. New York, Simon & Schuster, 1983
5. U.S. Department of Health, Education, and Welfare: Public Health Services: Bureau of Manpower Division of Nursing, 1967
6. U.S. Department of Health and Human Services: Public Health Services: Bureau of Health Professions: Division of Nursing. Unpublished data, 1984
7. Naisbitt J: Megatrends: Ten New Directions Transforming Our Lives. New York, Warner Books, 1982
8. Hodges C: The Master's Prepared Care Giver: Educational Aspects of Quality Care. Second National Invitational Conference. Practical Solidarity II, Styles and Processes of Mutual Effort in Nursing Service and Education, National Institute of Health, Bethesda, MD, October 1985
9. Poteet G: Risk management and nursing. In Nurs Clin North Am 18:3, September 1983
10. American Nurses Association: Facts About Nursing 84-85. Kansas City, MO, American Nurses Association, 1985
11. Andersen A: Health Care in the 1990's: Trends and Strategies. Chicago, Arthur Andersen/American College of Hospital Administrators, 1984

Index

The letter f after a page number indicates a figure; t following a page number indicates tabular material.